CURRENT THERAPY
IN NEPHROLOGY

DEVELOPMENTS IN NEPHROLOGY

Cheigh, J.S., Stenzel, K.H. and Rubin, A.L. (eds.): Manual of Clinical Nephrology of the Rogosin Kidney Center. 1981. ISBN 90-247-2397-3.

Nolph, K.D. (ed.): Peritoneal Dialysis. 1981 ed.: out of print. 3rd revised and enlarged ed. 1988 (not in this series). ISBN 0-89838-406-0.

Gruskin, A.B. and Norman, M.E. (eds.): Pediatric Nephrology, 1981. ISBN 90-247-2514-3.

Schück, O.: Examination of the Kidney Function. 1981. ISBN 0-89838-565-2.

Strauss, J. (ed.): Hypertension, Fluid-electrolytes and Tubulopathies in Pediatric Nephrology. 1982. ISBN 90-247-2633-6.

Strauss, J. (ed.): Neonatal Kidney and Fluid-electrolytes. 1983. ISBN 0-89838-575-X.

Strauss, J. (ed.): Acute Renal Disorders and Renal Emergencies. 1984. ISBN 0-89838-663-2.

Didio, L.J.A. and Motta, P.M. (eds.): Basic, Clinical, and Surgical Nephrology. 1985. ISBN 0-89838-698-5.

Friedman, E.A. and Peterson, C.M. (eds.): Diabetic Nephropathy: Strategy for Therapy. 1985. ISBN 0-89838-735-3.

Dzurik, R., Lichardus, B. and Guder, W. (eds.): Kidney Metabolism and Function. 1985. ISBN 0-89838-749-3.

Strauss, J. (ed.): Homeostasis, Nephrotoxicity, and Renal Anomalies in the Newborn. 1986. ISBN 0-89838-766-3.

Oreopoulos, D.G. (ed.): Geriatric Nephrology. 1986. ISBN 0-89838-781-7.

Paganini, E.P. (ed.): Acute Continuous Renal Replacement Therapy. 1986. ISBN 0-89838-793-0.

Cheigh, J.S., Stenzel, K. H. and Rubin, A.L. (eds.): Hypertension in Kidney Disease. 1986. ISBN 0-89838-797-3.

Deane, N., Wineman, R.J. and Benis, G.A. (eds.): Guide to Reprocessing of Hemodialyzers. 1986. ISBN 0-89838-798-1.

Ponticelli, C., Minetti, L. and D'Amico, G. (eds.): Antiglobulins, Cryoglobulins and Glomerulonephritis. 1986. ISBN 0-89838-810-4.

Strauss, J. (ed.), with the assistance of L. Strauss: Persistent Renal-genitourinary Disorders. 1987. ISBN 0-89838-845-7.

Andreucci, V.E. and Dal Canton, A. (eds.): Diuretics: Basic, Pharmacological, and Clinical Aspects. 1987. ISBN 0-89838-885-6.

Bach, P.H. and Lock, E.H. (eds): Nephrotoxicity in the Experimental and Clinical Situation, Part 1. 1987. ISBN 0-89838-977-1.

Bach, P.H. and Lock, E.H. (eds.): Nephrotoxicity in the Experimental and Clinical Situation, Part 2. 1987. ISBN 0-89838-980-2.

Gore, S.M. and Bradley, B.A. (eds.): Renal Transplantation: Sense and Sensitization. 1988. ISBN 0-89838-370-6.

Minetti, L., D'Amico, G. and Ponticelli, C. (eds.): The Kidney in Plasma Cell Dyscrasias. 1988. ISBN 0-89838-385-4.

Lindblad, A.S., Novak, J.W. and Nolph, K.D. (eds.): Continuous Ambulatory Peritoneal Dialysis in the USA. 1989. ISBN 0-7923-0179-X.

Andreucci, V.E. and Dal Canton, A. (eds.): Current Therapy in Nephrology. 1989. ISBN 0-7923-0206-0.

Current Therapy in Nephrology

Proceedings of the 2nd International Meeting on
Current Therapy in Nephrology
Sorrento, Italy, May 22-25, 1988

edited by
Vittorio E. Andreucci, M.D.
Antonio Dal Canton, M.D.
Department of Nephrology
University of Naples
Naples, Italy

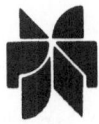

Kluwer Academic Publishers
Boston/Dordrecht/London

Distributors for North America:
Kluwer Academic Publishers
101 Philip Drive
Assinippi Park
Norwell, Massachusetts 02061 USA

Distributors for all other countries:
Kluwer Academic Publishers Group
Distribution Centre
Post Office Box 322
3300 AH Dordrecht, THE NETHERLANDS

Library of Congress Cataloging-in-Publication Data

International Meeting on Current Therapy in Nephrology
    (2nd : 1988 : Sorrento, Italy)
    Current therapy in nephrology.

    (Developments in nephrology)
    Includes bibliographies and index.
    1. Kidneys—Diseases—Treatment—Congresses.
I. Andreucci, Vittorio E. II. Dal Canton, Antonio.
III. Title. IV. Series. [DNLM: 1. Kidney Diseases—
therapy—congresses. W1 DE998EB / WJ 300 I593c 1988]
RC902.A2I566 1988   616.6'106   89–2447

ISBN-13: 978-1-4612-8209-9   e-ISBN-13: 978-1-4613-0865-2
DOI: 10.1007/978-1-4613-0865-2

CONTENTS

Nephrotic Syndrome

Miscellany

II. THERAPY IN RENAL FAILURE

Plasma Exchange in Acute Renal Failure

Medical Therapy in Chronic Renal Failure

Beta-2-Microglobulin

Miscellany

PREFACE

This book includes the proceedings of the 2nd International Meeting on Current Therapy in Nephrology held in Sorrento, Italy, May 22-25, 1988.

The book provides a comprehensive update on new therapeutic strategies in the broad field of Nephrology. The reader will receive information on advances in treatment of glomerulonephritis, new dialysis techniques and progress in renal transplantation. In addition, sections deal with provocative experimental approaches to treating renal disease.

Topics include: cyclosporine in treatment of nephrotic syndrome, plasma exchange in ARF, treatment of beta-2 microglobulin amyloidosis, nutritional assessment in patients on RDT, standards of dialytic adequacy revisited after development of biocompatible membranes, drug interaction with cyclosporine, renal transplantation in elderly recipients, and renal transplantation with elderly donors.

A special effort was made to recruit contributors among the most important scientific authorities in their respective fields: we are grateful to Drs. Cameron, Lamm, Isemberg, Meyrier, Niaudet, Brynger, Lundgren, Fauchald, Cockburn, Gotch, Kopple, Cheung and Horl for having accepted our invitation. We are also indebted to all other authors who participated in the meeting and submitted their original papers for publication.

I. GLOMERULAR DISEASES

Therapy of Nephritis: New Strategies

1. GLOMERULAR DISEASES

CELL MEDIATED IMMUNITY IN GLOMERULONEPHRITIS: PROSPECTS FOR TREATMENT

J STEWART CAMERON

Renal Unit, Department of Medicine, Guy's Campus, UMDS, London, UK

INTRODUCTION

During the 1960s and 1970s, a broad picture of the pathogenesis of glomerulonephritis emerged, depending on the one hand upon the binding of specific anti- kidney antibodies to glomerular structures or planted antigen; and on the other, upon the deposition of immune complexes already formed within the circulation to antigens unrelated to the kidney into the glomerulus. Thus, mechanisms of glomerular injury were pictured as relating primarily to the activation of antigen-bound IgG and other immunoglobulins, with subsequent release of chemotactic substances and secondary attraction and fixation of inflammatory cells. As concepts of the induction and regulation of the immune response evolved, antigen-presenting monocytes and helper T cells were perceived only as facilitating events which permitted B cell maturation, and their production in turn of pathogenetically important antibodies.

However, several workers noted a rather strange fact: although glomerulonephritis was pictured primarily as a glomerular event, in all progressive forms of the disease an extensive interstitial infiltrate was present, together with evidence of tubulo-interstitial damage. When these workers (and subsequently ourselves [1,2]) examined the relation between glomerular function at the time of biopsy, or the subsequent prognosis, correlations between interstitial damage and glomerular performance were much better than with the degree of glomerular damage. In general, although the utility of these observations was widely recognized, their possible implications for pathogenesis were ignored.

More recently, it has become possible to examine, using monoclonal antibodies, the phenotype of cells (both resident and infiltrating) in the interstitium and glomeruli; and the importance of cells within glomeruli and interstitium is being re-asessed [3-5] This brief article examines from these areas which suggests that cell-mediated immunity is directly important for the induction and particularly the progression of glomerulonephritis, and speculates on the implications for present and future therapies of this concept.

MONOCYTES IN GLOMERULONEPHRITIS

Cells of the monocyte- macrophage lineage have been shown to form
the major cell exaggerating glomerular cellularity and forming early
crescents [6], and are a major part of the interstitial infiltrate
[7-15] (Figure 1) in all forms of experimental and clinical human
"proliferative" glomerulonephritis. These observations, tentative at
first and based on optical microscopy as early as 1929, were
amplified first by glomerular culture of crescentic nephritis, then
identification with monocyte specific monoclonal antibodies, and
finally their origin in the marrow bone marrow was defined by
irradiation and transplantation experiments. It is now evident that
as well as the invasion of the glomerulus and the interstitium by
large numbers of fresh, marrow- derived monocytes during injury,
there is a long-term resident population of marrow- derived cells
forming perhaps 5% of glomerular cells, present also in the cortical
interstitium (dendritic cells) found in close apposition to
peritubular capillaries.

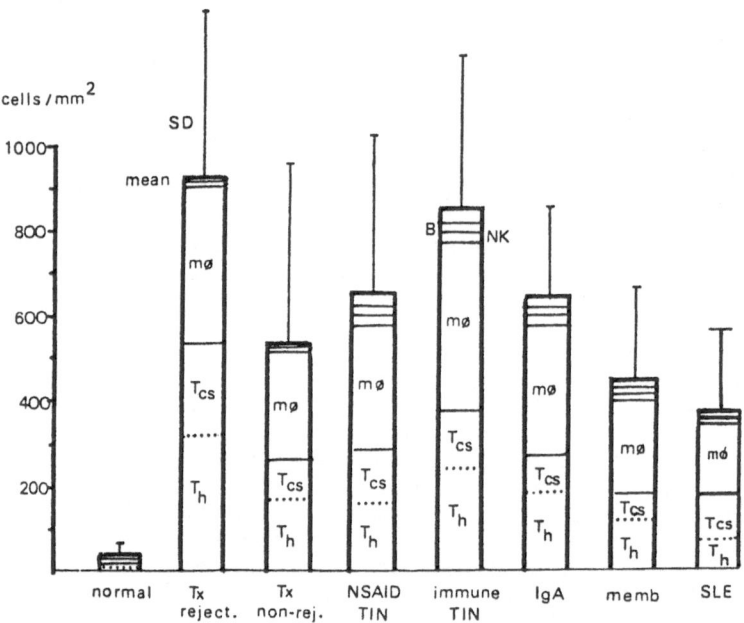

Figure 1: The composition of the interstitial infiltrate in various
renal pathologies, as revealed by phenotyping the infiltrating cells
using monoclonal antibodies. mo = monocyte/macrophage, Tcs =
cytotoxic/ suppressor cells, Th = T helper/inducer cells, B = B
cells, NK = NK cells.Tx = transplant, rej = rejecting, NSAID TIN and
immune TIN = tubulo- interstitial nephritis from non-steroidal
anti-inflammatory agents and systemic immune disorders respectively,
IgA = IgA nephropathy, memb = membranous nephropathy, SLE = systemic
lupus erythematosus

The invading monocytic cells were at first interpreted as secondary agents of damage and/or repair through the many active substances secreted by activated monocytes, but it is known now that in addition both resident and invading cells bear MHC antigens of class II on their surface and can function to present processed antigen to T helper cells and initiate the immune response. Thus an immune response to a foreign antigen can be induced locally in the kidney, even in the absence of an infiltrate.

T LYMPHOCYTES IN GLOMERULONEPHRITIS

The next step in induction of the immune reponse is the generation of specific T helper cells, committed against the antigen just presented to them in the context of MHC class II antigen. In human nephritis, 20 years ago, a number of investigators [3] using the crude technique of in vitro macrophage migration inhibition, showed the presence of cells committed against specific GBM or TBM antigens, or streptococcal antigens. These results however were generally ignored because the concomitant anti-GBM or anti- TBM antibody, (or circulating immune complexes) were then thought to be paramount, and it was not until 15 years later, when in experimental "immune complex" glomerulonephritis the presence of committed cells was demonstrated by lymph node transfer experiments, that interest in specific cell- mediated immunity revived.

It is known now that T cells form the predominant cell type in the interstitium of the kidney in all forms of human glomerulonephritis, both with and without glomerular proliferation, in numbers comparable to allograft rejection and interstitial nephritis in many cases [7-15] (figure 1); and that the majority of such cells bear the T helper/inducer cell phenotype CD4. The presence of intraglomerular T cells has been more difficult to demonstrate because of their small numbers, but it appears that T cells, both T helper and T suppressor, are present in excess in proliferative glomerulonephritides, especially those accompanied by crescent formation such as anti-GBM nephritis and vasculitis [16,17].

In experimental forms of nephritis, the role of T cells has been particularly well documented in anti-GBM nephritis, studied by Bolton and colleagues in chickens [18]. In birds, the maturation of B cells is dependent upon a para rectal organ, the bursa of Fabricius (hence B cells), and bursectomised birds have no humoral immunity. Nevertheless, bursectomised animals can develop crescentic nephritis in response to immunisation with GBM, and the disease is transferrable by T cells alone.

Not only T cells bearing the helper/inducer phenotype CD4, but also CD8- bearing cytotoxic /suppressor T cells are present in the interstitium in glomerulonephritis, although usually in lesser numbers (Th:Ts >2). However in lupus nephritis, alone amongst glomerulonephritides, T suppressor cells may equal or exceed T helper cells in the interstitium (16/34 in our own series [15], the majority in that of D'Agati and colleagues [11]). Within glomeruli, a CD4:CD 8 ratio about 1.5 is usual in most forms [16,17].

CD8 T lymphocytes are capable of direct cytolytic injury to target cells independent of antibody, by a mechanism still being worked out. What characterizes a target cell is also not yet clear, although expession of foreign viral or alloantigen are well-studied circumstances. What may be of importance in glomerulonephritis is that expression of Class I MHC antigens on the cell surface makes the cell more susceptible to injury by committed cytolytic CD8 T lymphocytes, since cytolytic attack is MHC class I restricted. On occasion one may see CD8 positive T lymphocytes within damaged tubular epithelium in glomerulonephrits, as in allograft rejection, suggesting cytolytic T cell mediated injury, and class I antigen expression is increased in renal inflammation (see below).

Recently we have studied activation markers on interstitial cell infiltrates, including the interleukin-2 and transferrin receptors. In rather few patients can interstitial cells be shown to display these receptors (6/34 and 9/34 patients with lupus nephritis respectively [15]), which are not present in large numbers even on activated T cells. Technical difficulties and lack of sensitivity interfere with study of this aspect at the moment. However the majority of interstitial cells in glomerulonephritis display abundant HLA-DR, an MHC class II antigen (Figure 2), normally present on monocytes and B cells but only displayed by T cells when activated.

POSSIBLE ROLE OF TUBULAR AND GLOMERULAR DISPLAY OF MHC II ANTIGENS

In the human kidney, several structures normally display MHC antigens of class II: HLA-DR, DQ, DP and DZ, of which DR has been most studied; our own studies of DP and DQ in the kidney do not differ much from DR. These structures are: the resident intraglomerular monocytes, the vascular endothelium of glomerular and peritubular capillaries, and the interstitial dendritic cells. All these structures are therefore at least potentially capable of presenting antigen on site within the kidney to induce comitted T cells as discussed above, and also inducing mature B cells to produce antibody, a process which is also MHC class II restricted.

Expression of class II antigens such as DR is however very variable, and in some circumstances epithelia can also display DR. The principal (but not the only) stimulator of normal DR display or inducer of "aberrant" DR display is interferon gamma, principally secreted by activated T lymphocytes. Aberrant tubular DR display is known to occur in transplant rejection, and recently we have studied HLA-DR expression in detail in primary tubulointerstitial nephritis [12], allograft rejection and in glomerulonephritis [13-15]. In general, tubular DR display was much lower than that observed in allografts or in primary tubulointerstitial disease, being similar to normal in membranous nephropathy, greater in IgA nephropathy and in lupus (Figure 2). However in lupus there was a correlation, as in primary tubulointerstitial nephritis, between tubular display of DR and numbers of activated cells, judged by DR expression, within the interstitium [15].

Although human renal tubular cells expressing MHC class II antigen
have not yet been shown to be capable of presenting antigen in
vitro, this has been demonstrated in an experimental model of
tubulointerstitial nephritis in which the antigen was identified
[19]. Clearly the potential for a vicious circle of increased DR
expression, increased generation of comitted cells, increased
generation of cytotoxic cells and further DR induction exists, in
both glomeruli and interstitium.

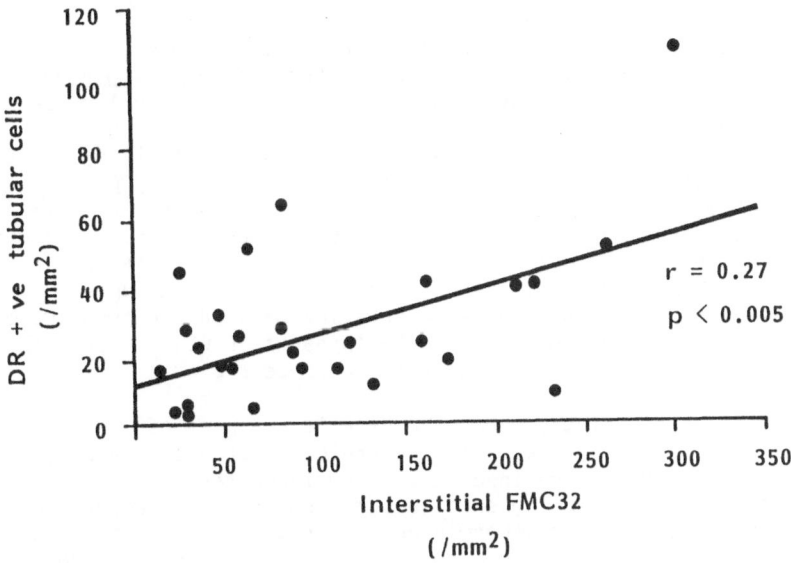

Figure 2. Nephritis of systemic lupus: relation between expression
of HLA-DR antigen (vertical axis) and numbers of monocytes/
macrophages (horizontal axis) (from reference 15).

MECHANISMS OF CHRONIC DAMAGE IN GLOMERULONEPHRITIS [2]

The major thesis of this article is that the progression of what
have been hitherto described as "glomerulonephritides" is to a
greater or lesser extent determined by events occurring in the
interstitium, and not by glomerular damage, glomerulosclerosis and
secondary tubular atrophy. The lack of correlation of outcome with
indices of glomerular damage [1], most evident and best studied in
lupus nephritis [11,15] and membranous nephropathy [13], together
with the correlations between tubulo- interstitial events and
outcome, supports this thesis.

The implication is that mechanisms of progression in glomerular
diseases are predominantly the same as those in tubulointerstitial
diseases. What mechanisms may operate in human glomerulo- and
tubulointerstitial nephritis? As indicated above and in figure 1,

the majority of cellular infiltrates in both instances are helperT cells and monocytes; this is the typical appearance of a _delayed hypersensitivity reaction_ , which presumptively is the major mechanism. In support of this idea we have found, in several forms of nephritis, a correlation between the numbers of T cells and monocytes in the interstitium and the GFR at the time of biopsy; even more interesting, in membranous nephropathy 5-year follow up status is correlated with the cellular infiltrate at the time of biopsy [13]. Lack of a similar correlation in lupus nephritis [15] may relate to the immunosuppression given.

However, many CD8 positive T cells are also present in the interstitium in glomerulonephritides, especially lupus [11,15], some infiltrating damaged tubules, so that direct _T cell- mediated cytotoxicity_ may well play a role. Some of these CD8 cells are, however, almost certainly playing a modulatory role. A third mechanism implicated in experimental tubulointerstitial injury is antibody- dependent cell- mediated cytotoxicity, or _ADCC_ for short. This involves reaction of natural killer cells (NK cells) bearing IgG Fc receptors, with IgG antibody bound to cells, leading to cytolysis. Few NK cells are present in any infiltrate (Figure 1) so this mechanism does not seem to be a major one. In lupus nephritis, however, we noted a correlation between the presence of tubular immune deposits of IgG ad C3 (present in 62% of patients) and the number of NK cells, and this deserves exploration.

Finally in considering damage, the genesis not just of acute reversible inflammation but of irreversible fibrosis, scarring and nephron loss must be examined. Activated monocytes and other activated cells- including endothelium- produce large amounts of interleukin 1, which is strongly chemotactic and stimulatory to fibroblasts. Other cationic mitogens such as platelet- derived growth factor (PDGF) and transforming growth factor B are also produced by monocytes, and could bind to the negatively- charged polyanion in the interstitium. The role of non-immunologic complement activation by interstitial ammonium as recently been recognized [20], and this may play a role is the chronic damage of glomerulonephritis as well.

IMPLICATIONS FOR TREATMENT

Various immunsuppressive agents such as corticosteroids and cytotoxic drugs have been given in the past to patients with glomerulonephritis with the idea that these drugs might modify the humoral events believed to determine glomerular damage. The thesis presented here would suggest that what benefit has accrued may well derive from an effect on tubulo- interstitial cell- mediated events. Non-specific agents which suppress monocytes (such as corticosteroids) or activated T helper cells (such as cyclosporin) may well be of benefit, but need careful monitoring. In the case of cyclosporin, data are few, and as yet no controlled data or long term followups are available.

In experimental tubulointerstitial nephritis, there is evidence of
suppressor cells which modify injury, and thus non-specific
immunosuppression is capable of worsening as well as ameliorating
disease. Equally, treatment with cyclophosphamide during antigen
presentation may facilitate the induction of suppressor cells. More
interesting are the implications for the future. The possibility
arises through the use of monoclonal antibodies of much more
specific treatment. First however, the problem of immunisation by
monoclonals, usually derived today from mouse or rat hybridomas,
will have to be solved. The appearance within two weeks of anti-
mouse antibody vitiates the use of current monoclonal antibodies in
a disease whose evolution is over years! However the engineering of
rodent-human monoclonals, or production of human hybridomas, would
eliminate this major difficulty, and should be achieved soon.

Already, moncolonal antibodies reacting with CD3 (T cells), CD4
(helper T cells), CD8 (supressor/sytotoxic cells) and a variety of
monocyte markers are available. In allografts and auto immune
disease in the mouse, anti- interleukin-2 receptor antibodies have
been shown to ameliorate rejection and the course of the autoimmune
disease. Further, Kelley, Strom and colleagues [21] have "spliced"
the gene for diphtheria toxin on to the gene for this antibody, and
produced a highly specific and effective suppression of delayed
hypersensitivity; it seems likely that such reagents will be useful
in so called idiopathic glomerulonephritides in the future, as well
as in transplantation and auto immune disorders.

REFERENCES:

1. Cameron, J.S. Interstitial changes in glomerulonephritis. In:
   Prevention in nephrology (Ed. Buccianti, G.) Masson, Milan, 1987.
   pp 8-18.
2. Cameron, J.S. Immunologically induced primary and secondary
   tubulointerstitial nephritis. Adv. Nephrol. 18 , (in press)
   1988.
3. Filit, H.M., Zabriskie, J.B. Cellular immunity in
   glomerulonephritis. Am. J Pathol. 109 , 227-243, 1982.
4. Bolton, W.K. The role of cell mediated immunity in the
   pathogenesis of glomerulonephritis. Plasma Ther. Transfus.
   Technol. 5 : 415-430, 1984.
5. McCluskey, R.T., Bhan, A.K. Cell mediated immunity in renal
   disease. Hum. Pathol. 17 , 146-153, 1986.
6. Various authors: Symposium: Monocyte- macrophage system in immune
   -related glomerulonephritis. Contr. Nephrol., 45 , 105-156,
   1985.
7. Stachura, I, Si, L., Madan, E., Whiteside, T. Nononuclear cell
   subsets in human renal disease. Enumeration in tissue sections
   with monoclonal antibodies. Clin. Immunol. Immunopathol., 30 ,
   362-373, 1984
8. Boucher, A., Droz, D., Adafer, E., Noel, L-H. Characterization of
   mononuclear cell subsets in renal cellular interstitial
   infiltrates. Kidney Int., 29 1043-1049, 1986

9. Brunati, C., Brando, B., Confalonieri, R., Belli, L.S., Lavagni, M.G., Minetti, L. Immunophenotyping of mononuclear cell infiltrates associated with renal diseases. Clin. Nephrol., 26 , 15-20, 1986.

10. Hooke D.H., Gee, D.C., Atkins, R.C. Leucocyte analysis using monoclonal antibodies in human glomerulonephritis. Kidney Int., 31 964-972, 1987.

11. D'Agati, V., Appel, G.A., Estes, D., Knowles, D.M., Pirani, C.L. Monoclonal antibody identification of infiltrating mononuclear leucocytes in lupus nephritis. Kidney Int., 30 , 573-581, 1986.

12. Cheng, H-F., Cameron, J.S., Nolasco, F., Hildreth, G., Neild, G., Hartley, B. Tubular damage in tubulointerstitial nephritis: a role for tubular DR expression? (submitted for publication) 1988; (abstract Kidney Int. 31 , 335, 1987)

13. Alexopoulos, E., Seron, D., Hartley, R.B., Cameron, J.S. Immune mechanisms in idiopathic membranous nephropathy; the role of the interstitial infiltrate. (submitted for publication) 1988.

14. Alexopoulos, E., Seron, D., Hartley, R.B., Nolasco, F., Cameron, J.S. The role of interstitial infiltrates in IgA nephropathy. A study with monoclonal antibodies. (submitted for publication) 1988.

15. Alexopoulos, E., Seron, D., Hartley, R.B., Cameron, J.S. The pathogenetic role of interstitial mononuclear cells in lupus nephritis. (submitted for publication) 1988.

16. Nolasco, F., Cameron, J.S., Hartley, B., Coelho, A., Hildreth, G., Reuben, R. Intraglomerular T cells and monocytes in nephritis: a study with monoclonal antibodies. Kidney Int., 31 , 1160-1166, 1987.

17. Bolton, W.K., Innes, D.J., Sturgill, B.C., Kaiser, D.L. T-cells and macrophages in rapidly progressive glomerulonephritis: clinicopathologic correlations. Kidney Int., 32 , 869-876, 1987.

18. Bolton, W.K., Tucker, W.L., Sturgill, B.C. New avian model of experimental glomerulonephritis consistent with mediation by cellular immunity. J. Clin. Invest. 73 , 1263-1276, 1984.

19. Hines, W.H., Kelly, C.J., Haverty, T.P., Neilsen, E.J. Recognition of antigen (Ag)- secretory renal epithelial cells by Ag- specific helper T cells. Kidney Int. 33 , 347, 1988 (abstract).

20. Hostetter, M.K., Nath, K.A., Tolins, J.P., Hostetter, T.H. Ammonia, the kidney and complement C3. In: Nephrology (Ed: Davison A.M.) Transmedica, London, 1988. pp 599 - 612.

21. Kelley, V.E., Pankewycz, O., Murphy, J., Strom, T. Chimeric interleukin-2 toxin selectively binds to its receptor and blocks delayed type hypersensitivity. Kidney Int 33 , 349, 1988 (abstract).

ENZYME THERAPY OF EXPERIMENTAL GLOMERULONEPHRITIS

STEVEN N. EMANCIPATOR and MICHAEL E. LAMM

Institute of Pathology, Case Western Reserve University
Cleveland, Ohio 44106, U.S.A.

INTRODUCTION

Glomerulonephritis (GN), resulting from the deposition or formation of immune complexes (IC) within glomeruli, is often progressive and represents a major public health problem worldwide (1). Although progress within the last decade has helped to elucidate the pathogenesis of GN, therapy remains limited. Several mechanisms and inflammatory mediators are capable of contributing to disease, apparently operative in different combinations in the various patterns of GN (2). Therapy directed at particular pathways is consequently restricted in scope and may be of limited potential.

We reasoned that digestion of glomerular immune deposits by enzymes could, to the extent that such deposits elicit GN, ameliorate the signs of disease and perhaps retard progression. Our earlier studies showed that non-toxic doses of proteolytic enzymes could markedly decrease IC deposits in the glomerular capillaries or mesangium in passive serum sickness GN models induced by injection of preformed IC of bovine gamma globulin (BGG) and rabbit antibody to BGG (3). Mice or rats treated systemically with mixtures of chymopapain and subtilisin did not display the intense immunofluorescence deposits seen in animals given the same amounts of IC but treated with saline instead of enzymes. The distribution of fluorescence intensities of rabbit antibodies in treated animals was significantly shifted to negative or low-grade scores compared to saline treated subjects, and antigen deposits were also significantly attenuated. We also quantified glomerular IC in rats given complexes of BGG antigen and radioactive rabbit anti-BGG and found that glomeruli from enzyme-treated rats contained only half the radioactivity present in rats treated with saline.

Extension of this principle to the heterologous and autologous phases of passive Heymann nephritis in rats, a model of membranous nephropathy, also proved fruitful (4). Proteases given during the heterologous phase, 1 to 7 days after injection of 5 mg of nephrito-genic rabbit anti-Fx1A antibody, significantly reduced glomerular deposits of rabbit IgG and rat anti-rabbit antibody. Perhaps even more promising results were obtained when higher doses of anti-Fx1A were given. Although proteinuria developed during the autologous phase (after day 10) among saline-treated rats, rats treated with enzymes had either no or significantly attenuated proteinuria. Enzymes not only prevented proteinuria if given on days 1-7 during the heterologous phase or started on day 6 before onset of the autolo-gous phase, but also were capable of reversing established protein-uria evident on day 14 when therapy was initiated on day 15. Ultra-structural morphometry in these animals showed that protease-treated rats had 33-50% fewer and smaller electron dense deposits than their saline treated counterparts, regardless of dose of anti-Fx1A anti-body or timing of enzyme therapy. Furthermore, the equal titers of serum anti-rabbit IgG developed in treated and control rats suggest that protease therapy is not acting via immunosuppression.

Our more recent work extends the previous observations along two avenues. First, we tested the ability of enzymes targeted to the sites of glomerular IC deposits to improve therapeutic efficacy. Second, we investigated whether digestion of macromolecules other than proteins might be of benefit in diseases where the antigen component of glomerular IC is not protein in nature.

MATERIALS AND METHODS
Induction of glomerulonephritis

Active serum sickness model. We prepared cationic BGG (cBGG) by substitution of BGG with ethylene diamine in the presence of carbo-diimide (3). The GN which results from immunization and challenge of mice and rats with cBGG over 2 to 3 wks has been described (5,6). For these experiments 200 g male Sprague-Dawley rats were primed subcutaneously with 1 mg cBGG in complete Freund's adjuvant followed by five progressive daily intravenous challenges of 1,2,4,6 and 8 mg cBGG starting 1 wk after the priming injection. Six h after the last injection, urine was collected for 24 h and rats randomly grouped.

Passive serum sickness model. Mesangial deposits containing IgA
or IgM anti-dextran antibodies were induced in 35 g male Swiss al-
bino mice by injecting soluble IC composed of either 2 mg J558 monoclonal IgA anti-dextran or 2 mg MOPC 104E monoclonal IgM anti-
dextran combined with five-fold excess 300 kD dextran sulfate via
tail vein, adapted from the work of Isaacs et al (7). Mice were
then randomly allocated to groups.

Treatment

Active serum sickness model. After initial urine collections,
rats were treated with 5 mg chymopapain and 2.5 mg subtilisin in 1
ml saline, given daily intraperitoneally for 5 days, in two divided
doses (3,4). In some cases we used chymopapain and subtilisin
substituted with biotin by incubation of enzyme at 5 mg/ml with
hydroxysuccinimidyl biotin at 25 mg/ml in 0.1 M sodium carbonate, pH
8.5, for 3 h at 25°, followed by dialysis. In addition, some rats
also received a single 5 mg dose of the cationic (pI = 9.8) biotin-
binding (10^{15} M^{-1}) protein, egg avidin A intravenously 1 h before
the first intraperitoneal injection of enzyme.

Passive serum sickness model. Some mice were given 5 intraperitoneal injections, at 10 min intervals, of 0.1 mg chymopapain
and 0.05 mg subtilisin in 0.1 ml saline. Other mice were given 5
doses of 200 U dextranase, also at 10 min intervals intraperitoneally, either alone or alternating with protease.

Analysis

After treatment a second 24 h urine collection was taken from
each rat, and rats were sacrificed under ether anesthesia. Serum
was harvested from venous blood. Renal cortex was snap-frozen in
liquid nitrogen and cryostat sections at 4 μm were stained by
immunofluorescence for rat IgG, BGG and rat C3 (6). Initial and
final protein excretion was determined by sulfosalicylic acid-
induced turbidimetry, and serum anti-BGG was assayed by ELISA (6).
Creatinine clearance was computed from the serum creatinine concentration and the creatinine content of 24 h urine samples, determined
by the picric acid method of Jaffe (8) in an automated procedure.
Serum cholesterol was assayed (9) in an automated procedure.

Mice were sacrificed under ether anesthesia, and renal cortex
snap frozen, sectioned, and stained for IgA and IgM (3,7). We used
indirect immunofluorescence with MOPC 104E and anti-mouse IgM to de-

tect dextran deposits in mice given IgA containing IC, and J558 and anti-mouse IgA to detect dextran in mice given IgM containing IC.

Quantitative proteinuria, creatinine clearance, serum anti-BGG and serum cholesterol were compared among groups of rats by analysis of variance, with intergroup comparisons by Fisher's protected t-test. After examination in "blind" fashion, immunofluorescence scores were evaluated by chi-squared analysis.

RESULTS

In the active serum sickness model, rats given targeted or untargeted enzyme therapy for 5 days had significantly less protein-uria than saline-treated controls (Table 1), despite the fact that protein excretion prior to treatment (84.6 ± 11.9 mg/day) was not different among the groups ($F = 1.3$). Rats given the naturally cationic avidin, which binds electrostatically to glomerular capil-laries, and then given biotinyl protease capable of binding tightly to the avidin, had significantly less proteinuria than rats given nontargeted proteases, either biotinyl protease alone or unmodified protease plus avidin. Moreover, rats given protease targeted to glomerular capillaries by avidin and biotin had the least intense glomerular deposits by immunofluorescence of all the groups (data not shown). The benefits of protease therapy are additionally evident in their amelioration of the hypercholesterolemia associated with the nephrotic syndrome in these rats (normal rat serum choles-terol is 98 ± 4.2 mg/dl). Again, targeted protease was significant-ly better than nontargeted protease (Table 1).

Table 1. Effects of protease on active serum sickness GN.

Treatment		No. of	Proteinuria	Serum Cholesterol
Protease	Avidin	Rats	(mg/day $\pm$ SD)	(mg/dl $\pm$ SD)
biotinyl	+	7	17.2 ± 13.2**	119 ± 5.5 **
native	+	7	38.8 ± 8.5*	126 ± 6.25*
biotinyl	–	4	37.8 ± 13.1*	not done
saline	–	7	51.3 ± 10.4	135 ± 7.5

* $p < 0.05$ vs saline group; ** $p < 0.01$ vs other protease groups, and $p < 0.001$ vs saline group, all by ANOVA.

15

We could detect increased protease activity in treated rats sera; nonetheless, serum protein electrophoresis patterns were not different from controls. Urine electrophoresis showed predominantly albumin, with no detectable cleavage products. Serum antibody specific for BGG was readily detectable in all rats; the slopes and intercepts of plots of ELISA optical density vs log serum dilution were identical in protease treated and saline treated rats. Enzymes did not influence creatinine clearance (all above data not shown).

In the passive serum sickness model, dextranase significantly reduced mesangial deposits of dextran antigen and either IgA or IgM anti-dextran, compared to mice given saline (Table 2). Protease had no significant effect given alone or when added to the dextranase regimen (data not shown).

Table 2. Effect of dextranase and protease on glomerular immune deposits in mice given dextran/anti-dextran IC.

Monoclonal Antibody Injected	Treatment	No. of Mice	Glomerular Immunofluorescence¶		
			IgA	IgM	Dextran
IgM	saline	10	0 (0)	10 (2.5)	10 (3.1)
IgM	dextranase	10	0 (0)	4 (1.2)*	4 (1.0)*
IgM	protease	10	0 (0)	7 (1.7)	9 (2.1)
IgA	saline	10	10 (1.5)	0 (0)	10 (2.3)
IgA	dextranase	10	3 (0.5)*	0 (0)	4 (0.8)*
IgA	protease	10	8 (1.2)	0 (0)	9 (2.0)

¶ Data are the number of mice positive (mean intensity on a scale of 1-4) for immune reactant.
* $p < 0.05$ vs saline group by chi-squared analysis.

There was no overt toxic effect of enzyme therapy in these experiments.

DISCUSSION

The results presented here in two models of GN, when considered in light of our previous work (3,4), provide additional evidence that systemic enzyme therapy can remove glomerular IC without obvious toxicity. Moreover, such enzyme therapy can improve glomeru-

lar function, ameliorating not only proteinuria but also attendant
hypercholesterolemia. Two additional findings in the current work
are noteworthy: (a) targeting of enzymes to the glomerular capillary
wall can improve the efficacy of therapy, and (b) enzymes other than
proteases can be useful in situations where non-protein antigens are
components of glomerular IC.

Dissolution of glomerular IC by giving excess antigen has been
applied successfully to therapy of experimental GN (10-13). Of
course, for solubilization of glomerular IC by excess antigen to be
effective, specific knowledge of the culprit antigen is required.
Likewise, inhibitors of inflammatory mediators are most useful when
the particular mediators involved are known. Such information,
often accessible in experimental systems, is not readily available
in spontaneous human disease. We hope that the approach of enzymatic digestion of glomerular IC might ultimately be adaptable for
therapeutic intervention in patients with GN. While such application
will require detailed studies of toxicity and of the long term effects of enzymes on progression of GN and development of strategies
such as genetic engineering of human enzymes to avoid immunological
"rejection" of the enzymes used for therapy, we believe the obsta-
cles can potentially be overcome, thereby offering a practical addition to the treatment of GN.

REFERENCES

1. Kalata, G.B. Science 208: 473-476, 1980.
2. Couser, W.G. Kid. Int. 28: 569-583, 1985.
3. Nakazawa, M., Emancipator, S.N. and Lamm, M.E. Lab. Invest. 55:
    551-563, 1986.
4. Nakazawa, M., Emancipator, S.N. and Lamm, M.E. J. Exp. Med.
    164: 1973-1987, 1986.
5. Gallo, G.R., Caulin-Glaser, T., Emancipator, S.N. and Lamm, M.E.
    Lab. Invest. 48: 353-362, 1983.
6. Rahman, M.A., Emancipator, S.N. and Dunn, M.J. Kid. Int. 31:
    1317-1326, 1987.
7. Isaacs, K. and Miller, F. Am. J. Pathol. 111: 298-306, 1983.
8. Wybenga, D.R., Pilleggi, V.J., Dirstine, P.H. and Di Giorgio J.
    Clin. Chem. 16: 980-992, 1970.
9. Owen, J.A., Iggo, B., Scandrett, F.J. and Stewart, C.P.
    Biochem. J. 58: 426-431, 1954.
10. Valdes, A.J., Senterfelt, L.B., Pollack, A.D. and Germuth, F.
    Johns Hopkins Med. J. 124: 9-16, 1969.
11. Wilson, C.B., and Dixon, F.J. J. Exp. Med. 134: 7s-19s, 1971.
12. Mannik, M. and Striker, G.E. Lab. Invest. 42: 483-489, 1980.
13. Haakenstad, A.O., Striker, G.E. and Mannik, M. Lab. Invest. 48:
    323-331, 1983.

DNA ANTIBODIES AND IDIOTYPES

D. ISENBERG MD MRCP

Bloomsbury Rheumatology Unit, University College And The Middlesex
Hospital Medical School. London UK.

INTRODUCTION

Systemic lupus erythematosus (SLE) is characterized by the
frequent detection of antibodies binding to DNA, especially in its
double-stranded form. Paradoxically it has been shown that DNA
itself is a poor immunogen, that anti-DNA antibodies may be found in
a variety of other conditions and that lymphocytes from normal
individuals have the capacity to produce anti-DNA antibodies.
Recent investigations have been concerned with the genetic origins
of anti-DNA antibodies and this in turn has focussed attention on
their idiotypes. I will review the results of studies analysing DNA
antibody idiotypes and show how they are leading to an increased
understanding of the origins of DNA antibodies and suggesting new
therapeutic approaches.

DEFINITION AND IDENTIFICATION

The variable regions of immunoglobulin molecules are
characterized by a variety of antigenic determinants which
constitute their idiotypes. At least two types of idiotypic determinants may be distinguished functionally; those at the antigen
combining sites and those adjacent to the combining sites which are
known as framework related idiotypes. In general, anti-idiotypes
directed against combining site related determinants will inhibit
the binding of antigen and antibody molecules bearing the relevant
idiotype, whereas antibodies directed against framework determinants
do not usually inhibit such inter-actions. The identification of
idiotypic determinants requires the production of anti-idiotypic
antibodies. This may be achieved, for example, by the immunization

of one species, such as a man. Such immunization will lead to the production of a rabbit antiserum directed against the antigen binding portion of a human antibody. After removal by absorption of all irrelevant antibodies, the rabbit antiserum may be used as an anti-idiotypic antibody.

CROSS REACTIVE IDIOTYPES

In general, a given idiotype on a particular antibody distinguishes this antibody from others. However, it is now widely recognised that immunoglobulin melecules may share idiotypes even if they have different antigen binding properties. These cross reactive idiotypes have been found amongst antibodies to foreign structures, including tetanus toxoid, rye grass pollen and hepatitis B surface antigen. Cross reactive idiotypes have also been demonstrated amongst autoantibodies form different individuals including anti-DNA antibodies and anti-Sm antibodies and a provisional report has suggested their existence on anti-Ro antibodies (reviewed in 1). These examples are taken form studies of serum from lupus patients or from the lupus mouse models. However, cross reactive idiotypes are also present on many other autoantibodies from different auto-immune diseases including anti-acetylcholine receptor antibodies, from patients with thyroiditis. These and many other reports suggest that a restricted number of germ line genes may encode the pathogenic antibodies in a variety of autoimmune disorders.

Idiotypic markers it must be emphasised, do not identify V genes but conformations on immunoglobulinsthat may occur in different anti-bodies. A particular idiotype could in theory originate from different V genes. Should this idiotype, however, be repeatedly detected on immunoglobulins from unrelated patients it is suggestive that these individuals do possess common germline genes.

SEROLOGICAL STUDIES

Many analyses of DNA antibody idiotypes in the lupus prone mouse models have been reported (2). There are in addition, a growing number of reports examining idiotypes from human anti-DNA antibody molecules. With the introduction of human hybridoma techniques to produce anti-DNA antibody molecules it was possible, by suitable immunization, to produce anti-idiotypic anti-DNA antibodies, and to screen 60 polynucleotide binding monoclonal lupus autoantibodies (3). Substantial idiotypic sharing was found with both polyclonal and monoclonal anti-idiotypic antibodies. Idiotype restriction was found on human autoantibodies to DNA derived from the serum of lupus patients by Zouali and Eyquem (4). Solomon et al (5) using a mouse monoclonal antibody which identified a framework determinant on anti-double-stranded DNA antibodies after suitable absorption, designated 3I, in the sera of 8 out of 9 lupus patients. I and my colleagues found that the serum levels of an idiotype designated 16/6 were elevated in 40 of 74 lupus patients and that there was a notable correlation with disease activity in several patients (6). This latter observation has been confirmed in a later study (7).

Two recent reports have demonstrated the presence of cross reactive idiotypes in healthy family members of lupus patients. Halpern et al found that 15 of 19 family members had high titred reactivity with an anti-idiotypic antibody measuring the 3I idiotype (8). My colleagues and I found idiotypes 16/6 and 32/15 in 24 % and 7 % respectively of 147 first degree relatives of 48 lupus patients (9). These observations seem to imply that common DNA antibody idiotypes cannot be pathogenic factors on their own. The differences between idiotype positive antibodies which bind DNA and those which do not, could in theory, help to distinguish subgroups of antibodies which are important in the pathogenesis of the disease. That the 16/6 and 32/15 idiotypes can mark antibodies which do have pathogenic significance is suggested by a study showing immunolobulins bearing there idiotypes on lupus kidney biopsy sections (10). We found that the frequency with which these common idiotypes are present amoung human monoclonal antibodies, serum lupus antibodies and tissue bound antibodies from lupus patients is much the same (40-50 % with 16/6 for example).

ORIGINS OF 16/6 ID

Although the 16/6 ID was first identified on IgM anti-DNA anti-

DNA antibodies, it has also been found in some normal sera, and in 23 out of 265 patients (8.7 %) with monoclonal gammapathies, few of whom had DNA binding properties (11). Datta et al (12) reported the in vitro production of this idiotype by lymphocytes of normal subjects and lupus patients. They suggested that the 16/6 ID exists on two populations of antibodies. The first population, conserved in normal idividuals, is of uncertain antigenic specificity though a recent study (13) strongly suggests they are on antibodies binding the klebsiella polysaccharide determinant (K-30). 16/6 ID is also found amongst SLE patients in relapse on antibodies binding to DNA.

SEQUENCE STUDIES

A striking similarity in the light chain amino acid sequences, was found between monoclonal antibody 16/6, bearing the 16/6 ID, and a monoclonal IgM (designated WEA) from a patient with Waldenstrom's macroglobulinaemia (14). WEA binds K-30 and subsequent studies showed that it also bound DNA and possessed the 16/6 ID. Furthermore nucleotide sequencing of heavy chain mRNA from the immunoglobulins of 2 SLE hybridomas expressing the 16/6 ID, showed more than 99 % homology to the VH26 germline gene sequence (15). This is a member of the human VH III gene family and the observation indicates that unmutated germ-line V genes can encode autoantibodies.

IMPLICATION FOR THERAPEUTIC STRATEGIES

Down regulation of antibodies bearing common idiotypes might have a beneficial effect for patients with SLE. Hahn and Ebling (16) reasoned that immunizing lupus prone mice with a syngeneic (from the same species) monoclonal anti-DNA antibody bearing a high frequency idiotype would induce the production of an immunoregulatory anti-idiotype antibody. Thus, they administered repeated injections of an IgG 2a monoclonal anti-DNA antibody to NZB/NZW fl female mice from the age of 6 weeks. The treatment resulted in the temporary suppression of circulating anti-DNA antibodies, a reduction in proteinuria, a reduction in the deposition of anti-DNA antibodies in the glomeruli, and fewer deaths from nephritis. Zouali et al (17) showed that by administering a syngeneic anti-DNA IgG together with

21

a synthetic immunoaduvant, a major reduction of both idiotype
expression and total DNA antibody levels could be achieved. In a
form of reciprocal experiment, Hahn and Ebling (18) were also able
to show temporary suppression of antibodies to DNA and significantly
prolonged survival due to a delay in the onset of nephritis by
innoculating NZB/NZW fl mice with a monoclonal anti-idiotypic antibody. However, as Bluestone et al (19) have commented, the in vivo
administration of xenogeneic (from a different species) anti-idiotypes induces the expression of idiotypic molecules rather than
suppressing them. For example, anti-idiotypic therapy in MRL lpr/
lpr mice, which was directed against the high frequency idiotype
H130, resulted in the augmentation of H130 idiotype and anti-DNA
antibody levels (20). In an effort to overcome this problem while
using the valuable targeting abilities of anti-idiotypes, Saski et al
(21) were able to selectively eliminate anti-DNA antibody producing
cells in in vivo experiments by conjugating an anti-idiotypic antibody with the cytotoxic agent, neocarzinostatin.

It is interesting to postulate whether passing lupus serum over
a column containing an anti-16/6 antibody might be of some benefit,
especially since the 16/6 ID has been found on anti Sm/RNP and anti-
Ro antibodies (22) which are also commonly found in SLE patients.

REFERENCES
1.   Isenberg, D.A. Acta Haemat: 76: 95-100, 1986.
2.   Isenberg, D.A., et al. Br Med Bull: 40: 262-266, 1984.
3.   Shoenfeld, Y., et al. J Exp Med: 158: 718-730, 1983.
4.   Zouali, M., et al. Immunol Lett: 7: 187, 1984.
5.   Solomon, G., et al. PNAS (USA): 80: 850, 1983.
6.   Isenberg, D.A., et al. Lancet: 2: 417-422, 1984.
7.   Isenberg, D.A., et al. Medicine (Balt): 66: 46-55, 1986.
8.   Halpern, R., et al. J Clin Invest: 70: 731, 1985.
9.   Isenberg, D.A., et al. Arthritis Rheum: 28: 999-1007, 1985.
10. Isenberg, D.A., and Collins, C. J Clin Invest:76: 287-294, 1985.
11. Shoenfeld, Y., et al. J Clin Immunol: 6: 194-203, 1986.
12. Datta, S.K., et al. Clin Immunol Immunopathol:38: 302-308, 1986
13. El Roiey, A., et al. Clin Exp Immunol: 67: 507-515, 1987.
14. Atkinson, P.M., et al. J Clin Invest: 75: 1138-1143, 1985.
15. Dersimonian, H., et al. J Immunol 139: 2496-2501, 1987.
16. Hahn, B. and Ebling, F. J Clin Invest: 71: 1728-1736, 1983.
17. Zouali, M., et al. J Immunol: 135: 1091-1096, 1985.
18. Hahn, B. and Ebling, F. J Immunol: 132: 187-190, 1984.
19. Bluestone, J.A., et al. Immunol Rev: 90: 5-27, 1986.
20. Teitelbaum, D., et al. J Immunol: 132: 1282-1285, 1984.
21. Saski, T., et al. J Clin Invest: 77: 1382-1386, 1986.
22. Kaburaki, J. and Stollar, B.D. J Immunol: 139: 385-392, 1987.

REDUCTION OF PROTEIN EXCRETION BY ALLOPURINOL IN RATS WITH
ADRIAMYCIN NEPHROSIS.

F.GINEVRI,G.M.GHIGGERI,R.OLEGGINI,G.CANDIANO,R.BERTELLI, F.PER-
FUMO,R.GUSMANO.
Nephrology and Dialysis Department, G.Gaslini Institute, Genoa,
Italy.

INTRODUCTION

The kidney is a target organ for Adriamycin (ADR) toxicity
in rats producing renal changes which are similar in many ways
to the human minimal change nephropathy (1). Hystorically DNA
was considered the major site for ADR cytotoxicity in several
organs and tissues. Studies are now in progress to elucidate the
possible contribution of other mechanisms, mainly tissue damage
induced by oxygen free radicals. It is well known that ADR can
be converted "in vitro" to semiquinone unstable radicals (2)
that eventually give rise to superoxide anion (O_2^-) and hydro-
gen peroxide (H_2O_2).

In order to evaluate the possible implication of free radicals
in ADR nephrotoxicity "in vivo", experiments were performed with
the administration of specific and unspecific scavengers of
unstable radicals in rats. We hereby present data which demonstrate a marked inhibitory effect of allopurinol on proteinuria.

MATERIALS AND METHODS

Twenty-eight Sprague-Dawley rats weighing 200 to 300 g were
used in this study and divided into 4 experimental groups, 2 of
which served as control animals (groups A and B). In all rats
ADR nephrosis was induced by single intravenous injection of ADR
(5 mg/Kg). Groups A and B were given ADR plus saline or 0.25 M
NaOH (to simulate the pH of the allopurinol solution); group C
was pretreated with allopurinol (100 mg/Kg) 4 hours before ADR;
group D was treated with the same dosage of allopurinol immediately after ADR administration. Rats were maintained in metabolic

cages and proteinuria was evaluated every 5 days with the
Coomassie dye binding assay (3).

RESULTS AND DISCUSSION

ADR induces in rats a progressive increment of proteinuria
which reaches values of nephrotic syndrome 10-15 days after the
drug administration. When allopurinol was given 4 hours before
ADR failed to prevent the progression of the renal disease :
proteinuria in this group was only moderately lower than in the
untreated rats on day 10 and day 15 (Tab. I, group C). A different outcome of proteinuria was observed when allopurinol was
given immediately after ADR injection (Tab I, group D). In this
case proteinuria was only moderately increased above the normal
range on day 10 from ADR administration and was significantly
lower compared to the nephrotic groups on day 15 (p<0.05 vs
groups A and B).

Tab. 1. Outcome of proteinuria in ADR rats in relation to
allopurinol treatment.

Days from ADR injection

ADR treated rats	N·	5	10	15
a) Saline	(10)	51±9	251±54	395±42
b) NaOH 0.25 mM	(5)	53±7	324±42	481±94
c) Allopurinol 100 mg/Kg 4 hr before ADR	(8)	33±6	181±25	269±52
d) Allopurinol 100 mg/Kg immediately after ADR	(5)	39±7	91±38·*	159±54·*

· p<0.05 vs a.
* p<0.025 vs b.

At least two hypotheses can be put forward to explain such an
inhibitory effect of allopurinol on ADR nephrotoxicity. Allopurinol could effectively prevent proteinuria first of all by
acting as a general scavenger of free radicals, which may arise
from ADR renal metabolism. Indeed, the generation of free radicals has been from time proposed as the main mechanism for ADR
cytotoxicity in other organs and tissues such as the heart and
cultured cells of various origins (4). A second speculative

possibility is that ADR could produce free radicals via the xanthine-oxidase system. In this case kidney protection by allopurinol would derive from the well known inhibitory effect of the drug on the xanthine-oxidase enzyme. Very few data are so far available to support such an implication, however ADR is able to induce a marked decrease of ATPase activity on rat GBM (5) that could in turn increase the supply of substrates for the adenosine-uric acid pathway. Although these data need further evaluation we think that the inhibition of proteinuria by allopurinol in this experimental model could be relevant to the future developements in this area of research.

REFERENCES

1. Bertani T., Poggi A., Pozzoni R., Delaini F., Sacchi G., Thova Y., Mecca G., Remuzzi G., Donati M.B. Lab. Invest. 46:16-23, 1982.

2. Minnaugh E.G., Trush M.A. In: Oxyradicals and scavenger systems,vol. I: Molecular aspects (Eds. Cohen G., Greenwald R.A.) New York, Elsevier Biomedical, pp 300-303, 1983.

3. Read S.M., Northcate D.M. Anal. Biochem. 116: 53-64, 1981.

4. Doroshow J.H., Locker G.Y., Ifrim I., Myers C.E. J. Clin. Invest. 68: 1053-1064, 1981.

5) Bakker W.W., Kalicharan D., Donga J., Hulstaert C., Hardonk M. Kidney Int. 31: 704-709, 1987.

CLINICAL EXPERIENCE WITH AN ANTITHROMBOTIC AGENT (DEFIBROTIDE) IN GLOMERULAR DISEASES. PRELIMINARY RESULTS.

G.M. FRASCA', B. STAGNI, C. RAIMONDI, A.VANGELISTA, V.BONOMINI.

Institute of Nephrology, St.Orsola Univ.Hosp., Bologna, Italy

INTRODUCTION

Anticoagulants and/or antiplatelet agents have been previously investigated in the treatment of glomerular diseases on the basis of observations suggesting that the coagulation mechanisms are involved in glomerular injury and may play an important role in the persistence and/or progression of glomerular lesions (1). Although they are frequently associated with undesirable side effects, several studies have reported a beneficial effect from such treatment. (2,3).

The present study deals with our experience in treating primary glomerular diseases with Defibrotide, a polydeoxyribonucleotide salt which has a profibrinolytic and deaggregating activity based on its ability to induce a release of plasminogen activator factor and prostacyclin from vascular tissue and to decrease concentration of plasmin inhibitors (4).

PATIENTS AND METHODS

27 patients aged 32±14 years were included in the study. They all had a primary glomerular disease demonstrated by renal biopsy, unresponsive to steroids and cytotoxic drugs. The histological diagnosis was: membranous GN in 5 patients, focal segmental glomerulo-sclerosis in 6, IgA nephritis in 8, membrano-proliferative GN in 8. All patients had persistent proteinuria, which was in the nephrotic range in 16 of them (59.2%); 10 patients had abnormal renal function before treatment (37%) and 6 were hypertensive (22.2%).

TABLE I. Effect of Defibrotide on proteinuria.

Diagnosis	Pt.n.	Proteinuria (g/day) before	after	p value
Membranous GN	5	3.0±0.9	1.3±1.0	< 0.04
Focal segmental GS	6	4.2±1.1	1.9±1.7	n.s.
IgA nephritis	8	1.0±0.6	0.4±0.3	n.s.
Membrano-Prolif. GN	8	3.6±1.1	1.2±0.8	< 0.01
All patients	27	2.8±1.6	1.2±1.1	< 0.001

Before entering the study all patients had been treated with steroids, associated with cytotoxic drugs in 15 cases, for an average period of 27 months. During the study 10 mg/kg/day of Defibrotide were administered orally for 18±9 months; this regimen was the only treatment in 5 patients, while in the remainder it was associated with low-dose steroids (0.14-0.20 mg/kg/) on alternate days; 4 patients received an additional course with cyclophosphamide. After withdrawal of Defibrotide the patients were followed for 21±11 months and treated with steroids associated with cytotoxic drugs in 7 patients.

RESULTS AND DISCUSSION

16 patients (59%) were considered "responders" on the basis of a reduction in proteinuria exceeding 50% of the pre-treatment values. In these patients the improvement was maximum after 3 to 6 months of treatment and it does not seem that extending the therapy could result in any further reduction in proteinuria. The daily protein excretion significantly reduced after treatment (Table I) and showed a progressive increase after Defibrotide was withdrawn, although it did not reach the pre-treatment values. When the data are analysed in the light of histological diagnosis, it seems that patients with membrano-proliferative GN are the most susceptible to Defibrotide (Table I).

No significant change in serum creatinine was observed after treatment when all patients were considered (1.1 vs. 1.3 mg/dl), but an improvement was evident in patients with abnormal renal function (1.5 vs. 2.0 mg/dl; p < 0.01).

The success rate we observed in patients treated with Defibrotide, was similar to that reported in previous studies where anticoagulant and/or antiplatelet agents were used (2,3,5); unlike that trial, however, no significant side effect was associated with Defibrotide administration, even after prolonged periods.

The precise mechanism by which Defibrotide treatment induces a clinical improvement in chronic glomerular diseases is not known. It is probably related to the antithrombotic and deaggregating activity of the drug, through a reduction in platelet-vascular wall interaction. The possibility that Defibrotide could interfere with the prostaglandin balance is extremely attractive, since experimental studies have demonstrated that prostanoids can act as mediators of glomerular injury (7). The improvement we observed in patients with abnormal renal function could indeed be related with an increase in prostacyclin production induced by Defibrotide.

In conclusion, our preliminary results confirm that drugs interfering with coagulation mechanisms may be useful in patients with glomerular diseases, but deeper studies on a larger number of patients are desirable in order to identify the precise nephropathies and patients who may benefit from treatment.

REFERENCES
1. Vassalli,P., McCluskey,R.T. Adv. Nephrol.1:49-63,1971
2. Zimmerman,S.W., Moorthy,A.V., Dreher,W.H., Friedman,A., Varanasi,U. Am.J.Med. 75:920-927,1983.
3. Donadio,J.V.,Anderson,C.F.,Mitchell,J.C.,Holley,K.E., Ilstrup,D.M.,Fuster,V.,Chesebro,J.H. N.Eng.J.Med.310:1421-1426,1984.
4. Bonomini,V., Frascà,G.M., Raimondi,C., Liviano,G., Vangelista,A. Nephron 40:195-200,1985.
5. Ueda,N., Kawaguchi,S., Niinomi,Y., Nonoda,T., Ohnishi,M., Ito,S., Yasaki,T. Nephron 44:174-179,1986.
6. Lianos,E.A. Nephron 37:73-77,1984.

DEFIBRINATION WITH ANCROD IN CRESCENTIC GLOMERULAR LESIONS :
PRELIMINARY OBSERVATION.

Mauri J.M., Poveda R., González M.T., Carrera M., Carreras J.,
Díaz C., Ferrer P.

Hospital de Girona (Girona).
Hospital de Bellvitge (Hospitalet de Ll. Barcelona).

INTRODUCTION

   The activation of the coagulation mechanisms plays an important role in the sequence of events triggered by humoral immunological factors leading to glomerular damage. In this context,
wide epithelial proliferation -affecting a 50% or more of the
glomeruli- and some diffuse proliferative nephritis secondary
to collagen or systemic diseases are situations where the intraglomerular fibrin formation is currently agreed.

   Both, previous experimental and clinical reports, have stimulated to us for studying the effects of ancrod defibrination on
a group of patients with diverses unselected glomerulopathies
which common trait consisted in the presence of epithelial crescents in the 50% or more of the glomeruli studied.

PATIENTS AND METHODS

   Written consent was obteined. This study had previously been
approuved by the Ethics and Research Committee and by the Medical Director of the Institution.

   Thirteen patients, 8 males and 5 females aged 15-73 y.o., ful-
filling the following criteria, were introduced in the study :
Severe or proggresive loss of renal function of glomerular ori-
gen, presence of crescents in a 50% or more of the glomeruli,
abscence of recent bleeding or hemorrhagic dyathesis.

   This patients were randomly distributed into two groups. One
group of 6 patients, received ancrod alone. In the second group
ancrod was initially institued and subsequently immunosuppression with Prednisone (P) 1 mg/k.b.w. and Cyclophosphamide (CY)

2 mg/k.b.w. -either with or without plasma exchanges- was started.

Initial doses of 1-1.5 units/k.b.w. of ancrod (KNOLL-MADE S.A. LABORATORIOS, MADRID, ESPAÑA) were administered in a slow infusion with dextrose 5%. The first dose was infused in 4 hours. On later administrations ancrod doses were empirically stablished between 0.6-1.5 units/k.b.w. in order to keeps blood fibrinogen at less than 100 mg% and the infusion time was shorted to two hours.

Out of the case 4, in all improved patients an antiaggregating treatment with aspirin 0.5 gr/d. and dypiridamol 200 mg/d. was undertaken 72 hours before ancrod suppression.

Statistical analysis have been performed by using an HP 3000 computer and the SPSS programs package. A bivariate correlation between serum creatinine level and disease evolution time by using the scattergram and pearson-corr procedures, was performed.

RESULTS

In the group of patients receiving ancrod followed by P and CY -with/without plasma exchanges- significative changes of creatinine values during ancrod administration could not be seen. Creatinina in these patients changed towards steady state levels lower than the values seen before rebound took place. Only one out of four patients presenting HD requirements dit not improve and remained under HD assistancies. In the other three patients -all of them with histological pattern of severe acute tubular necrosis but without significent interstitial fibrosis- a sharp fall of the serum creatinine values associated to the recovery of diuresis was seen. Thereafter, a progressive improvement of creatininemias was observed.

DISCUSSION

The striking improvement of the renal function and glomerular changes observed in 5 over 6 patients receiving ancrod alone strongly suggests a cause-effect relationship roughly similar to that observed in experimentally induced immunologic nephritis.

It is difficult to evaluate the role played by desfibrination in the satisfactory evolution observed in 3 out of 4 patients with hemodialysisi requirements that received immunosuppression after ancrod. Only the pathological changes -improvement of the epythelial proliferation and marked reduction of the glomerular and capsular fibrinogen fluorescence- would argue in favor of an effectiveness of the desfibrination. On the other hand the association of severe morfological changes of acute tubular necrosos present in all 3 cases could explain the absece in them of any early improvement of their renal function.

It is noteworthy than the serum creatinine rebound when seen in immunosuppressed patients was lesser and that improvement ocurred without changes in the immunosuppressive regime applied in spite of an hiperaggregative platelet state similar to that observed in patients that received ancrod alone. It seams probable that the immediate immunosuppression therapy, started when hypofibrinogenemia was still present, could have had a protective effect by means of an action on the installed immunological events.

Further studies are required to recognize in which way the enhancement of the glomerular fibrinolisis mechanisms favorized by the interruption of fibrin generation may participate in the favorable responses seen after ancrod therapy.

1) Ancrod reduced effectively the epythelial proliferation and the glomerular fibrinogen staining.

2) The improvement of the serum creatinine levels seen when ancrod was administered alone could be related to the suppression of fibrin formation per se or to an enhancement of the fibrin clearing mechanisms. In our interpretation changes in blood viscosity could not explain but might have contributed to the renal function improvement observed.

3) Ancrod immediately followed by immunosuppression with P and CY -with/without plasma exchanges- offers better perspectives to steadly improve the renal function in this kind of patients.

PAF INDUCED GLOMERULAR AND VASCULAR ALTERATIONS IN THE ISOLATED PERFUSED RAT KIDNEY.

Ullrich Schwertschlag, Vincent Dennis and Giovanni Camussi*
Department of Medicine, Duke University Medical Center, Durham, North Carolina and Department of Microbiology and Pathology*,
SUNY, Buffalo, New York

INTRODUCTION

PAF is a proaggregatory and proinflammatory mediator with potent vasoactive properties [1, 2]. At low doses, some of its vasodilating properties are attributable to a direct action on vascular smooth muscle cells; at higher doses, extravasation of labeled albumin has been observed. These changes in vascular permeability result in part from the release of vasoactive mediators from inflammatory cells and to direct effects on vessel walls. PAF infusion in rabbits causes reversible proteinuria concomitant with an accumulation of platelets and PMN in capillary lumens and the deposition platelet- and PMN-derived cationic proteins in the glomerular capillary wall [3]. These events coincide with a loss of fixed negative charges of glomerular capillary wall. Because resident glomerular cells can produce PAF [4], it seems important to test the hypothesis that PAF might act directly on glomerular permeability. The aim of the present study was to determine whether PAF may increase glomerular permeability in the isolated rat kidney perfused with a cell-free medium and, if so, whether such effect was related to glomerular hemodynamic alterations or to neutralization of fixed anionic charges.

MATERIALS AND METHODS

Native horse spleen ferritin was dialyzed against 1 mM EDTA and phosphate buffered saline. The final concentration in the perfusate was 0.1mg/ml. Polyethylenimine (MW 1800) was dissolved in perfusion fluid and infused at 0.05 mg/ml. Perfusion procedure and measurement of renal function were as described [2]

Experimental Protocols

Kidneys were perfused with various concentrations of L-PAF (1nM to 1 uM) for 5 minutes. Changes in glomerular permeability were assessed morphologically using native ferritin infused into the perfusion system for 5 minutes. PAF (1 nM-100 nM) was infused with ferritin for 5 minutes and then the kidneys were fixed by perfusion for 3 minutes. Changes in anionic glomerular charges were assessed in two ways. First, lysozyme was used to stain polyanionic sialoglycoproteins of glomerular epithelial cells [5]. Second, fixed negative charges of GBM were quantified with polyethylenimine [6]. The degree of penetration of the glomerular basement membrane (GBM) by native ferritin was assessed on unstained or lead citrate stained sections. Comparisons were by Dunnett's t-test or unpaired t-test as appropriate.

RESULTS

Effect of PAF on Renal Functional Parameters

Platelet activating factor produced a dose-dependent decrease in renal vascular resistance and GFR (Fig. 1). r-PAF had no effect (not shown).

Histological Changes Induced by PAF

Fig. 1. Changes in RVR and GFR during control and L-PAF infusions. Comparisons were made between preinfusion and infusion periods. (n, 8)

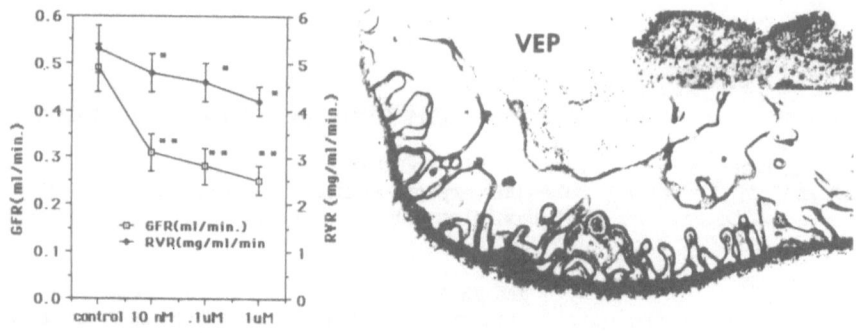

Fig. 2. Electron micrograph of a portion of glomerular capillary of a kidney perfused with 10 nM L-PAF followed by infusion of lysozyme. Lysozyme can be seen as a dense layer on the epithelial cell coat and on GBM (x 26,000; n, 6). VEP:visceral epithelial cells. L: lumen. Inset: Portion of glomerular capillary of a kidney perfused with 10 nM L-PAF stained with PEI to detect anionic site of GBM. The electron-dense granular aggregates of polyethylenimine are seen along the laminae rara interna and externa (arrow heads) with a regular distribution (x 53,000).

L-PAF at concentrations ranging from 1 nM to 100 nM markedly increased penetration of ferritin in GBM (Table 1). In kidneys perfused with r-PAF, no significant penetration of native ferritin in the GBM was observed for concentration of 10 nM or 100 nM (Table 1). The glomerular binding of lysozyme in kidneys perfused either with s-PAF (10 nM) or r-PAF (10 nM) or the perfusion buffer alone was similar to that previously reported [3]. Lysozyme bound to the epithelial cell coat (glycocalix) forming a dense layer approximately 30 nm thick (Fig. 2) and to the GBM usually at the level of the lamina rara externa. Thus L-PAF did not detectably reduce epithelial cell sialoglycoprotein polyanions. In addition, quantitation of fixed negative sites of GBM by PEI showed no differences between kidneys perfused with 10 nM s-PAF (32.2 ± 2.9 [SE] sites/1000 nm of GBM length), or with 10 nM r-PAF (35.4 ± 3.6 sites/1000 nm), or with perfusion buffer alone (33.8 ± 3.3 sites/1000 nm).

	CONTROL	D-PAF (10^{-8}M)	D-PAF (10^{-6}M)	L-PAF (10^{-9}M)	L-PAF (10^{-8}M)	L-PAF (10^{-7}M)
GBM (#/um2)	1.2 ± 0.9	8.0 ± 2	70.4 ± 60	43.1 ± 21.7	86 ± 4.1	830 ± 41
LRE (#/um2)	0.2 ± 0.06	5 ± 2	20 ± 16	21.4 ± 5.1	80 ± 12	88 ± 19

Table 1: Native ferritin particles in the glomerular basement membrane (GBM) and lamina rara externa (LRE) (# Particles/um^2)

DISCUSSION: The present study demonstrates three actions of L-PAF on the isolated rat kidney: 1) renal vasodilation, 2) decreased GFR, and 3) increased glomerular permeability. Glomerular filtration is determined by glomerular pressure gradients, by the hydraulic conductivity of the glomerular basement membrane and possibly by the contractile state of the glomerulus itself. Because PAF reduced both renal vascular resistance and GFR, a postglomerular vasodilation by PAF would explain the fall in GFR. Filtration fraction decreased by about 50% although RVR decreased by only 15%. This suggests that PAF may affect GFR by mechanisms other than hemodynamic actions.

33

The present study indicates that PAF may directly increase glomerular permeability but does not alter the electrostatic properties of the glomerular capillary wall (Fig. 2). In the absence of inflammatory cells such as macrophages and polymorphonuclear leukocytes, it is possible that s-PAF acts directly on glomerular cells. In isolated rat glomeruli, PAF decreases planar surface area [4], perhaps from mesangial cell contraction. PAF also increases the permeability of endothelial cells in vitro [7]. PAF increases glomerular permeability in the isolated perfused rat kidney as indicated by the increased penetration of native ferritin particles in the glomerular basement membrane. The quantitation of fixed negative charges in the laminae rarae interna and externa of GBM by PEI did not show any differences in s-PAF-infused kidneys versus controls. Within the limitation of these methodologies, PAF-induced increases in glomerular permeability are thus not associated with alterations of glomerular electrostatic barriers.

In conclusion, the possible candidates to explain the fall in GFR are postglomerular vasodilation, mesangial and endothelial contraction, and increased permeability. The effect of s-PAF is specific, since r-PAF does not produce the same effects. These results suggest that, in vivo, two concomitant mechanisms are responsible for PAF-induced proteinuria. The first is related to the release of inflammatory mediators that may neutralize glomerular anionic charges. The second mechanism, consistent with the results of this study, is the direct effect of PAF on glomerular capillary walls independent of changes in the glomerular electrostatic barrier. This not only includes endothelial and mesangial cell contraction but also production of secondary mediators from these cells such as PGE2 and TXB2 from mesangial cells [4]. Further studies are needed to investigate if PAF may alter the size selectivity of GBM.

1. Camussi G: Potential role of platelet-activating factor in renal pathophysiology. Kidney Int. 29: 469-477, 1986.
2. Schwertschlag US, Scherf H, Gerber J, Mathias MP and Nies AS: L-platelet activating factor induces changes on renal vascular resistance, vascular reactivity, and renin release in isolated perfused rat kidney. Circ. Res. 60: 534-539, 1987.
3. Camussi G, Tetta C, Coda R, Segoloni GP and Vercellone A: Platelet activating factor-induced loss of glomerular anionic charges. Kidney Int. 25: 73-81, 1984.
4. Schlondorff D, Goldwasser P, Neuwirth R, Satriano JA, and Clay KL: Production of platelet-activating factor in glomeruli and cultured glomerular mesangial cells. Am. J. Physiol. 250: F1123-F1127, 1986.
5. Barnes JL, Radnik RA, Gilchrist EP and Venkatachalam MA: Size and charge selective permeability defects induced in glomerular basement membrane by a polycation. Kidney Int. 25: 11-19, 1984.
6. Schurer JW, Hoedemaeker and Molenaar I: Polyethylenemine as tracer particle for (immuno) electron microscopy. J. Histo Chem Cytochem. 25: 384, 1977.
7. Bussolino F, Camussi G, Aglietta M, Braquet P, Bosio A, Pescarmons G, Sanavio F, D'Urso M, and Marchisio PC: Human endothelial cells are targets for platelet activating factor (PAF), I. PAF induces changes in cytoskeleton structures. J Immunol., (In press).

HISTOGENESIS OF GLOMERULAR CRESCENTS IN IDIOPATHIC PROLIFERATIVE EXTRACAPILLARY GLOMERULONEPHRITIS. CLINICAL ASPECTS.

J. DIEZ [*], F. J. PARDO-MINDAN [**]

Departments of Nephrology (*) and Pathology (**), Clínica Universitaria, Universidad de Navarra, Pamplona, Spain.
This work was financed by a Grant of the FISS.

INTRODUCTION

The histogenesis and cellular constituents of glomerular crescents in proliferative extracapillary glomerulonephritis (PEGN) is controversial: so the presence of parietal and visceral epithelial cells (1), and monocytes (2) have been demonstrated in the crescents, and each one responsabilized of their histogenesis. A study was undertaken to determine the histogenesis of the glomerular crescents. It is the purpose of this paper to identify the cells which form crescents in idiopathic immuno-complex mediated PEGN, using immunohistochemical methods and electron microscopy, and to discuss their formation and evolution.

MATERIALS AND METHODS

Twenty cases of idiopathic immuno-complex mediated PEGN with crescents were evaluated. Selected biopsies were from patients, in which renal symptoms had started the month prior to the biopsy, so that the crescents were predominantly cellular.

Biopsies were studied by light, immunohistochemical and electron microscopic study. A panel of antibodies against Igs, complement fractions, fibrin, types III and IV collagen, laminin, fibronectin, keratin, vimentin, lisozyme, $alpha_1$-antitrypsin, OKT_3, and Leu M_3 was used in avidin-biotin immunohistochemical technique.

RESULTS

Two types of PEGN may be demonstrated: PEGN with crescents formed predominantly by proliferation of parietal epithelial cells (ty-

pe PE-PEGN) and PEGN with crescents predominantly formed by proliferation of visceral epithelial cells (type VE-PEGN).

Twelve biopsies with type PE-PEGN had an average of 55% of glomeruli with crescents. Periglomerular inflammation was frequently pre
sent. The glomerular tufts were focally necrosed and the capillaries
collapsed. Proliferation of mesangium was mild. Tubular atrophy, interstitial inflammatory infiltration of macrophages, lymphocytes,
plasma cells, polymorphonuclear leukocytes and perivascular inflamma
tion were common. Organization with fibroblasts and collagen deposition occurred in focal areas. Fixation of C_3 in a granular pattern
could be demonstrated in all cases with varying intensity. Type III
collagen was present in the crescents. By electron microscopy the
crescents were formed by a proliferation of cells with morphological
features of parietal epithelial cells, particularly by the presence
of many desmosomes and the absence of foot processes. Clinical onset
was insidious (Table 1) and only half of the patients were in hemodialysis after an average follow-up of 24 months.

Table 1. Nephrological data

Type of PEGN	Time from clinical onset (weeks)	Oliguria Anuria (%)	Edema (%)	Hematuria (%)	MAP (mmHg)	Protei- nuria (g/d)	C_{Cr} (ml/min)
PE N=12	40 80-136	16	33	100	110 73-145	1.06 0.1-3.9	29 6-66
VE N=8	7 2-28	37	64	100	110 88-140	2.54 0.3-5.7	15 2-38

(%): Percent of patients with the manifestation

Eight biopsies with type VE-PEGN had an average of 72% of glome
ruli with crescents, and a prominent mesangial proliferation. Type IV
collagen, fibronectin, and laminin were present in crescents. By
electron microscopy, the crescents were formed by a proliferation of
cells with morphological features of visceral epithelial cells which
showed cytoplasmic proccesses similar to podocytes and microvillis.
Patients had a more abrupt clinical onset with a greater proteinuria

and a lesser clearance of creatinine than patients with type PE-PEGN (Table 1). Most of the patients were in hemodialysis after an average follow-up of 15 months.

DISCUSSION

Immunohistochemical methods (3, 4) and the ultrastructural study (5) of early predominantly cellular crescents allow to distinguish between different cells of the kidney, and of the cells which form the crescents and it gives a morphological base to make a clear differentiation between two types of PEGN (5). Type PE-PEGN has a mo re protracted course, because glomerular sclerosis, due to emigration and proliferation of fibroblasts and subsequent collagen deposition may cease without reaching a total renal sclerosis. Clinically, this type of PEGN is less agressive at presentation, patients have an indolent course to renal failure, and medical treatment appears to exert a protective role against the total loss of renal function. This group of patients could present the "not so rapidly progressive form" of crescentic glomerulonephritis which has been clinically identified by some authors (6). In contrast, type VE-PEGN has a more agressive course and a worse prognosis, since crescents end in total glomerular hyalinization by deposition of fibronectin and type IV co llagen. Clinically,most patients with this type of PEGN pursue a rapid course with total loss of renal function despite treatment.

REFERENCES

1. Salant, D.J. Immunopathogenesis of crescentic glomerulonephritis and lung purpura. Kidney Int. 32:408-425, 1987.
2. Thomson, N.M., Holdsworth, S.R., Glasgow, E.F., Atkins, R.C. The macrophage in the development of experimental crescentic glomerulonephritis. Am. J. Pathol. 94:223, 1979.
3. Courtoy, P.J., Timpl, R., Farquhar, M.G. Comparative distribution of laminin, type IV collagen and fibronectin in rat glomerulus. J. Histochem. Cytochem. 30:874, 1982.
4. Scheinman, J.L., Foidart, J.M., Michael, A.E. The immunohistology of glomerular antigens: V. The collagenous antigens of the glomerulus. Lab. Invest. 43:373,1980.
5. Norgaard, J.O.R. Rat glomerular epithelial cells in culture. Parietal or visceral epithelial origin?. Lab. Invest. 57:277-290, 1987.
6. Baldwin, D.S. et al. The existence of a protracted course in crescentic glomerulonephritis. Kidney Int. 31:790-794, 1987.

PREMISES FOR AN ANTIOXIDANT THERAPY IN PREGNANCY INDUCED NEPHROPATHY

P.Stratta*, C.Canavese*, L.Gurioli*, M.Porcu*, M.Dogliani*, F.Bel-
liardo°, E.Garbo°, G.Artuffo°, A.Vercellone*

Department of Nephrology* and Science and Tecnology of Drugs°,
University of Torino, Italy

INTRODUCTION

Different experimental and clinical observations support an
imbalance between oxidant and antioxidant factors in preeclampsia
(PE): a) an increased concentration of lipid peroxides, and by-
products of peroxidation due to free-radicals (1); b) a reduced
ability to produce Prostacyclin by the fetal and maternal endothelial
cells (2); c) the preeclamptic-like syndrome induced in pregnant rat
by a vitamin E deficient diet (3); d) the directly reduced placental
Prostacyclin production due to a deficit of Vitamin E (4).

Even in normal pregnancy an increase in polyunsaturated fatty
acids,which are the most favourable substrate for peroxidation (5-6)
seems to constitute a background requirement for an increase of antioxidant defenses able to overwhelm the greater risk of peroxidation.

The aim of this study was to evalute if the behaviour of the main
components of the antioxidant defense mechanism (Vitamin E, ceruloplasmin and transferrin) is able to provide useful information about
the oxidant/antioxidant balance in normal pregnancy and in PE.

PATIENTS AND METHODS

The study was undertaken on 40 normal pregnancy monitored monthly
from the first trimester until birth, and on 14 cases of PE. We evaluated: plasma Vitamin E (HPLC, Perkin-Elmer 3B liquid chromatogr-

aph), serum transferrin and ceruloplasmin (radial immunodiffusion) serum uric acid and total proteins (standard techniques).

RESULTS

In normal pregnancy, Vitamin E is below normal (10±mg/dl) in the first weeks,and progressively increases until a maximum is reached in the third trimester, but still in normal ranges.Transferrin continuously increases until birth, while ceruloplasmin increases until the beginning of the third trimester, and after remains stable.(Table 1).

TABLE 1 - Vitamin E, Transferrin and Ceruloplasmin kinetics in normal pregnancy

Vitamin E (mg/l)	6.3± 1.8	7.7± 2.7	8.3± 3.1	9.1± 2.8	9.9± 3.2	9.4± 2.9
Transferrin (mg/dl)	49± 15	62.8± 17	67.7± 16	68.9± 20	64.4± 19	68.2± 16
Ceruloplasmin mg/dl	299± 95	337± 85	366± 66	408± 100	431± 72	466± 79
	<12	13-19	20-24	25-29	30-34	>35
			GESTATION WEEKS			

In PE transferrin and Vitamin E are significantly reduced (respectively 339±99 mg/dl and 6.5±1.3 mg/l),whereas ceruloplasmin is not significantly different (62.8±18 mg/dl). Total serum protein in PE was also significantly reduced (5.3±1.4 vs 6.3±1.9 g/dl), but the transferrin decrease was more than that of total serum protein percentage - wise (-26.0±3% vs -16.6±3%). In 7 patients in which Vitamin E (100-300 mg/day per os) was administered as therapy, the Vitamin E value itself increases, while transferrin and/or ceruloplasmin continued to decrease at the same time as uric and levels went up.

CONCLUSIONS

The behaviour of transferrin and ceruloplasmin in normal pregnancy clearly demonstrates that they are intentionally produced, because their constant increase is in direct opposition to the 10-20%

serum protein decrease which is known to occurr in the same time (7, 8). Also the Vitamin E increase (perhaps due to a greater gastro-intestinal absorption or to an increased disponibility from tissue stores) could have a biological goal in order to increase the anti-oxidant defenses. Also in PE, the variations observed in transferrin and ceruloplasmin seem to be directly related to specific biological features, instead of being merely consequences of changes in total protein concentration. In fact, transferrin decrease is greater than what was expected following total protein decreas, thus speaking in the favour of an a selective actual consumption. Furthermore, the absence of ceruloplasmin decrease as total protein may support the hypothesis of an active compensatory effort to overcame the oxidant stress. Nevertheless, in our preliminary therapeutic approach, although Vitamin E is also reduced, Vitamin E supplementation does not seem to be able to avoid a further decrease in one or both the two other plasma antioxidant agents.

In sum,while our results confirm the existence of premises for an antioxidant therapy in PE,the dosages, and perhaps also the times and the ways of somministration of this therapy et remain to be defined.

REFERENCES
1) Halliwell, B., Gutteridge, J.M.C. Lancet i: 1396-1397, 1984
2) Ongari, M., Ritter, J.M., Orchard, M.A., Waddel, K.A., Blair, I.A., Lewis, P.J. Am. J. Obstet Gynecol 149: 455-460, 1984
3) Stamler, F.M. Am. J. Path. 35: 1207-1231, 1959
4) Spitz, B., Deckmyn, H., Van Bree, R. Pijnemborg, R., Vermylen, J., Van Assche, F.A. Am. J. Obstet Gynecol. 151: 116-120, 1985
5) Rosing, V., Johnson P, Alund A., Samsive G. Gynecol. Obstet. Invest. 14: 225-235, 1982
6) Erkkola, R., Grönrons, M., Ekblad, U., Haataya, M., Nieminen, A.L. Leukotrienes Med. 13: 311-314, 1984.
7) Oian, P., Maltau, J.M., Noddelan,H., Fadnes, H.O. Gynaecol 93: 235-239, 1986
8) Oian, P., Maltan, J.M., Noddelan, H., Fadnes, H.O. Brit. J. Obstet. Gynecol. 97: 1113-1119, 1985.

PULSE THERAPY WITH CYCLOPHOSPHAMIDE IN PRIMARY AND SISTEMIC
GLOMERULOPATHY RESISTANT TO STEROID TREATMENT

D. Grekas, H. Kalekou, G. Karkavelas, L. Settas, P. Alivanis,
M. Pyrpasopoulos. First Renal Unit, University of Thessaloniki,
AHEPA Hospital, Thessaloniki, Greece.

INTRODUCTION

If the addition of cytotoxic agents to methyilprednisolone pulse
therapy improves survival and morbidity in systemic nephrites is
controversial (1,2). Intermittent boluses of cyclophosphamide have
been shown to reduce the adverse effects observed with daily chronic
administration (3,4,5,6). To our knowledge, cyclophosphamide pulse
therapy has never been tested on idiopathic glomerulonephropathy with
or without nephrotic syndrome.

PATIENTS, METHODS AND RESULTS

Twelve patients, seven with multisystem glomerular disease and
five with idiopathic nephropathy were included in the study. The
initial clinical and renal pathology findings are shown in Table 1.
All patients were given 1-2 mg/kg body weight methylprednisolone
daily reducing the dosage within two months. 3/7 patients with systemic glomerular disease, 2 with lupus nephritis and the patient with
cryoglobulinemic nephritis were also given pulse methylprednisolone
of 1 gr daily for 3-4 consecutive days. Because no response was
obtained we decided to give pulse therapy with 0.5-1 gr cyclophosphamide every four weeks. 3/5 patients with primary nephrotic syndrome
showed full remission (clinical and laboratory), 1/5 partial remission
and the patient n.3 no remission; 5/7 patients with systemic glomerular disease showed full remission, 1/7 partial remission and 1/7 no
remission (Table1). The final outcame of patients after 1-5 years
of follow-up is shown also in Table 1.

DISCUSSION

Lupus Nephritis. The current method of approach to patients with
lupus

41

nephritis is to detect the disease early and to treat it as rapidly as posible. Corticosteroids and cyclophosphamide have been valuable in helping to increase the survival of patients with renal lupus, but when the patients receiving cyclophosphamide in any regimen compared with those receiving prednisone only the 10 year probability on no renal failure was significantly greater in the first group than the second. It is also accepted that this kind of treatment after the kidneys are scarred is not very effective when compared with the treatment begun carlier (6).

Cryoglobulinemic nephritis. Successful pharmacologic treatment with corticosteroids and/or cytotoxic drugs has not been uniformely achieved in cryoglobulinemia associated with systemic autoimmune diseases, but our case showed a dramatic responce to cyclophosphamide pulse therapy.

Idiopathic nephropathy. Because in our five patients with nephrotic syndrome proteinuria did not change by oral or iv methylprednisolone we used the new protocol of pulse cyclophosphamide treatment. The results were satisfactory at the end of the therapy as well as at the final follow up. Side effects were not observed by this mode of therapy.

So, pulse therapy with cyclophosphamide should be yet considered experimental, and randomized clinical trials to confirm its efficacy are needed. Our observations to date suggest that this mode of treatment retards immune-mediated destruction better than oral or bolus therapy with methylprednisolone.

REFERENCES

1. Cameron, J.S. In: 9th Int. Congress Nephrology (Eds R.R. Robinson), Springer-Verlag, Los Angeles 1984, pp. 1445-1463.
2. Bolton, W.K. In: 9th Int. Congress Nephrology (Eds. R.T.Robinson), Springer-Verlag, Los Angeles 1984, pp. 1464-1473.
3. Steinberg, A.D. N. Engl. J. Med. 310:458, 1984.
4. Dinant, H.J., Decker, J.L., Klippel, J.H., Balow, J.E., Plotz,P.H. and Steinberg, A.D. Ann. Intern. Med. 96:728, 1982.
5. Austin, H.A., Klippel, J.H., Balow, J.E., LeRiche, N.G., Steinberg, A.D., Plotz, P.H. and Decker, J.L. N. Engl. J. Med. 314:614-619, 1986.
6. Steinberg, A.D. Kidney Intern. 30:769-787, 1986.

Clinical and renal pathology data, pharmacologic therapy and outcome of studied patients with primary and systemic glomerular disease

No	Patient Age/sex	Clinical presentation	Renal pathology	Pharmacologic therapy methyl-prednisolone	Cyclophosphamide	Follow-up (years)	Final outcome
1	KP 31/Male	nephrotic syndrome renal function normal	membranous nephropathy	80mg/d/2mo.	1g/mo/6 doses	4	Remission
2	KK 37/Male	nephrotic syndrome renal function normal	membranous nephropathy	2mg/kg/d/2mo.	1g/mo/7 doses	5	Relapse
3	HC 27/Male	nephrotic syndrome renal function impaired	focal glomerulosclerosis	2mg/kg/d/2mo. 1g/d/3 doses	1g/mo/7 doses	3	Dialysis
4	TN 25/Male	nephrotic syndrome renal function normal	mesangio-proliferative nephritis	2mg/kg/d/2mo.	1g/mo/8 doses	1	Remission
5	SE 22/Female	nephrotic syndrome renal function normal	minimal change nephropathy	2mg/kg/d/2mo.	1g/mo/6 doses	1	Remission
6	AP 19/Female	SLE,nephritis,hypertension,renal function normal	diffuse proliferative nephritis	2mg/kg/d/2mo.	1g/mo/6 doses	5	Remission
7	MT 43/Female	SLE,nephrotic syndrome, hypertension, CRF(?)	focal glomerulosclerosis	2mg/kg/d/2mo. 1g/d/3 doses	0.7g/mo/8 doses	5	CRF
8	ME 41/Male	SLE,nephrotic syndrome hypertension, CRF (?)	membranous nephropathy	80mg/d/2mo. 1g/d/4 doses	0.5g/mo/6 doses	5	Remission
9	KG 56/Female	SLE,nephrotic syndrome thromboembolic episodes	mesangio-proliferative nephritis	80mg/d/2mo.	1g/mo/8 doses	3	Death
10	VE 26/Female	SLE, nephrotic syndrome	membranous nephropathy	2mg/d/2mo.	1g/mo/8 doses		
11	RK 25/Female	SLE,nephrotic syndrome	diffuse proliferative nephritis	80mg/d/2mo.	1g/mo/9 doses	1	Remission
12	MA 56/Female	Cryoglobulinemia, nephritis purpura	diffuse membrano proliferative nephritis	80mg/d/2mo. 1g/d/3 doses	1g/mo/6 doses	4	Remission

IgA Nephropathy

CLINICAL PRESENTATION OF IGA NEPHROPATHY IN SOUTHERN ITALY

M. BALLETTA, G. FUIANO, P. STANZIALE, M. VISCIONE, G. MARINELLI, A. SELLARO, N. COMI, G. COLUCCI, V. SEPE.

Department of Nephrology II Faculty of Medicine Naples Italy

INTRODUCTION

First discovered by Berger (1-2), primary IgA nephropathy has been recognized as a distinct glomerulonephritis and defined as a disease with prominent mesangial IgA deposits in the absence of clinical signs of associated disease.

The clinical presentation is usually characterized by one or more episodes of gross hematuria; however asymptomatic microscopic hematuria, asymptomatic proteinuria, nefrotic proteinuria are sometimes the sole laboratory signs.

To investigate if any correlation exists between the presence of gross hematuria and the clinico-morphological findings at presentation,we analyzed data from 36 adults with IgA nephropathy presenting with or without gross hematuria.

PATIENTS AND METHODS

The study was carried out in 36 adults with IgA nephropathy (22%) selected among 162 patients with primary glomerulonephritis who underwent a renal biopsy in the last six years: in all cases criteria for performing renal biopsy were presence of microhematuria and/or proteinuria > 1 gr./24 h, two or more episodes of gross hematuria, " nephrotic" proteinuria.

The specimens were processed for optical microscopy using conventional technics, immunohistochemical studies were performed using a direct immunofluorescence method on frozen tissue. Renal histology was reviewed by three of us (MB, GF, PS.) glomerular changes were scored as mild, moderate and severe.

The patients were divided in two groups according to the presence (group 1) or absence (group 2) of gross hematuria and compared for sex, age, interval between clinical onset and biopsy, blood pressure, 24 hours proteinuria, blood hemoglobin, serum IgA, serum albumin, creatinine clearance, histological and immunohistological changes by Student's t test and Fisher's Exact test.

RESULTS

Tables 1 and 2 summarize the main clinical and morphological data in our 36 patients at the biopsy time.

Table. 1   Clinical findings at biopsy time

	Mean	SD	Pos.	Range
Sex M:F			1.7:1	
Age at biopsy (yrs)	28.7	11.2		16-52
Upper respir. tract inf.			20(56%)	
Gross hematuria			24(67%)	
Microhem. and/or prot.			12(33%)	
Mean blood pres. (mmHg)	95.9	12.6		74-122
Blood hemoglobin (g/dl)	14.2	1.6		10-19
Serum IgA > 350 mg/dl			16(52%)	
Serum albumin (g/dl)	3.9	0.5		3-4.8
Proteinuria (g/24h)	1.6	1.5		0-5.8
Creatinine cl. (ml/min)	107	31		62-166

Table 2.   Histological findings at biopsy time

	Total tested	Positive	%
Glomerular changes:			
mild	31	6	19.4
moderate	31	5	16.1
severe	31	20	64.5
Tubular atrophy	31	11	35.5
Interstitial fibr.	31	10	32.2
Interstitial inf.	31	8	25.8
Arteriolar scler.	31	1	3.2

The two groups showed no significant differences when
compared for age (25.8 ± 10.9 vs 34.4 ± 8.6 yrs),
interval between clinical onset and biopsy (42.6 ± 56.8
vs 88.4 ± 79.6 months), mean blood pressure (91.5 ± 11.2
vs 104.6 ± 9.6
mmHg), blood hemoglobin (14.5 ± 1.0 vs 13.4 ± 2.2 g/dl),
serum albumin (4.0 ± 0.4 vs 3.8 ± 0.5 g/dl), 24 hours
proteinuria (1.38 ± 1.5 vs 1.97 ± 1.2 gr) and incidence
of patients with serum IgA > 350 mg/dl (50% vs 55%).
Creatinine clearance was higher in group 1 (116.0 ± 28.8
vs 81.1 ± 20.3 ml/min p < 0.01). Males predominated in
group 1 (M:F ratio = 3:1) and females in group 2 (F:M
ratio = =1.4:1).

Severe glomerular changes were prevalent in
patients of group 2 (52% vs 90% p < 0.05). Tubular
atrophy was present in 5 patients of group 1 (23.8%) and
in 6 patiets of group 2 (60%). No significant differences
in the distribution and intensity of immunodeposits were
observed between the groups.

DISCUSSION

Primary IgA nephropathy is one of the most common
forms of glomerulonephritis in Italy as it is in France
(2), in Australia (3) and in Japan (4). All ages and both
sex were affected although male adults aged 16-52 years
comprised 63.9% of our adult patients. As reported in
many papers gross hematuria either isolated or recurrent
was present in most of patients, whereas microscopic
hematuria and/or proteinuria were the only clinical
features in the others.

Since its presentation is so variable and its
definition is purely descriptive, many investigators
suggested that primary IgA nephropathy may comprise
different disease forms with the same epiphenomen of
mesangial IgA deposits.

According to this hypothesis, we evaluated if any

correlation exists between the presence of gross
hematuria and the the clinico-morphological findings at
presentation.

The two groups showed no rilevant differences when
compared for age, interval from onset to biopsy, mean
blood pressure, blood hemoglobin, serum albumin, 24 hours
proteinuria and incidence of high levels of serum IgA.
The only significant clinical difference was a lower
creatinine clearance in the group presenting with
microscopic hematuria and/or proteinuria. "Severe"
glomerular involvement and tubular atrophy were prevalent
in patients presenting with microscopic hematuria and/or
proteinuria.

This data suggest that at least two subentities in
primary IgA nephropathy exist : the first represented by
patients presenting with gross hematuria and a mild renal
involment, the second by patients without gross hematuria
but with a worse renal involment. Alternatively, a
different renal involvement at presentation could be
related to an earlier diagnosis in patients with gross
hematuria. In this study no significant differences were
observed between the groups when compared for age and
interval from onset to diagnosis but, notwithstanding
this,it is possible that asymptomatic hematuria and/or
proteinuria may date from many months before the
"apparent onset".

References
1. Berger, J. and Hinglais, N. J. Urol. Nephrol. 74:
   694, 1968.
2. Berger, J. Transplant Proc. 1:939-944, 1969.
3. Clarckson, A.R., Seymour, A.E., Thompson,A.J., Haynes,
   W.D.G., Chan, Y.L., Jackson, B., Clinical Nephrol. 8:
   459, 1977
4. Chida, Y., Tomura, S., Takeuchi, J. Nephron 40:
   189-194, 1985

INTERLEUKIN-2 PRODUCTION AND ABNORMALITIES OF IMMUNE REGULATION IN
PATIENTS WITH PRIMARY IgA NEPHROPATHY.
F.P. SCHENA, G. MASTROLITTI, A.R. FRACASSO, L. AVENTAGGIATO

Chair of Medical Therapy, University of Bari, Italy.

IgA nephropathy (IgAN) is characterized by the presence in the
blood of increased IgA-specific helper T cell activity with the receptor for the Fc region of IgA (Tα cells) (1), decreased IgA-specific
suppressor T cell activity (2) and increased number of peripheral B
lymphocytes with IgA Fc receptor (Bα cells) (3). Since interleukin
2 (IL-2) is a polypeptidic hormone which plays an important role in
immunoregulation and lymphocyte activation, we thought it opportune
to study the production of IL-2 from peripheral blood mononuclear
cells (PBMC) of patients with IgAN. Furthermore, we studied the
distribution of IL-2R on PBMC surface.

MATERIALS AND METHODS
      PBMC were isolated from heparinized peripheral blood of 13
patients with IgAN, 9 patients with chronic glomerulonephritis without mesangial IgA deposits and 7 healthy subjects. Purification of
T and non-T cell populations was obtained by rosette formation with
neurominidase-treated sheep red blood cells. Enriched OKT4[+] lymphocyte
subpopulations were obtained by depleting OKT4[+] and OKT8[+] cells from
the purified T cell population using OKT4 and OKT8 monoclonal antibodies
and fetal calf serum. OKDR[+] and OKT8[+]M1[+] surface phenotypes were
detected using OKDR monoclonal antiserum (Technogenetics) in purified T
cell population and OKM1 monoclonal antiserum (Ortho Diagnostic) in
OKT8 enriched cell subpopulation. IL-2 production was quantitated in

the supernatant of PBMC stimulated with phytohaemaglutinin (PHA)
(5 µg/ml) for 24 hours at 37° C in a 5% CO_2-95% air atmosphere. The
commercially available enzyme immuno assay kit (Inter-test 2) was used
to measure the IL-2 production. The distribution of IL-2 receptor
(IL-2R) on the PBMC was studied using monoclonal antibody (IgG1) to
TAC (Technogenetics).

RESULTS

Spontaneous significant IL-2 production was generated in cultures
of PBMC from patients with IgAN (p < 0.025). In contrast, no significant production of IL-2 was observed in cultures of PBMC from non-
IgAN patients and from healthy subjects. Increased production of IL-2
was observed in healthy subjects and patients after PHA stimulation.
IL-2 production was increased significantly in IgAN patients (p < 0.005).

IgAN patients had significantly higher expression of IL-2R on the
surface of PBMC than did the healthy subjects (p < 0.001). A significant increase of IL-2R expression was observed on the surface of
PBMC from patients with IgAN after PHA stimulation (p < 0.01).

To investigate the TAC^+ cell subset involved in the regulatory
role of T cell system we separated T cells from non-T cells in 4 patients with IgAN by E-rosette technique. A high percentage of TAC^+
cells was detected in the purified T cell population. Moreover,
purified T cells revealed a high percentage of $OKDR^+$ cells. This
suggests the presence of "in vivo" activated T cells.

Since it is well known that $OKT8^+$ cells exerting suppressor function on B cell activity bear M1 antigen, the frequency of $OKT8^+M1^+$
cells was evaluated in enriched $T8^+$ cells from both IgAN patients and
healthy subjects. Results provide evidence that a low percentage of
$OKT8^+M1^+$ cells was found in the purified $T8^+$ cell population from IgAN
patients when compared to controls (p < 0.025).

51

CONCLUSIONS

The present study indicates that the spontaneous production of IL-2 by PBMC occurs in patients with primary IgAN. Mitogen-stimulated PBMC produce large amounts of IL-2. In addition, an increased number of IL-2R is expressed by PBMC in resting conditions and after PHA stimulation. There is evidence that the spontaneous IL-2 hyperproduction seen in the patients in this study may be the cause of the observed increased activity of helper T cells since IL-2 is a polypetide hormone produced by T cells, and is critically involved both during the initial stage of T cell-dependent B cell activation and in the final stage of B cell differentiation.

Initial reports (4,5) on the detection of IL-2R by monoclonal antibody (anti-TAC) indicated that IL-2R is expressed by activated human T cells. To further investigate this point we have evaluated the expression of another activation antigen, such as DR, on unstimulated purified T cells from IgAN patients. The increased DR^+ cell frequency, observed in these subjects, fully supports this hypothesis. On the other hand, a similar mechanism may be also explained by the increased spontaneous synthesis of IL-2.

Since the production of IL-2 may be related to the hyperactivity of helper T cells as a consequence of an imbalance of Th/Ts ratio, we studied the number of suppressor T cells. It is well known that suppressor T cells can be divided into two different subsets according to M1 antigen expression. The suppressor activity on B cell function is confined to the subset expressing M1 antigen. Therefore, we have studied the $OKT8^+M1^+$ cell frequency in purified T cell population from IgAN patients. Our data support the hypothesis that the oversynthesis of Ig may be explained by the overactivity of helper T cells since the number of these suppressor T cells ($OKT8^+M1^+$) is significantly reduced in IgAN.

REFERENCES

1. Morgan, D.A., Ruscetti, F.W. and Gallo, R.C. Science 193: 1007-1008, 1976.
2. Nakagawa, N., Nakagawa, T., Volkman, D.J., Ambrus, J.L., Jr. and Fauci, A.S. J. Immunol. 138:795-801, 1987.
3. Ting, C.C., Yang, S.S. and Hargrove, M.E. J. Immunol. 133: 261-266, 1984.
4. Robb, R.J., Munch, A. and Smith, K.A. J. Exp. Med. 154:1455-1467, 1981.
5. Uchiyama, T., Broder, S. and Waldmann, T.A. J. Immunol. 126: 1393-1397, 1981.

IN-VITRO STUDY OF T LYMPHOCYTE ACTIVATION IN IgA NEPHROPATHY (GN)

K.N. Lai, J.C.K. Leung, P. Li, F.M. Lai. Departments of Medicine
and Morbid Anatomy, The Chinese University of Hong Kong, HONG KONG.

INTRODUCTION

Recent studies have suggested a defective T lymphocyte
immunoregulatory function in patients with IgA GN (1). The human
lymphocytic interleukin-2 receptor [IL-2R] plays a critical role
in the growth of T cells and is required for full expression of
the normal immune response (2). The present study was undertaken
to examine the in-vitro expression of IL-2R in T lymphocytes in
patients with IgA GN. In addition, the effect of cyclosporin A
(CyA), a fungal peptide that inhibits activation of T lymphocytes,
on the expression of IL-2R was studied in patients with IgA GN.

MATERIALS AND METHODS

Twenty-six patients with primary IgA GN, not on immunosuppressive therapy, were studied. All patients had been free from infections or macroscopic hematuria for at least 4 weeks before the
initial investigation. Seven patients received CyA (5 mg/kg/day)
for 3 months. The dosage was adjusted according to the plasma CyA
trough levels. Seventeen healthy subjects with normal renal
function were used as donors of control lymphocytes.

The separation of lymphocytes and lymphocyte culture were performed as previously described (3). The T and B cell markers and
the expression of IL-2R on individual lymphocytes were studied with
double immunofluorescence technique using Phycoerythrin conjugated
anti-leu-2a, anti-leu-3a, or anti-leu-12 and Fluorescein conjugated
anti-IL-2R murine monoclonal antibodies [Becton-Dickson].

RESULTS

The sex ratio, age, and lymphocyte counts of the patients were comparable to those of the controls. The mean percentages of CD4+ (T-helper/inducer) and CD8+ (T-suppressor/cytotoxic) lymphocytes, CD4/CD8 ratio in peripheral blood from IgA nephritic patients were not different from those of the control subjects. With double direct immunofluorescence technique, there was a paucity of IL-2R on the cell surfaces of peripheral lymphocytes and lymphocytes cultured with no mitogen. With pokeweed mitogen stimulation, there was a significant increase of activated lymphocytes with IL-2R on their cell surface. Nevertheless, no difference in the total percentage of cultured lymphocytes bearing IL-2R was demonstrated between IgA nephritic patients and healthy controls. Twenty-five percent CD4+ (helper/inducer) lymphocytes from IgA nephritic patients demonstrated cellular activation with expression of IL-2R after culturing with pokeweed mitogen and the value was significantly higher than the 19.8 percent observed in the controls $[p < 0.05]$. IgA nephritic patients had increased activated CD4+ lymphocytes (with IL-2R) $[p < 0.025]$ and reduced activated CD8+ lymphocytes $[p < 0.025]$ compared with controls [Figure 1]. CyA therapy resulted in a reduction of total activated T cells [CD25+]

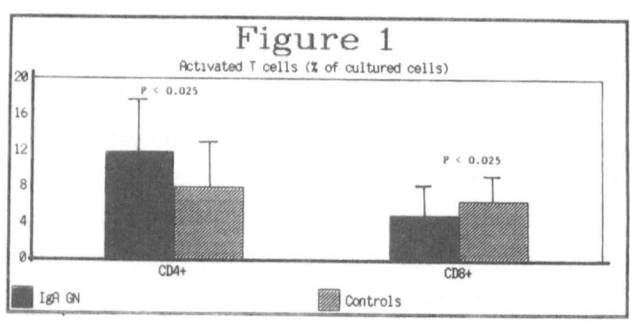

Figure 1. Increased activated CD+ and reduced activated CD8+ lymphocytes in IgA nephropathy.

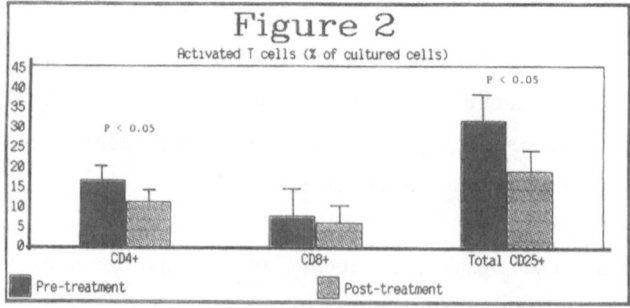

Figure 2. Effect of Cyclosporine on lymphocyte activation.

[p< 0.05] due to an absolute reduction of activated CD4+ cells [p<
0.05] but not the CD8+ cells [Figure 2].

DISCUSSION

Recent studies reveal that the immunoregulatory function of T
lymphocytes is related to the disease activity of IgA GN (1,4,5).
We have previously studied the activation of lymphocytes
indirectly by measuring the number of lymphoblastoid cells
expressing the IL-2R upon mitogen stimulation (4). Similar to our
recent report (4), we did not demonstrate an overall increase in
number of activated T lymphocytes in our 26 patients with IgA GN
during clinical quiescence compared with the healthy controls.
When the individual T cell subpopulation was studied with double
immunofluorescence technique, it became apparent that IgA
nephritic patients had increased activated helper/inducer T
lymphocyte and reduced activated suppressor/cytotoxic T lymphocyte
compared with controls upon pokeweed mitogen stimulation. These
findings are in accordance with the previous observation that an
increased number of CD4+ cells and CD4/CD8 ratio, and reduced
number of CD8+ cells were found in peripheral blood during
clinical exacerbation with synpharyngitic hematuria (4,5).
Furthermore, CyA therapy reduced the number of activated CD4+
cells in IgA nephritic patients and this may play a role in the
immunoregulatory function of IgA GN by CyA (6). In conclusion, we
have revealed intrinsic abnormalities in the immunoregulatory T
cell subpopulations in patients with IgA GN. Upon antigenic
stimulation, either in vitro by pokeweed mitogen or in vivo by
bacterial infection of mucosal surface, the CD4+ lymphocytes
demonstrate an increased proliferative activity whereas the CD8+
lymphocytes have a reduced proliferative activity.

REFERENCES
1. Linne, T., Wasserman, J. Clin Nephrol 23: 109-111, 1985.
2. Cantrell, D.A., Smith, K.A. Science 224:1312-1316, 1984.
3. Lai, K.N., Chui, S.H., Lai, F.M., Lam, C. Kidney Int 33:
   584-589, 1988.
4. Feehally, J., Beattie, T., Brenchley, P. et al., Kidney Int
   30: 924-931, 1986.
5. Lai, K.N., Lai, F.M., Chui, S.H. et al. Clin Nephrol 28:
   281-287, 1987.
6. Lai, K.N., Lai, F.M., Li, P. et al. BMJ 2: 1165-1168, 1987.

HLA CLASS II HISTOGLOBULINS INVOLVEMENT IN MESANGIAL IgA GLOMERULONE-PHRITIS (BERGER'S DISEASE).

A. VOLPI, L. SALVANESCHI*, A. SESSA, M. MARTINETTI*, P. SERBELLONI, M. CUCCIA BELVEDERE**.

Unità Operativa di Nefrologia e Dialisi, Ospedale di Vimercate, Italy; *Centro Trasfusionale A.V.I.S. di Pavia, Italy; **Dipartimento di Genetica e Microbiologia dell'Università di Pavia, Italy.

INTRODUCTION

Berger's disease is characterized by mesangial granular deposits of IgA, with or without other immunoglobulin or complement protein deposits, and no evidence of systemic diseases. This form of glomerulonephritis has an unclear pathogenesis, but it is considered to be the consequence of immunological injuries. The diagnosis is based on the immunofluorescent examination of renal biopsy, laboratory data, and clinical findings. HLA histoglobulin frequency data, available from several studies, show that B35 (1,2) and B12 (3,4) seem to have a significant association with this disease. Fauchet (5) reported a statistical decrease of the DR3 frequency among the Berger's patients. However,there is evidence of heterogeneity in these data: multiple reports from Japanese (6,7,8) and French (9,10) investigators show also a positive association with HLA-DR4 antigen.

The aim of our work was to identify in our group of Italian patients, from the same geographic area (Northern Italy), the possible association with HLA markers. We also looked for an explanation of some clinical heterogeneity of this disease on the basis of a particular genetic background.

MATERIALS AND METHODS

We studied a group of 48 patients affected with IgA nephropathy (Berger's disease) according to the following clinical and histologi cal criteria: age, sex, microscopic or macroscopic hematuria, blood pressure, plasma creatinine concentration, serum IgA levels, immuno- fluorescence microscopy and light microscopy of the renal biopsy.

All patients were typed with the microlymphocytotoxicity tech-

nique, for class I (A,C,B) and class II (DR,DQ) histoglobulins. The
HLA phenotype frequencies of patients were compared with those obtained in a group of controls (400 healthy Italian blood donors from
the same geographic origin Northern Italy). Fisher's exact test was
used to calculate the significance of the deviations. Strength of
the associations was measured by the estimate of the relative risk
(RR). The associations presented in Table 1 are only those that are
statistically significant.

RESULTS

The mean age of our population was 41 years (range 15-68); we
studied 35 males and 13 females 99% presented persistent microscopic
hematuria (18% of these patients had also episodes of macroscopic hematuria), 1% had only macroscopic hematuria; 51% of the patients was
hypertensive (blood pressure > 150/95 mmHg); 28% presented a plasma
creatinine > 1.4 mg/100 ml (8 mg/100 ml in 1 patient); serum IgA levels were higher than 250 mg/100 ml in 77% of patients.

Deposits of IgA, as the predominant immunoglobulin class, were
always found in the mesangium of all the glomeruli in the typical di
stribution with less frequent extension along the capillary basement
membrane. Light microscopy showed focal segmental proliferative glomerulonephritis in all the patients.

Table 1 represents the positive and negative associations of
Berger's disease patients with HLA class II genetic markers. We noti
ced a higher occurence of DR5 and a lower incidence of DR3 in the to
tal number of patients than in our control.

Table 1. Positive and negative significant associations.

HLA histoglobulins	phenotype frequency		uncorrected Fisher's p value	RR
	Patients n=48	Control n=400		
DR3	8.33%	21.41%	< 0.001	0.22
DR5	52.08%	31.49%	< 0.01	2.36

Considering the decreased frequency of DR3, our results agree
with the previous work of French investigators (5). On the contrary,

our data on the increased frequencyof DR5 are original, probably reflecting an ethnic heterogeneity rather than a new marker of susceptibility to Berger's disease, which appears as a unique clinical entity characterized by different markers in different populations.

It is known that HLA DR genes influence various aspects of humoral and cellular immune functions including immune responsiveness; in literature the DR3 seems to be associated to immune hyporesponsiveness (11), while the DR5 has an opposite trend. In this way we might explain the excess of circulating immune complexes and immunoglo bulins in Berger's disease in which DR5 is overrepresented.

The phenotype frequency distribution of DR3 and DR5 did not mark one particular clinical subgroup. We did not show any relationship between gross hematuria, hypertension, plasma creatinine levels, serum IgA levels, immunofluorescent glomerular patterns and a particular HLA class II marker. We did not find any significant association between HLA class I molecules (coded by genes at A, C, B loci) and Berger's disease.

REFERENCES

1. Berthoux, F.C., Gagne, A., Sabatier, J.C., Ducret, F., Le Petit, S.C., Marcellin, M., Mercier, B. and Brizard, C.P. New Engl. J. Med. 298: 1034-1035, 1978.
2. Noel, L.H., Descamps, B., Jungers, P., Bach, J.F., Busson, M., Suet, C., Hors, J. and Dausset, J. Clin. Immunol. Immunopathol. 10: 19-23, 1978.
3. Richman, A.V., Mahoney, J.J. and Fuller, T.J. Ann. Intern. Med. 90: 201, 1979.
4. Savi, M;, Neri, T.M., Silvestri, M.G., Allegri, L. and Migone, L. Clin. Nephrol. 12: 45-46, 1979.
5. Fauchet, R., Gueguen, M. and Genetet, B. New Engl. J. Med. 302: 1033-1034, 1980.
6. Hiki, Y., Kobayash i, Y., Tateno, S., Sada, M. and Kashiwagi, N. Nephron 32: 222-226, 1982.
7. Kashiwabara, H., Shishido, H., Tomura, S., Tuchida, H. and Miyajima, T. Kidney Int. 22: 377-382, 1982.
8. Kashiwabara, H., Shishido, H., Yokoyama, T. and Miyajima, T. Tissue Antigens 16: 411-412, 1980.
9. Fauchet, R., Le Pogamp, P., Genetet, B., Chevet, D., Gueguen, M., Simon, P., Ramée, M.P. and Cartier, F. Tissue Antigens 16: 405-410, 1980.
10. Le Pogamp, P., Chevet, D. and Simon, P. Néphrologie 2: 43, 1981.
11. Reeves, W.G., Gelsthore, K., Van Der Minne, P., Torensma, R. and Tattersall, R.B. Clin. Exp. Immunol. 57: 443-448, 1984.

VARIATIONS IN T LYMPHOCYTE SUBSETS IN IgA NEPHROPATHY

M.SANNA,R.PISTIS,R.FAEDDA,A.SATTA,E.SULIS,G.SERRA,G.VARGIU,E.BARTOLI.
Istituto di Patologia Medica,Università di Sassari,Italy.

INTRODUCTION

Berger's disease is an IgA nephropathy characterized by irregular
hematuria and variable proteinuria (1).Generally considered as benign,
it may neverthless progress towards chronic renal failure (2).Though
its pathogenesis is unknown,IgA serum levels are important.This immunoglobulin acts on the mucosal surface protecting towards the anti-
gens.The mechanism leading to deposition of IgA containing immune com
plexes at renal level and activation of C3 and properdine factors is
not known (3).Recently,several authors investigated some aspects of
the immune regulation of these patients and discovered a reduced acti
vity of T-suppressor cells,a high activity of the T-helper IgA specific cells,and consequently an altered OKT4/OKT8 ratio (4,5).These results are controversial because of the different variables involved
in immune regulation.To evaluate this aspect, we studied the lymphocyte subsets in patients with IgA nephropathy before,during and after
immunosuppressive treatment.

PATIENTS AND METHODS

The study was performed on six patients (4 male,2 female) affected
by IgA nephropathy diagnosed by immunological clinic and histological
studies.Urinary protein loss was variable,from 0.130 gr/24 hr to 1.40
gr/24 hr.The renal biopsy showed a remarkable increase in mesangial
matrix with focal or diffuse mesangial proliferation and IgA and C3
immunefluorescence positivity in all patients.The electron microscopy

confirmed the diagnosis.The patients were treated with Prednisone for six months administered every other day (1.18+0.11 mg/Kg/day) and Cyclophosphamide (1.03+0.16 mg/Kg/day) or Chorambucil (0.08+0.005 mg/Kg /day).Hematological tests were controlled frequently and urine protein and erythrocyte loss monthly.The lymphocyte subset was estimated at the moment of the diagnosis,after 45 days from the beginning of treatment and 30 days after discontinuation of therapy.The results were statistically analized by paired "t" test.

RESULTS

The immunosuppressive treatment determined a remarkable reduction of the protein loss.Consequently,serum concentration of proteins was normalized.The hematuria remained unchanged.The lymphocyte subset was not significantly correlated with the clinical development of the disease.Indeed,in basal condition there was no difference in the subjects with respect to the normal group.OKT4/OKT8 ratio was 1.4+0.7 (n. v. 1.4+0.5,P>.05).During immunosuppressive treatment we observed 1) an increase of the OKT4,not statistically significant, 2)a significant reduction of OKT8 both as percent and absolute value (from 747.3+381. 8 to 314.3+133.0,P<.05) and 3) a significant increase in the OKT4/ OKT8 ratio. This result was mainly due to the fall in the OKT8 during immunosuppressive therapy.Thirty days after withdrawal of therapy these changes had reverted to normal.(Fig.1,Fig 2.For explanation,see text).

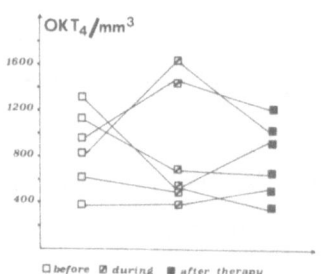

Fig. 1

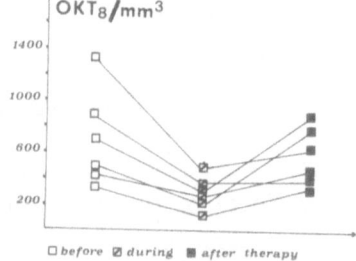

Fig.2

DISCUSSION

This study shows that patients treated with immunosuppressive therapy have an altered OKT4/OKT8 ratio determined by a remarkable increa
se of the T helper with respect to T suppressor activity.In basal conditions and 30 days after drug withdrawal the lymphocyte subset was
not different with respect to normal subjects.Probably this altered
regulation is due to the therapeutic agents used rather than to the
stage of the disease.There is no agreement on this issue in the literature because of the complexity of immunoregulation.In conclusion,
we believe that in Berger's disease there are no peculiar significant
modifications in the T,B IgA specific cells which may modulate the
clinical development of renal damage.The changes observed by some authors could be due to the stage of the disease or to allergic reaction
towards external antigens or dietary proteins.The modification in
OKT4/OKT8 ratio may be due to the drugs used in blocking the development of the nephritis rather than to the particular stage of Berger's
disease.Therefore,this findings cannot be used as a diagnostic test
although it seems important in monitoring the effectiveness of therapy.

REFERENCES

1. Berger,J.,Hinglais,N. Nephrol. 74 : 694-695 , 1968
2. Berger,J.,Yaneva,H.,Crosmier,J. Nouv.Press.Med. 9 :219, 1980
3. Valentijn,R.M.,Kauffmann,R.H.,Brutel de la Riviere,G.,Daha,M.R.,
    Van Es,E.A. Am.J.Med. 74: 375-381,1983
4. Cagnoli,L.,Beltrandi,E.,Pasquali,S.,Biag,R.,Casadei-Maldini,M.,
    Rossi,L.,Zucchelli,P. Kidney Intern.28 :648-651,1985
5. Egido,J.,Blasco,R.,Sancho,J.,Lozano,L.,Gutierrez-Millet,V.
    Clin.Exp.Immunol. 54 : 532-538,1983

ACUTE RENAL FAILURE (ARF) AS EXPRESSION OF A IgA NEPHROPATHY (IgAN).

S. Cigarrán, J. Avedillo, A. Pereira

Renal Unit. Montecelo Hospital. 36071 Pontevedra. Spain

INTRODUCTION

IgAN is the commonest glomerulonephritis in the world, and it was described in 1968 by Berger and Hinglais[1]

It is defined inmunohistologically by mesangial deposits of IgA, often accompanied by less intense staining for IgM and/or IgG and C3, in absence of a sistemic disease.

Its incidence is about 20 - 40 % of patients with primary glomerulonephritis who undergo biopsy in Western Europe, Asia and Australia, and it is the underlying disease in about 10 % of patients who receive renal replacement therapy.[2]

The most common clinical expression is macroscopic haematuria coincident with the early symtomps of an upper respiratory tract infection in young man, with normal renal function and blood pressure. However, some authors noted ARF associated with macroscopic haematuria is a rare mode of presentation.[3]

We report a case with ARF and macroscopy haematuria whom needed renal replacement therapy.

CASE

A 19 years old boy was admitted in our Hospital by macroscopic haematuria and impaired renal function. Two days prior admission, developed shore throat, low grade fever and gross haematuria. He had not history of rash, haemodinamic damage and/or nephrotoxicity agents.

Physical examination was unremarkable. B.P.: 100/60 mmHg. Diuresis: less 100 cc/day.

Laboratory data in admission.- Hto: 35 %, Hb: 12 grs/dl. BUN: 100, SCr: 13.6, IgA: 430 (40-400), IgG: 1960 (700-1900), IgM: 101 (20-250), C3: 103, C4: 44 (mgrs/dl). ESR: 45 mm/h. Na: 135, K: 5.5 (mEq/l). Urinalisys: Prot.: 5 grs/24 h. WBC: 5-10 hpf. Red cell casts: Presents. NaO: 15, KO: 35 (mEq/l). Culture: Negative. ANA, ENA, LE, Anti-GBM, HBsAg, ASLO: Negatives.

He needed two HD sessions of 4 hours each. Biopsy was performed on twelve admission day.

Light microscopy: Red cells were present into the tubular lumen (Photo 1). Immunofluorescence showed diffuse
and granular deposits of IgA in the messangium, and granular deposits of C3 in the glomerulous (Photo 2).

He was discharged at the 31th day with normal renal
function.

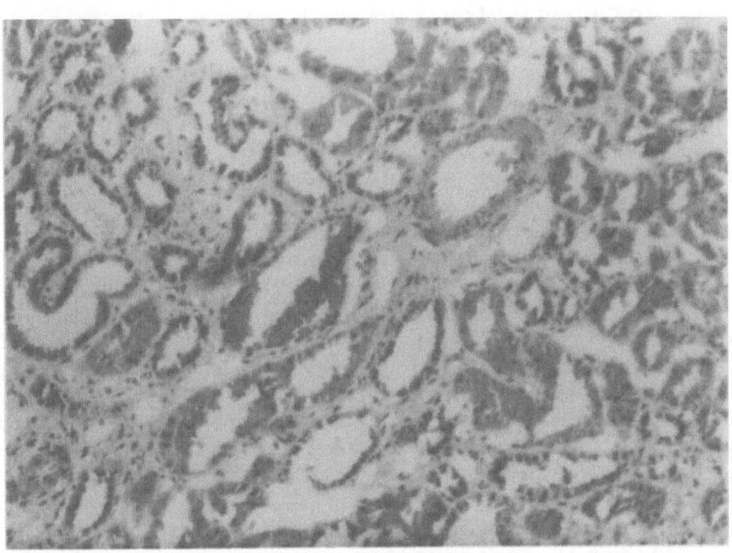

Photo 1 : Red cells into the tubular lumen (x 100)

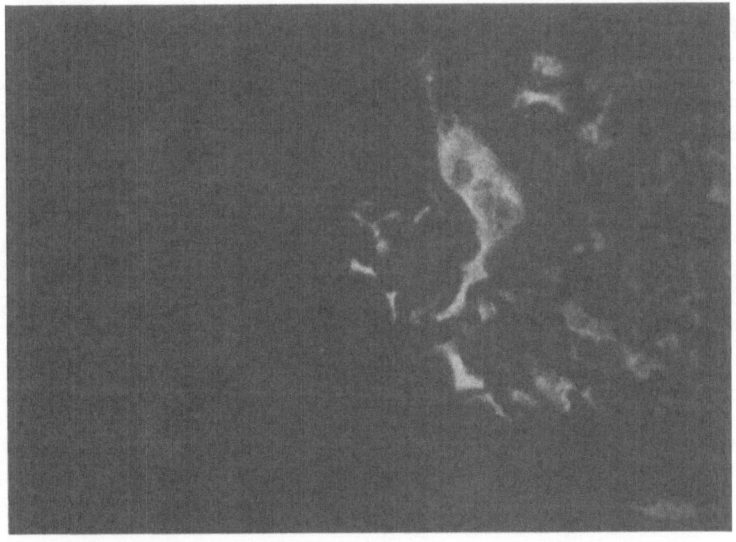

Photo 2 : IgA and C3 deposits in the glomerulous (x 200)

DISCUSSION

ARF in mesangial IgAN may ocurr in association with diffuse crescentic lesions or where there is acute tubular necrosis associated with massive glomerular bleeding in absence or little abnormalities of glomeruli.

Several mechanisms are involved in the pathogenesis of this clinical expression. By one hand, the blood in the tubules and phagocytosis of red cells by renal tubular epitelial cells may play a part in the tubular necrosis. Obstruction in renal tubules by red cells casts may contribute to acute tubular necrosis.(4,5) The findings of tubular necrosis correlates closely with the presence of red cell casts, and only the tubules with those in its lumen, shows signs of tubular damage.(5,6)

By another way, by analogy with animal systems, the messangial IgA deposits are likely to be either IgA polymers or IgA class immunocomplexes. If the latter, they may be formed in situ or be derived from circulating antigen — antibody complexes. Once lodged in the messangium, the IgA causes damage by fixing complement "via alternative" pathway, and probably by other mediators system. Macrophages may contribute to the messangial proliferative lessions. The best hypotesis is that messangial deposits are derivated from circulating antigen — IgA class antibody complexes and this is supported on clinical grounds.

Anyway, one or another clinical expression depend of several factors: enviromental, virus, and quantity of immunocomplexes may be formed. The prognosis of ARF over IgAN evolution is unknown.

REFERENCES

1.- Berger J., Hinglais N. J. Urol. Nephrol. 74: 694-695, 1968.
2.- Woodroffe A.J., Clarkson A.R., Seymour A.E., Lomax-Smith J.D. Springs Sem. Immunol. 5: 321-332, 1982.
3.- Bruce A.J., Bryson W., Abdalla R., Jiri M. Am. J. Med. 84: 129-132, 1988.
4.- Kincaid-Smith P., Nicholls K. Am. J. Kidney Dis. 3: 90-102, 1983.
5.- Rodicio J.L. Kidney Int. 25: 717-729, 1984.
6.- Praga M., Gutierrez Rullet V., Navas J.J., Ruilope L.M., Morales J.M., Alcazar J.M., Bello I., Rodicio J.L. Kidney Int. 28: 69-74, 1985.

ABNORMAL INTESTINAL PERMEABILITY IN IGA NEPHROPATHY

C. PECORARO, M.T. SARAVO*, P. STANZIALE*, M.M. BALLETTA*, G. PARRIL-
LI**, G. BUDILLON**.

Department of Pediatrics, *Department of Nephrology and **Center of
Hepatology, Second Faculty of Medicine, University of Naples, Italy

INTRODUCTION

IgA Nephropathy is the most common glomerulonephritis in the
mediterranean area (1).

Several observations have recently pointed out the possible role of
dietary antigens in the pathogenesis of IgA Nephropathy. Antibodies
against dietary antigens have in fact been detected in serum (2),
in circulating immune complexes (3) and in renal-biopsy eluates from
patients with IgA Nephropathy (4).

Aim of this study was to investigate if an abnormal small intestinal permeability is a feature of children affected by IgA Nephropathy.

PATIENTS AND METHODS

-14 children affected by immunohistologically proven IgA Nephropathy
(6 boys and 8 girls, mean age 10.5 yr, range 7.5-23.3 yr)
-12 age-matched children affected by coeliac disease on gluten containing diet
-15 age-matched normal controls.
Renal function, assessed by creatinine clearance, was normal in all
subjects.

After an overnight fast an isotonic load containing 2.5 g lac-
tulose (Lacl), 0.5 g L-Rhamnose (L-Rh) in 125 ml water, was given

orally. All urine passed in the subsequent 5 hr was collected, the volume recorded and an aliquot preserved with merthiolate was kept at -20°C until analysis. Urinary concentrations of both sugar were measured by gas-liquid chromatography, according to Menzies (5). Data in the different groups were compared using the unpaired Student's t-test.

RESULTS

Fig. 1: Lacl (A) and L-Rh (B) urinary recovery and Lacl/L-Rh urinary excretion ratio (C) in normal controls, patients affected by IgA Nephropathy (IgAN) and patients affected by coeliac disease.

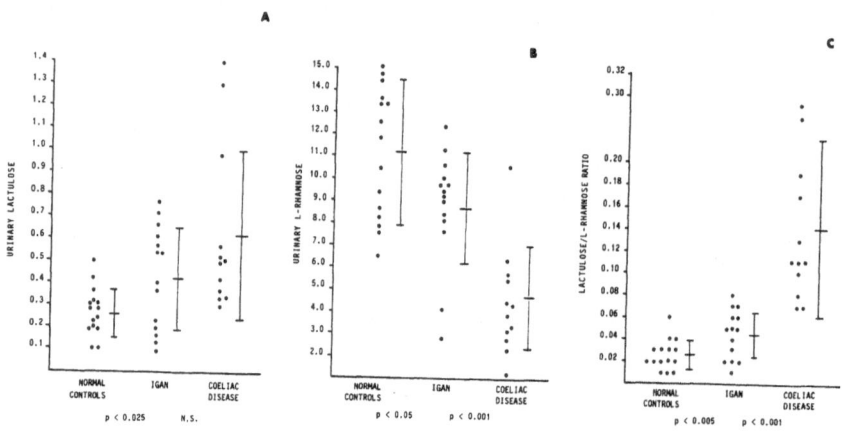

Lacl urinary recovery (expressed as percent of the oral load) was significantly higher in IgAN (mean ± SEM: 0.42 ± 0.23) than in normal controls (0.26 ± 0.11); it was comparable to that found in coeliac disease (0.52 ± 0.38). On the contrary L-Rh urinary recovery was lower in IgAN (8.72 ± 2.5) than in normal controls (11.2 ± 3.31); the L-Rh urinary recovery was not as reduced as in coeliac disease

(4.7 ± 2.3). The Lacl/L-RH ratio was higher in IgAN (0.044 ± 0.02) than in controls (0.026 ± 0.013).

These findings indicate that both the increased absorption of larger molecules (Lacl) and the reduced absorption of the smaller ones (L-Rh) contribute to the higher sugar ratio found in IgAN.

CONCLUSIONS

An abnormal intestinal sugar permeability is present in children affected by IgA Nephropathy. Both an increased absorption of larger probe molecules and a reduced absorption of smaller sugars have been observed.

SPECULATIONS

The increased intestinal permeability may represent a primary defect of the mucosal barrier, responsible of the abnormal immune response to dietary antigens in IgA Nephropathy.

Alternatively it may be the result of a deranged mucosal immunity.

REFERENCES
1. Colasanti G. Contr. Nephrol.; 40: 147, 1984
2. Woodroffe A.J., Gormly A.D., Mc Kenzie P.E. Kidney Int. 18:366-374, 1980
3. Sancho J., Egido J., Rivera F., Hernando L. Clin. Exp. Immunol. 54:194-202, 1983
4. Galla J.H., Russel M.N., Hammond D., Spotswood M., Mastecky J. Kidney Int. 27:210 abstract
5. Menzies I.S., Laker M.F., Pounder R. Lancet ii, 1107-1109, 1979

Nephrotic Syndrome

EFFICIENCY AND TOLERANCE OF CYCLOSPORINE TREATMENT
IN ADULT NEPHROSIS

A. MEYRIER

Service de Néphrologie, Hôpital Avicenne, 93009 Bobigny, France

INTRODUCTION

The term "Nephrosis" encompasses two varieties of glomerular disease leading to the nephrotic syndrome (NS), namely "minimal change" or "nil" glomerular disease (MCD), and focal segmental glomerulosclerosis (FSG). The incidence of nephrosis in the adult is in the order of 34% of all cases of NS. MCD is usually responsive to corticosteroid therapy, but it often follows a multirelapsing course. FSG is distinctly less corticosensitive than MCD, and corticoresistance is the best predictive factor of progression of FSG to end-stage renal failure. Patients (pts) with nephrosis may unpredictably develop corticodependency or corticoresistance. Dependency on high doses of steroids invariably leads to steroid toxicity. Such cases are indications for immunosuppressive therapy, especially with alkylating agents. In case of failure of such treatment (Rx), NS evolves to chronicity and complications.

In 1985 several pilot trials demonstrated that cyclosporine A (CyA) was able to suppress proteinuria in cases of corticodependent or corticoresistant nephrosis which often had also resisted Rx with alkylating agents. In 1986 we undertook a collaborative study of CyA in the Rx of nephrosis. Fifty-six pts were included in this trial. In this paper we shall discuss the three following issues: 1) What are the results of CyA Rx in adult nephrosis? 2) What is the long-term tolerance of such Rx given the nephrotoxicity of CyA? and 3) What is the mechanism of action of CyA in nephrosis?

PATIENTS AND METHODS

The pts were enrolled on the following criteria: idiopathic NS; corticoresistance or corticodependency or contraindication to corticosteroid Rx; MCD or FSG proven by recent renal biopsy. Pts with blood pressure (BP) > 180/100 mmHg, creatinine clearance < 50 ml/min, liver disease, pregnancy or infection were excluded.

After an 18-day placebo period, CyA alone (i.e., without concomitant corticosteroid Rx) was started at an initial dosage of 5 mg/kg/day, subsequently titrated for target whole blood trough levels of 200-800 ng/ml (12-hour post-dose, radioimmunoassay, polyclonal antibody). The main goals of the study were to assess the efficacy of CyA Rx at 3 months and the incidence of relapses after discontinuation, i.e., "CyA dependency." In those cases where Rx had been effective but where relapse occurred, investigators were free to resume CyA or to return to any other form of therapy.

There were 56 pts, aged 31.8 ± 14 yrs (range 14 to 69). NS had evolved 54 ± 63 months before the trial. Thirty-two were corticoresistant, 19 were corticodependent and 5 had some contraindication to corticosteroid Rx. Twenty-seven had at some time been treated with conventional immunosuppressive drugs. There were 23 pts with MCD and 33 with FSG. Of 23 MCD cases, 15 were corticodependent and 8 corticoresistant. Of 33 FSG cases, 6 were corticodependent and 27 were corticoresistant. Before treatment, systolic BP was 126.4 ± 15.7 mmHg, diastolic BP was 78.4 ± 10.4, serum creatinine was 104 ± 45 umol/L and creatinine clearance was 92 ± 35 ml/min.

RESULTS

1) Results at 3 months.

Fifty-one pts completed the 3-month course of Rx. The 5 withdrawals were due to death of one pt, hypertension or reduced renal function in 2 and sepsis in 2. The response to Rx in the remaining 51 is shown in Table 1. At this stage systolic BP was 134.8 ± 19.3 (p=0.002), diastolic BP was 82.7±12.4, serum creatinine was 110.4 ± 54 (NS) and creatinine clearance was 91 ± 30. These values were not significantly different from those recorded before CyA Rx. Complete remission was achieved within 5.12 ± 2.75 weeks (1 to 10).

Table 1. Results of 3-month CyA Rx.
(Dep=corticodependent. Res= corticoresistant)

	Response to CS Rx	Completed protocol: 51			Withdrawals: 5	
		Complete Remission	Partial Remission	Failure	Side Effects	Death
MCD	Dep	10	1	4	0	0
(23)	Res	3	1	4	0	0
FSGS	Dep	2	1	1	2	0
(33)	Res	3	2	19	2	1

In all cases, CyA was stopped abruptly. Of 15 remissions, 4 persisted and the other 11 cases relapsed within 3 weeks and were classified as CyA dependent. Resuming Rx was followed by new remission in all but one case.

Results at 6 months.

At 6 months 4 remissions were long-lasting without further Rx. CyA was resumed or continued in 25 pts, with or without additional corticosteroid Rx. It is noteworthy that in 5 cases of FSG classified as failure at 3 months, continuing Rx was followed by partial remission at 6 months. Conversely, in 3 cases with FSG continuing Rx did not lead to any improvement, and in 2 of these increasing serum creatinine levels were attributed to both progression of glomerular lesions and probable CyA nephrotoxicity. Of 14 pts with MCL, 11 were in complete and 3 in partial remission.

Results at 12 months or more.

To date, data on pts treated for 12 months or more are available in 20 cases. The longest Rx is 26 months. In 2 pts with FSG no remission had ever been obtained and rising serum creatinine levels should have led to a study end point at 6 months; these 2 cases must be excluded from consideration. In the remaining 18 cases, serum creatinine was 87.3 ± 33 umol/L, as compared with pretreatment values of 110.6 ± 53. Thirteen cases were in complete remission, with CyA alone in 6 and with an association of CyA and low-dose corticosteroid therapy in 7. In addition, 5 pts were in partial remission, including 3 with CyA + corticosteroids. In thirteen pts repeat renal biopsy was done after at least a year of Rx. The initial diagnosis was FSG in 5 and MCL in 8. Of these 8 cases with

MCL repeat biopsy showed progression of glomerular lesions to FSG in 3. In 2 cases initial interstitial and/or vascular lesions had been observed on pretreatment biopsy and were less marked on repeat examination. In 4 other cases repeat biopsy showed minor but definite tubulointersitital and/or vascular lesions which could be attributable to incipient CyA toxicity.

COMMENTS

This study showed that in pts with MCL, the rate of complete + partial remission at 3 months was 73% in corticodependent and 50% in corticoresistant cases. Conversely, in pts with FSG and corticoresistance, 8/10 cases were failures. Thus, initial glomerular histology and previous response to corticosteroid therapy were the best predictors of response to CyA Rx in these two forms of adult nephrosis. Nonetheless, remission with CyA was somewhat unpredictable and it is noteworthy that 8 cases of corticodependent or resistant FSG evolved to complete or partial remission with CyA. In cases where CyA had not obtained remission at 3 months continuing Rx and, in most cases, adding low-dose corticosteroid therapy led to an increased number of remissions. The overall impression was firstly that CyA exerted a suspensive but not a curative effect on the nephrotic syndrome, and secondly that the best results were achieved with a combination of relatively low dose CyA and a small daily dosage of prednisone. In other terms, CyA seemed to restore corticosensitivity in some cases and more generally had the major advantage of drastically reducing the threshold of corticosensitivity.

The mechanism of action of CyA in nephrosis is probably not simple. The postulated mechanism of nephrosis is loss of membrane negative charges due to lymphokine(s) secretion by activated T lymphocytes. CyA could intervene as an immunosuppressive agent, as it interferes with IL-2 and gamma IFN action in the immune recognition machinery. On the other hand, CyA has many nonimmune pharmacologic effects, especially on renal hemodynamics and prostaglandins. It is probable that the diminution of proteinuria leading to par-tial remission could be due in part to such nonspecific effects on the kidney. We nonetheless reject the hypothesis that such a me-

chanism was operational in inducing <u>complete</u> remission of nephrosis. When obtained, remission was slow and progressive; stopping Rx
induced relapse long after CyA had dropped to unmeasurable blood
levels and remission was accompanied by definite improvement of GFR
in the majority of cases. Nonetheless, such arguments do not exclude some form of direct action of the CyA molecule on membrane
and/or serum albumin negative charges, independently of any effect
on T cell cytokines.

The major concern of investigators who participated in this
study was the risk of CyA nephrotoxicity. The one-year data were
definitely reassuring on this issue. Nephrotoxicity with serum
creatinine values rising to unacceptably high levels was observed
only in cases with FSG where Rx had been maintained despite both
absence of remission and declining GFR. In the other pts, renal
function was remarkably stable and even exhibited a trend to improved GFR as compared with pretreatment values. This finding is
only superficially paradoxical, as most of these cases were severely nephrotic when Rx was initiated, and CyA-induced remission was
followed by suppression of functional renal failure. This favorable
impression was substantiated by repeat renal biopsy which confirmed
the paucity of histologic features of CyA toxicity.

This should not lead to the conclusion that CyA is a routine
and harmless Rx of corticoresistant or corticodependent nephrosis.
The overall good renal tolerance of CyA in our series was certainly
explained both by the use of low dosage and of meticulous weekly
monitoring of circulating levels, which in the majority of cases
were maintained in the range of 500 ng/ml of whole blood. In our
opinion, nephrologists intending to treat nephrosis with CyA
should strictly adhere to the following guidelines: 1) Exclude pts
with FSG + serum creatinine levels > 250 umol/L + interstitial and
vascular lesions on renal biopsy; 2) Avoid CyA whole blood trough
levels over 500 ng/ml; 3) Discontinue Rx when no definite remission has been obtained at 6 months with combined CyA + low-dose
prednisone; 4) Discontinue Rx when serum creatinine levels rise
by 50% > baseline values; 5) Perform systematic renal biopsy after
one year of CyA before deciding to continue Rx.

CICLOSPORINE TREATMENT OF CHILDHOOD IDIOPATHIC NEPRHOSIS.

P. NIAUDET, M. BROYER and R. HABIB.

Service de Néphrologie Pédiatrique and INSERM U 192, Hôpital Necker-Enfants Malades, 149 rue de Sèvres, 75015 Paris, France.

INTRODUCTION

Children with idiopathic nephrosis are usually treated with corticosteroids and, in the vast majority of cases, nephrosis is steroid responsive. However, some 60% of cases relapse as soon as steroid therapy is withdrawn or when the dosage is decreased. This constitutes steroid dependant nephrosis where patients may develop serious side effects of steroid therapy. Immunosuppressive drugs, mainly alkylating agents, are effective in these situations but their long term toxic effects also limit their use. Few children with idiopathic nephrosis fail to respond to steroids. In these patients, the effectivness of immunosuppressive drugs have not been demonstrated. In the past few years, several reports have claimed that ciclosporine (CSA) could be beneficial in such patients (1-7). We shall report here our experience with Ciclosporine in 51 children, 37 steroid dependant and 14 steroid resistant.

CICLOSPORINE IN STEROID DEPENDANT NEPHROSIS

Thirty seven children, 8 girls and 29 boys, aged 1.5 to 12 years at onset of disease, received CSA, 4 to 11 mg/kg BW, for at least 3 months before tapering. They all had steroid dependant nephrosis with serious side effects of steroid therapy. Renal biopsy had shown minimal change disease in 32 cases, diffuse mesangial proliferation in 2 cases and focal and segmental glomerulosclerosis in 3 cases.

Twenty nine of the 37 patients either went into remission or did not relapse at all during the period of full dose CSA despite the fact that prednisone was withdrawn. Among the 29 patients, 25 relapsed at CSA tapering or soon after CSA withdrawal and 4 had not relapsed at last examination but they were still receiving CSA. CSA was ineffective in 6 patients who relapsed when prednisone was tapered and in 2 patients who relapsed as soon as alternate day prednisone was started. The subsequent course was evaluated in 23 patients who had relapsed when CSA had been tapered or withdrawn and who had been treated again with CSA. Eight patients went into remission on CSA alone whereas in 11 patients, the addition of prednisone was necessary to induce the remission. In 2/3 of these 19 patients, low doses of CSA or of CSA and prednisone have been effective for periods of up to 2 years. In the remaining 4 patients, CSA and prednisone were unable to induce a remission.

The treatment with CSA has been well tolerated in these patients. Three children experienced a transient impairment of renal function during a relapse. Blood pressure was elevated in 6 patients who were all receiving steroid therapy. Hypertrichosis was noted in 28 children and gum hypertrophy in 20. One patient had seizures while on CSA and prednisone.

CICLOSPORINE IN STEROID RESISTANT NEPHROSIS.

Fourteen children, 5 girls and 9 boys, aged 8 months to 14 years at onset of disease, were treated with CSA. Three patients although they had initially been steroid responders had failed to respond to steroids during a subsequent relapse. The duration of disease before CSA therapy varied from 3 months to 7 years and 9 months.

Seven patients had previously received immunosuppresive agents. No renal biopsy was performed in one patient, a late non responder. The remaining 13 cases were classified by light microscopy as minimal change disease (5 cases), diffuse mesangial proliferation (2 cases) and focal and segmental glomerulosclerosis (6 cases).

The dose of CSA varied from 4.3 to 17 mg/kg. CSA alone induced a remission in one patient, a late non responder. The remission was obtained during the first month of treatment and the patient was still protein free 2 years after CSA withdrawal. CSA induced a partial and transient remission in 4 patients and the remaining 9 patients failed to respond to the treatment. Ciclosporine was associated with Prednisone in 4 patients, 2 of whom went into complete remission.

Renal side effects of CSA were more pronounced in these patients. Indeed, 6 of the 14 patients experienced an alteration of renal function. In one patient, renal function was impaired after 2 months of CSA and further deteriorated after CSA withdrawal. In 4 patients, the impairment of renal function was transient and reversible after tapering the CSA dosage. In the remaining patient, the impairment in renal function was only partially reversible. Four children had blood hypertension, in all cases with renal function impairment. Hypertrichosis was observed in 6 cases and gum hypertrophy in 5 cases.

SERIAL RENAL BIOPSIES.

Among the side effects of CSA, nephrotoxicity is the most worriing. In order to document the real incidence of nephrotoxicity, serial renal biopsies have been performed in 25 cases, 22 patients with steroid dependant nephrosis and 3 patients with steroid resistant nephrosis, 6 to 14 months after initiation of CSA. The specimen have been compared to pretreatment biopsies. There were no significant changes in 8 cases whereas, in 14 cases, there were few groups of atrophic tubules within stripes of interstitial fibrosis. It should be stressed that in 6 of these 14 cases these tubulo interstitial lesions were associated with lesions of focal and glomerular sclerosis. More severe tubulo interstitial lesions were observed in 3 cases. The changes consisted of numerous atrophic tubules within interstitial fibrosis. There were also isometric vacuolisations of proximal tubules and in one patient calcifications of tubular epithelium.

The analysis of serial renal biopsies have shown that patients who responded to CSA did not developped severe lesions of nephrotoxicity. The most severe lesions were observed in steroid resistant patients who failed to respond to CSA. There were no correlation between the severity of histological lesions and the duration of treatment, trough CSA levels or the dose of CSA. Finally, histological lesions of nephrotoxicity may be seen in patients who have no alteration of renal function.

CONCLUSION

The response of patients with idiopathic nephrosis to CSA is well correlated with initial steroid responsiveness as 84% of steroid responders responded to CSA whereas only 21 of steroid non responders did so. We also found a good correlation between the response to treatment and the histological findings on initial biopsy. 72% of patients with minimal change disease responded to CSA but only 20% of patients with focal and segmental glomerulosclerosis responded to CSA. Ciclosporine has been effective in most cases of steroid sensitive nephrosis and has allowed to stop prednisone therapy in cases with steroid intoxication. However, patients relapse at CSA tapering or withdrawal. Studiens are in progress to see if an association of low doses of

CSA and prednisone could be effective for long periods of time without the risk of nephrotoxicity.

Conversely, CSA alone has not been effective in steroid resistant patients. Preleminary results show that the association of CSA and prednisone may be beneficial, particularly if undertaken early in the course of the disease.

Serial renal biopsies show that after 4 to 16 months of CSA at doses of 6 to 7 mg/kg, CSA is not nephrotoxic in steroid sensitive patients. Conversely, severe histological lesions of nephrotoxicity were found in 3 steroid resistant patients. These lesions may occur in patient without alteration of renal function.

REFERENCES

1. Hoyer, P.F., Krull, F. and Brodehl, J. Lancet 2 : 335, 1986

2. Capodicasa, G., De Santo, N.G., Nuzzi, F. and Giordano, C. Int. J. Pediatr. Nephrol. 7 : 69-72, 1986.

3. Niaudet, P., Habib, R., Tête, M.J., Hinglais, N. and Broyer, M. Pediatr. Nephrol. 1 : 566-573, 1987.

4. Brandis, M., Burghard, R., Leititis, J., Zimmerhackl, B., Hildebrandt, F. and Helmcher, U. Pediatr. Nephrol. 1: C42, 1987.

5. Waldo, F.B. and Kohaut, E.C. Pediatr. Nephrol. 1: 180-182, 1987.

6. Brodehl, J., Ehrich, J.J.H., Hoyer, P.F., Lee, I.J., Oemar, B.S. and Wonigeit, K. Korean J. Nephrol. 6 : 26-33, 1987.

7. Tejani, A., Butt, K., Trachtman, H., Suthanthiran, M., Rosenthal, C.J. and Khawar, M.R., Kidney Int. 33 : 729-734, 1988.

ACUTE RENAL EFFECTS OF INTRAVENOUS HIGH DOSE METHYLPREDNISOLONE (P)
THERAPY IN NEPHROTIC SYNDROMES

G. PATERNOSTER, A. BIONDA, N. CAPORALI, V. PANICHI, R. PALLA
2nd Medical Clinic, University of Pisa, Pisa, Italy

INTRODUCTION

P "pulses" are often used as a first therapeutic step in clinical
transplantation, in autoimmune diseases and proteinuric nephropathies.
Conflicting observations have been published on nonimmunologic effects
of steroids on renal hemodynamics, tubular transports, and proteinuria
increase or fluctuation which, however, does not necessarily mean resistance to treatment. The study was undertaken to evaluate, in
patients with nephrotic syndrome, the acute effects of P on the following: urinary flow rate (V), renal plasma flow (RPF), filtration fractions (FF), endogenous creatinine clearance (CrCl), fractional clearances (FCl) of sodium (Na), potassium (K), albumin (Alb), transferrin
(TF) and immunoglobulin G (IgG), urinary excretion of Thromboxane B2
(UTxB2), quantitative and qualitative urinary protein excretion.

MATERIALS AND METHODS

Plasma and urinary concentrations of creatinine, NA, K and urinary
enzymes (γGT, LDH, α-glucosidase, N-acetyl-β-glucosaminidase) were
assayed by using standard methods. Serum and urinary IgG, Alb, TF, were
measured by radial immunodiffusion using LC-Partigen plates (Behring).
Selectivity of proteinuria (S) was calculated by the ratio of IgG and
TF clearances. Urinary protein excretion (UProt) was measured by
BIORAD Protein assay. Molecular weights and electrophoretic patterns

of urinary proteins were determined by sodiumdodecylsulfate 10% poly-crylamide gel electrophoresis (SDS-PAGE). UTxB2 was measured by radio-immunoassay (N.Engl.Nucl.Dupont) after extraction by Bond-Elut SI column chromatography. RPF was evaluated by plasmatic I^{131} hippuran clearance using single injection. The clinical characteristics of the patients are depicted in the following Table:

Patient/ Age*/sex	B.D.	Lasting **	Cr Cl ml/min	UProt g/24h	SProt g/dl	ALB g/dl
LA 36 M	MGN	120	38	4.1	5.0	2.97
RP 33 F	MLGN	9	147	3.6	5.5	3.39
SL 43 F	FGS	9	25	11.2	4.0	1.71
PG 62 M	MGN	7	106	7.7	4.1	1.78
FM 24 F	MGN	90	168	6.1	4.6	2.22
RE 33 M	FGS	130	40	17.8	4.7	2.91
BA 35 F	MGN	14	113	5.6	5.2	3.35

*years; **months: the time of clinical onset was that time when signs of glomerulonephritis were definitely present. M=male; F=female; BD=biopsy diagnosis; GN=glomerulonephritis; MGN=membranous GN; MLGN=minimal change GN; FGS=focal glomerulosclerosis. S/Prot=total serum protein; ALB=serum albumin.

All patients were treated with a course of steroids and enrolled in the study one month or more after suspension of all other therapy except a 80 mEq/d diet. Blood samples and spontaneously collected urines were analyzed at 3 steady-state conditions: "baseline" = 24 hrs before the day of the study; Phase I and Phase II = two 40 min. clearances and Phase III and Phase IV = two 50 min. clearances started 40 min. after 1/g body surface P injection. The study lasted 7 hrs with 3/l oral water loading and 1.7 l continuous I.V. saline infusion.

RESULTS

During the study, the hematocrit, Na and K serum levels, and SProt were unchanged. The hydratation occurred at Phase I changed the V from

a mean of 1.1±3.2 to 9.5±5.1 ml/min (P<0.001), CrCl from a mean of
91±57 to 164±96 ml/min (P<0.001) and UV Prot from a mean of 5.4±3.4 to
7.7±4.3 mg/min (P<0.001). At Phase II,V decreased to a mean of 8.3±4.5
ml/min, CrCl to a mean of 103±47 ml/min and UV Prot to a mean of
5.3±2.3 mg/min. A comparison between "control" and "experimental" period parameters is shown in the following Table:

	CrCl ml/min	V ml/min	UNA V μ Eq/min	UK V μ Eq/min	UTxB2 μ ml/min	F F %	UVProt mg/min
MB	141±78	9.3±4.7	151±84	75±35	2.1±1.3	.138±4	6.4±3.9
MA	101±62*	4.5±4.8**	96±88***	71±33	2.1±1.4	.137±4	6.7±3.6

*P < 0.01; **P < 0.01; ***P < 0.01. Values are the means ± SD of the two
consecutive determinations obtained before (MB), after (MA) P.
UNA V = sodium excretion rate; UK V = potassium excretion rate.

Comparing the parameters of Phases II and III, the decreases in V
(from 8.3±4.5 to 2.9±1.7ml/min) and UNaV (from 176±92 to 96±100
mEq/min) were more couspicuous; moreover, a significant FeNa decrease
(P<0.05) was found. Between Phases II and IV the UV Prot changed from
5.3±2.9 to 7.4±4.4 mg/ml (P<0.01). After P, the increase of proteinuria
was present in 5 patients who did not ameliorated in the follow up with
daily steroid treatment; of the 2 patients showing a decreasing in
proteinuria, one was affected by MLGN and had a clinical remission of
the disease; no clinical information are available about the follow up
of the other. No variations in RPF and UTxB2 were seen between the
control and experimental periods. The SDS-PAGE urinary molecular
patterns showed no change after P, either with respect to the "control"
period or to the "baseline". After P, the clearances of Alb and TF
slightly increased while that of IgG decreased (MB = 0.052±.04; MA =
0.036±.03); the S index was significantly (P<0.05) less. The urinary
enzymes considered showed no significant variations. The study shows
that P pulse infusion produces immediate and considerable interference
with tubular transports and variations on renal hemodynamics.

SHOULD STEROID THERAPY BE USED IN NEPHROTIC SYNDROME [NS] RELATED
TO HEPATITIS B VIRUS [HBV] ASSOCIATED NEPHRITIS?

K.N. Lai, J. Tam, F.M. Lai, H.J. Lin. Departments of Medicine,
Microbiology, and Morbid Anatomy, Chinese University of Hong Kong
and Clinical Biochemical Unit, University of Hong Kong, Hong Kong.

INTRODUCTION

   Nephrotic syndrome remains the commonest clinical presentation
of HBV associated glomerulonephritidies (1). Although spontaneous
remission of nephrotic syndrome in these HBsAg carriers has
occasionally been observed, most patients remain symptomatic for a
long period despite diuretic therapy. Steroid had previously been
given to some nephrotic patients with HBV associated nephritis
before the renal biopsy was performed (2,3) while other patients
with biopsy-proven HBV associated membranous nephropathy received
steroid as a therapeutic trial for symptomatic NS (2,4). The
present study is conducted to investigate the value of steroid
therapy in these nephrotic patients with HBsAg.

MATERIALS AND METHODS

   The criteria of patient selection have previously been reported
(1).The HBV antigens were screened two to four months before, and
at the time of renal biopsy. HBsAg, anti-HBs, anti-HBc, HBeAg,
and anti-HBe were assayed with commercial kits. The HBV DNA in
serum was detected by dot blot hybridization using an oligonucleo-
tide probe as previously described (5). Frozen sections of renal
biospies were studied by indirect immunofluorescence technique for
HBsAg, HBcAg and HBeAg using polyclonal monospecific rabbit
anti-human antisera. The initial regimen of prednisolone was 60
mg/day. The dosage of steroid was reduced by half after 8 weeks
and was further reduced gradually over the following 8-12 weeks.

RESULTS

   Eleven patients were studied and their pathologic findings are shown in Table 1. The clinical evolution for each patient is depicted in Figure 1. Six patients had remission of NS or protein-uria after steroid therapy. The symptoms usually improved within 6 months in those responders. Transient rise of alanine aminotrans-aminase [ALT] was observed in 2 patients after commencement of steroid despite the patients remained symptom-free. Elevated ALT was not observed after stepwise steroid withdrawal. Three patients became hypertensive with treatment. One patient died of intracerebral hemorrhage and the other died of septic peritonitis.

The serum HBeAg concentration increased with steroid therapy. The post-treatment HBeAg concentration remained elevated in 2 patients with persistent proteinuria and one patient with frequent relapses. HBV DNA was elevated in 5 patients with steroid therapy but decreased when steroid was withdrawn (Figure 2). The 3 patients with detectable HBV DNA after steroid withdrawal also had persistent elevation of HBeAg in their serum.

TABLE 1. HISTOPATHOLOGY OF THE PATIENTS

Case	LM	IgG	IgA	IgM	HBsAg	HBcAg	HBeAg	EM
1	MGN	$+^c$	−	−	−	−	−	subepithelial EDD
2	MPGN	$+^c$	$+^m$	−	$+^m$	$+^c$	−	subepithelial EDD
3	normal	−	−	−	−	−	−	fusion of FP
4	MGN	$+^c$	−	−	$+^c$	$+^c$	−	subepithelial EDD
5	MGN	$+^c$	−	−	−	−	−	subepithelial EDD
6	MGN	$+^c$	−	−	−	$+^c$	−	subepithelial EDD
7	MPN	−	$+^m$	$+^m$	−	−	−	↑mesangial matrix
8	MPN	−	$+^m$	−	−	−	−	mesangial EDD
9	MGN	$+^c$	−	−	$+^c$	$+^c$	−	subepithelial EDD
10	MGN	$+^c$	−	−	−	$+^c$	−	subepithelial EDD
11	normal	−	−	−	−	−	−	fusion of FP

+, present; −, absent; c, capillary; m, mesangial; MGN, membranous nephropathy; MPGN, mesangioproliferative nephropathy; FP, foot process; EDD, electron-dense deposits.

DISCUSSION

The NS was reported to regress spontaneously in 30 to 60 percent of HBV associated membranous nephropathy, but these patients could remain symptomatic for twelve months or longer (2,6,7). The remaining patients had persistent proteinuria with fluid retention. As some patients remained symptomatic despite albumin infusion and diuretic therapy, the steroid regimen used in idiopathic membranous nephropathy was administered to some

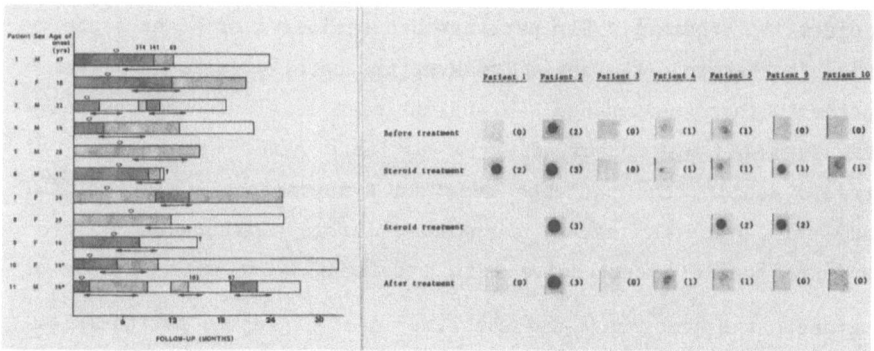

Figure 1: ▨▨▨ nephrotic syndrome; ▨▨▨ proteinuria; ☐ complete remission; ◇ renal biopsy; ◄─► steroid treatment, † deceased. The numbers above the bar represent the value of ALT.
Figure 2: Radioautogram of nylon membrane to which sera were tested for HBV DNA. The density of the dot was scored 0, 1, 2, 3, and 4.

patients as a therapeutic trial for symptomatic relief [2]. Our study suggested the nephrotic syndrome may regress earlier with steroid treatment compared with untreated patients. Nevertheless, the complications of liver dysfunction and hypertension remained significant. The effect of steroid on HBeAg and HBV DNA has not been previously studied in HBV associated glomerulonephritis. Steroid therapy in these patients was associated with active viral replication with increased HBeAg and HBV DNA concentrations, despite clinical evidence of liver impairment may not be obvious. Hence, the usage of steroid may apparently reduce the duration of NS but it could potentiate the risk of viral replication. Our results do not support the earlier notion (4) that short-term steroid, given at the onset of the nephrotic syndrome, does not seem to interfere with the favorable outcome of the infection or the related renal disease.

REFERENCES
1. Lai, K.N., Lai, F.M., Chan, K. et al. Q J Med 63: 323-333, 1987.
2. Kleinknecht, C., Levy, M., Peix, A. et al. J Pediatrics 95: 946-952, 1979.
3. Brzoko, W. et al. Lancet 2: 476-482, 1974.
4. Cadrobbi, P. et al. Arch Dis Child 60: 583-585, 1985.
5. Lin, H.J., Wu, P.C., Lai, C. J Virol Methods 15: 139-149, 1987.
6. Ito, H., Hattori, S., et al. Lab Invest 44: 214-220, 1981.
7. Hsu, H.C., et al. Clin Nephrol 20: 121-129, 1983.

CICLOSPORIN A THERAPY IN NEPHROTIC ADULTS

M. Laville, E. Boussema, J. Finaz, O. Madonna, S. Colon, M. Labeeuw, P. Zech

Département de Néphrologie, Université Claude-Bernard-Lyon I, Hôpital Edouard-Herriot, 69437 Lyon FRANCE

INTRODUCTION

The effects of Ciclosporin A (CsA) upon lymphokine production by activated T-lymphocytes (1) had raised its clinical use for the treatment of steroid-resistant idiopathic nephrotic syndromes (NS), which account in adults for about 20% of minimal change glomerulonephritis (MCGN), 65% of focal glomerulosclerosis (FGS) and 35% of membranous glomerulonephritis (MGN) (2, 3, 4). With regards to the encouraging results reported in these glomerulopathies from several pilot studies (5, 6, 7), and the absence of clinically relevant nephrotoxicity we observed in lupus patients treated by CsA for at least 10 months (8), we started in May 1986 to treat steroid-resistant NS by CsA (as a part of multicentric trials involving most of Nephrology centers in France).

PATIENTS AND METHODS

Patients

Patients were selected according to the following criteria: age over 15 yr; idiopathic nephrotic syndrome from biopsy-proven MCGN, FGS and MGN; lack of remission after 6 weeks of treatment with prednisolone 1mg/kg/day (defining resistance) or at least 3 relapses occuring in the 2 weeks after prednisolone reduction to 20 mg/day (dependence); absence of known contra-indication to CsA especially uncontrolled hypertension; fully informed consent. Relevant data on clinical course before the start of CsA treatment are summarized in the following table.

Methods

Oral CsA was started alone at 2,5 mg/kg twice daily after previous steroid treatment had been stopped and at least 4 months after the last cyclophosphamide treatment. Dosage adjustements were made to maintain CsA through levels in the range of 200-800 ng/ml (whole blood, RIA) or 50-200 ng/ml (serum, RIA), as measured 12 h after the last dose. The result was judged after 3 months as the remission or the persistance of NS on the usual criteria: when CsA failed to obtain partial or complete remission it was abruptly and definitively stopped.

PATIENT	SEX	AGE (years)	TYPE	DURATION OF NS (months)	LAST BIOPSY months)	PREVIOUS TREATMENT	RESPONSE
BP	M	21	MCGN	10	7	PRED	resistant*
DJ	F	36	MCGN->FGS	64	1	PRED+CY	dependent
LM	F	23	MCGN->FGS	17	2	PRED	dependent
MA	M	19	FGS	18	4	PRED	resistant
GC	F	17	FGS	7	7	PRED+CY	resistant
TA	M	47	MCGN	10	2	PRED	resistant
CE	F	38	MGN	24	24	PRED	resistant
GB	F	63	FGS	9	9	PRED	resistant**
Mean		32,8		20,0	7,0		
±SD		16,2		18,8	7,6		

* : initially steroid-sensitive   ** : initially steroid-dependent

RESULTS

Nephrotic syndrome

Minimal change glomerulonephritis . Among the 2 patients with MCGN, there was 1 failure (TA) and 1 success (BP). In the later, highly nephrotic, partial remission occured during the 3nd month then completed thereafter. CsA dosage was gradually reduced to 140 mg/day after 12 months then definitively stopped at 24 months because of the occurence of a T-cell lymphoma of Ki-1 type. This patient has actually, while receiving cytostatic drugs, no proteinuria and normal plasma protein and creatinine levels.

Focal glomerulosclerosis . Among the 5 patients with FGS, only 1 (GC) had a partial remission occuring in the first month. CsA was gradually reduced to 220 mg/day after 12 months. At the 18th month of treatment, proteinuria is about 1g/day, and she has normal plasma protein and creatinine levels. Proteinuria decreased in 2 patients (MA and DJ) but insufficiently to obtain even a partial remission.

Membranous glomerulonephritis . In the only patient with MGN (CE), a partial remission occured at the end of the 3rd month and is actually sustained after 15 months of treatment. CsA dosage is being reduced to 260 mg/day, proteinuria is about 0.5 g/day and plasma proteins are in normal range. GFR (inulin clearance) and RPF (PAH clearance) are increased from 27 and 166 ml/min/1.73 m2 respectively before CsA to 51 and 314 ml/min/1.73 m2 after 1 year of treatment.

Adverse effects

Using CsA dosages in the range of 3,7-5,8 mg/kg/day (4.76±0.65), a slight reversible increase in plasma creatinine level occured in 3 patients (DJ, MA, TA) while in 2 others (GB, LM) a slow continuous functional impairement was likely related to the treatment-unresponsive underlying nephropathy. The occurence of a T-cell lymphoma of Ki-1 type cannot be related undoubtedly to CsA treatment, since immunosuppressive drug-induced lymphomas generally share B-cell antigens. Some benign and transient adverse effects were noted such as gastro-intestinal disorders (3 patients), hypertension (2 patients), hyperuricaemia (2 patients), and hirsutism (1patient), but no treatment had to be withdrawn because of it.

CONCLUSION

These cases added to already published series emphasize the usefulness of CsA treatment in steroid-resistant nephrotic syndromes from minimal change glomerulo-nephritis. As previously reported most of patients with focal glomerulosclerosis are CsA-resistant. Some patients with membranous glomerulonephritis could beneficiate from CsA but the analysis is more hazardous given the high frequency of spontaneous remissions. Overall, there are as yet no reliable predictive parameter of CsA efficiency in nephrotic patients.

REFERENCES
1. Borel, J.-F., Ryffel, B., In: Ciclosporin in autoimmune diseases (Eds. R. Schindler), Springer-Verlag, Berlin, 1985, pp 24-32.
2. Meyrier, A., Simon, P. In: Actualités Néphrologiques de l'Hôpital Necker (Eds. J. Crosnier, J.-L. Funck-Brentano, J.-F. Bach and J.-P. Grünfeld), Flammarion Médecine-Sciences, Paris, 1987, pp 121-140.
3. Collaborative Study of the Adult Idiopathic Nephrotic Syndrome New Engl. J. Med. 301: 1301-1306, 1979.
4. Zech, P., Colon, S., Pointet, P., Deteix, P., Labeeuw, M., Leitienne, P. Clin. Nephrol. 18: 232-236, 1982.
5. Adhikari, M., In: Ciclosporin in autoimmune diseases (Eds. R. Schindler), Springer-Verlag, Berlin, 1985, pp 323-328.
6. Lagrue, G., Laurent, J., Belghiti, D., Robeva, R. Lancet 2: 692-693, 1986.
7. Meyrier, A., Simon, P., Perret, G., Condamin-Meyrier, M.C. Brit. Med. J. 292: 789-792, 1986.
8. Deteix, P., Lefrançois, N., Laville, M., Colon, S., Zech, P., Traeger, J. In: Ciclosporin in autoimmune diseases (Eds. R. Schindler), Springer-Verlag, Berlin, 1985, pp 361-365.

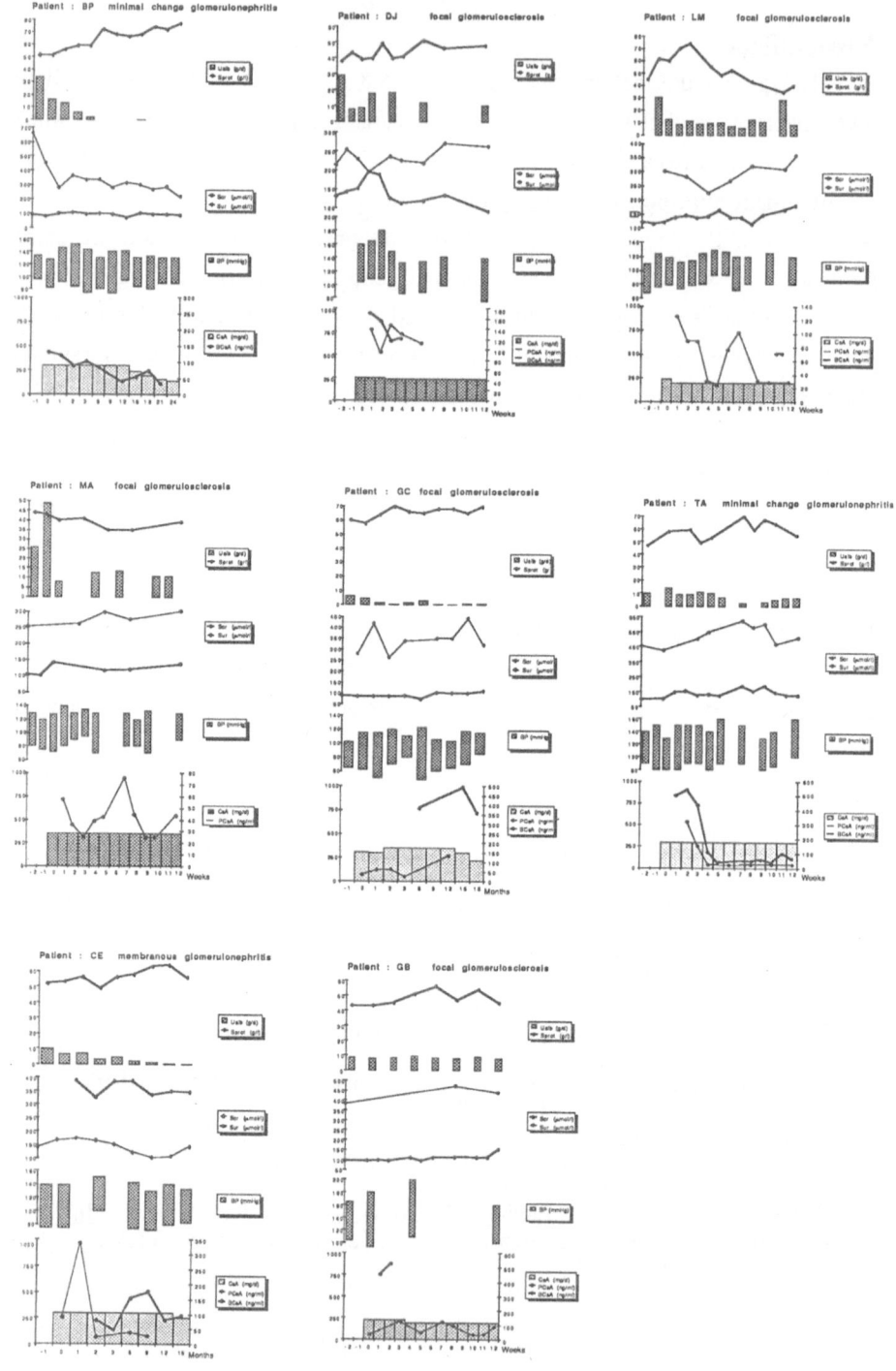

CYCLOSPORINE EFFECT ON CORTICORESISTANT NEPHROTIC SYNDROME IN PRIMARY GLOMERULONEPHRITIS

R. CONFALONIERI, L. RADAELLI, G. CIVATI, E. MINETTI, A. MONTOLI, B. BRANDO, L.MINETTI

Renal Unit, Ospedale Niguarda - Ca' Granda, Milano, Italy.

INTRODUCTION

Cyclosporine (CsA) efficacy in nephrotic syndrome (NS) from primary glomerulonephritis (GN) other than minimal changes GN is still controversial (1) ; moreover CsA has been generally employed at high doses and / or associated to steroids (2, 3). Its interference with lymphokines more than haemodynamic effect has been emphasized (4, 5). In order to test CsA efficacy in NS and in the attempt to avoid dose-related or steroid associated side effects, we started an open self-controlled therapeutic trial with low-dose CsA alone.

PATIENTS AND METHODS

10 adult patients (age ranging 24 - 64), 7 males , 3 females have been so far included. All had steroid-resistant NS due to biopsy proven primary GN with creatinine clearance (CCr) higher than 60 ml/min. NS was defined as the presence of proteinuria higher than 3.5 g/day and serum albumin less than 3.5 g /dl. Steroid resistance was assessed by a previous treatment with prednisone (1 mg /kg b.w./day) for at least 8 weeks consecutively. A 2 months wash out period was established before starting CsA treatment. 8 patients had membranous GN (MGN) with different type of lesion, and 2 had membranoproliferative GN of the first type (MPGN). Table 1 summarizes the main clinical features and laboratory findings of this series before starting CsA therapy. Proteinuria ranged 5 -15 g/day (mean 8.3) , serum albumin 2.2 - 3.4 g/dl (mean 2.6). 5 patients were moderately hypertensive . The duration of disease ranged 5 -145 months (mean 37). We considered as responders (R) patients with serum albumin over 3.5 g/dl and at least halving of proteinuria with disappearence of edema .

CsA was given at the daily dosage of 4 mg/ kg b.w. refracted in 2 oral administrations for 6 months consecutively, then stopped. The dosage was never changed during the treatment period. In patients showing nephrotoxicity or other main side effects CsA was withdrawn. CsA efficacy was assessed by regular monitoring of proteinuria, serum proteins and clinical observation; side effects were controlled by measurement of plasma creatinine (PCr), CCr , liver enzymes, haemocromocitometry, blood pressure. CsA BTLs were regularly determined.

Lymphocyte subsets were studied before and at the end of the treatment. Relapsing patients were admitted to a second course with CsA lasting 1 year with the same modalities after a therapy free period of 3 months.

Table 1 - Main clinical features and laboratory findings before CsA treatment

Patient	Sex	Age	Histol- ogical diagnosis	Plasma creat- inine mg/dl	Serum albumin g/dl	Protein- uria g/24h	Mean blood pressure mmhg	Duration of disease months
1) B.M.	M	38	GNM II	1.2	2.2	11.0	102	28
2) T.A.	F	64	GNM II	1.0	3.4	7.5	130	24
3) M.R.	F	26	GNM I	0.6	3.1	5.0	87	15
4) M.L.	M	57	GNM II	1.1	2.7	12.0	127	5
5) P.A.	M	59	GNM II	1.6	2.4	7.0	120	37
6) F.D.	M	34	GNM III	1.7	2.7	15.0	97	145
7) Z.V.	M	56	GNM II	0.9	2.9	5.0	97	27
8) V.R.	M	36	GNMP	1.2	2.8	6.0	112	47
9) F.P.	M	24	GNMP	1.1	3.2	7.0	107	28
10) B.M.	F	40	GNM IV	0.9	3.2	9.5	102	16
Mean		43		1.1	2.9	8.6		37

RESULTS

2 patients with MPGN and 4 with MGN were considered as responders (R), 3 had no improvement and 1 was withdrawn after 3 months for nephrotoxicity (CCr= 42 ml/min). This patient (M.L.) recovered a normal renal function (RF) a month after the drug had discontinued. In this patient CsA BTL average was 590 ng/ml while in the others it ranged 160 - 440. Table 2 summarizes the clinical and laboratory findings at the end of the 6 month therapy.

Table 2 - Main laboratory findings at the end of 6 month CsA course
(R = Responder, NR = Non responder, D = dropout)

Patient	Plasma creat- inine (mg/dl)	Mean CsA BTL (µg/ml)	Serum albumin (g/dl)	Protein- uria (g/24h)	Halving t. of potein- uria (weeks)	Histol- ogical diagnosis	Outcome
1) B.M.	1.4	306	3.8	3.2	12	GNM II	R
2) T.A.	1.8	277	4.3	2.8	5	GNM II	R
3) M.R.	0.9	440	3.9	1.3	2	GNM I	R
4) M.L.	-	590	-	-	-	GNM II	D
5) P.A.	1.8	215	2.6	10.0	-	GNM II	NR
6) F.D.	1.7	311	3.6	6.0	6	GNM III	R
7) Z.V.	0.9	159	3.3	3.6	-	GNM II	NR
8) V.R.	1.5	256	3.6	2.0	8	GNMP	R
9) F.P.	1.0	232	3.7	2.8	5	GNMP	R
10) B.M.	1.0	330	2.4	7.9	-	GNM IV	NR
Mean	1.3		3.6	4.6	6		

Serum albumin of R significantly increased from a mean of 2.6 to 3.8 g/dl (p< 0.005) and proteinuria decreased from 8.6 to 3.0 g/24h (p< 0.005). Time needed for halving of proteinuria ranged 2-12 weeks (mean 6). Mean PCr of R and nonresponders (NR) was the same before treatment (1.13 mg/dl) and at the end it was 1.38 and 1.23 respectively (p = ns). Mean Csa BTL in R was 303 and in NR 234 (p = ns). All 5 hypertensive patients required increasing of hypotensive drugs; 4 further patients developed hypertension, quite easily controlled by therapy. 5 out of 6 R relapsed within 6 weeks; 4 of them have been admitted to a second CsA course lasting 1 year (not yet concluded) .

DISCUSSION

CsA alone at low dosage had a beneficial effect on steroid-resistant NS although no complete remission occurred during the 6 month therapy; clear-cut decrease of proteinuria in R could not be explained only by haemodynamic mechanism since a mild impairment of RF occurred. Neither different type of GN or histological stage of MGN correlated to CsA response, though patient M.R., affected by MGN I, had a very early response in both CsA courses and a complete remission within 6 weeks during the second one. Early relapse of 5 out of 6 R, while giving support to CsA efficacy, rises the question if long term treatment could be proposed in front of possible side effects due to chronic immune suppression or renal toxicity. The analysis of T lymphocyte subsets indicated that the baseline patterns were maintained throughout the study in each patient, although our series appeared very heterogeneous as starting values. Mechanisms of action of CsA on immune complex mediated GN like MGN and MPGN could be explained by the interference with lymphokine-mediated response of humoral immunity (5, 6) or by GBM electric charge restoration from IL-2 inhibition (6). Early relapsing of quite all patients suggests that the latter hypotesis could be more suitable. In spite of low CsA doses 1 patient had acute reversible nephrotoxicity ; chronic toxicity, though mild and statistically not significative should be taken in account as well. Hypertension, though very frequent, has been well dominated by therapy.

REFERENCES

1. De Santo N.G., Capodicasa G., Giordano C., Am. J. Nephrol., 7, 74-76 (1987)
2. Balcke, P. ,Derfler, K., Stockenhuber, F. et al., Wien.Klin.Wschr. 99, 242-245 (1987)
3. Chan, M.K. and Cheng, I.K.P., Postgrad.med.J. 63, 757-759 (1987)
4. Capodicasa,G.,De Santo,N.G.,Nuzzi,F. et al, Int.J.Pediat. Nephrol. 7, No.2, 69-72 (1986)
5. Tejani, A.,Butt, K.,Trachtman, H. et al.,Kidney Int. 33, 729-734 (1988)
5. Hess, A.D.,Prog Allergy 38, 198-221 (1986)
7. Koenig, P.,Defregger M, Dittrich P.,2nd Int. Congress on Cyclosporine (Abst.),Washigton, 79.

EFFECTS OF CYCLOSPORINE A ON RENAL FUNCTION AND PROTEINURIA IN PATIENTS WITH NEPHROTIC SYNDROME AFTER A SINGLE ORAL ADMINISTRATION

G. Fuiano, P. Stanziale, M. Balletta, V. Sepe, G. Conte*, C. Libetta, B. Guida, V. Bisesti, R. Alfieri^, P. Cianfrone

Chairs of Nephrology, of 2nd Faculty of Medicine of Naples and *Catanzaro and ^Dept. of Biochemestry of Naples, Italy

Cyclosporine A (CyA) is probably the most important advance in the immunosuppressive management of transplants, reducing the incidence of acute rejections without relevant incidence of haematologic and infective complications as observed with "traditional" therapy. This encouraged to evaluate the effectiveness of Cy in the treatment of several immunological diseases. In Nephrology, Cy has been mostly experimented -besides in renal tranplants- in the treatment of nephrotic syndrome secondary to different forms of glomerular diseases, with conflicting results. However, in the last few years many authors have pointed out that Cy can acutely impair renal function by inducing renal vasoconscriction or by reducing Kf (1-4) or both. Since systemic and renal haemodynamics is often impaired in nephrotic patients (NP), the detrimental effect of Cy on GFR could be magnificated in these patients, with dangerous clinical consequences (5).
Moreover, it is also possible that such a fall in GFR, lowering the protein filtered load, may partly account for the reduction of proteinuria reported in some studies.

To test this possibility, we have studied the effects induced by Cy on renal haemodynamics and on proteinuria after a single oral administration in nephrotic patients.

METHODS

The study was carried out on 7 nephrotic patients and on 8 healthy volunteers (Controls, C). All subjects gave informed consent. Any medications was discontinued at least 1 week before the study; all were also requested of not drinking coffee, tea, alcohol and of not smoking during the 24 hours preceding the test.

The normal subjects were young physicians (age: 25-36, mean: 28 yrs) of our Unit. The clinical features of the nephrotic patients (NP) are reported in Table I.

TABLE 1. CLINICAL AND LABORATORY FEATURES OF PATIENTS.

	Age	Blood Pressure	Plasma Proteins	C_{Inul}	Blood Volume*
	yrs	mmHg	g/dl	ml/min	ml/kg
Mean	47	133/76	5.0	97	56
SD	18	21/12	1.4	31	10

* Normal values: 67 ml/Kg b.w.

All subjects were studied by renal clearance methods. Briefly, water diuresis was induced by 20 ml/min of water/kg/ b.w. per os and maintained by 20 ml/min of 5% glucose i.v. infusion. As a steady urinary volume was reached, the renal clearances were started. Two consecutive 30-min control clearance periods were performed. In controls, a commercially available solution (containing Cy 100 mg/ml in an olive oil vehicle and peglicol 5 oleate vehicle with 12.5 % alcohol) of Cy was administered orally at the dosage of 12 mg/kg, with some milk; in NP the dosage was lowered to 10 mg/kg on the basis of the presence of oedema overestimating the actual body weight and of hypoprotidemia increasing Cy bioavailability. Oral administration was preferred to i.v. route to avoid the

risk of anaphylactoid reaction. Inulin and PAH were
infused by infusion pump throughout the study to achieve
and maintain respective plasma concentrations of 15-20
and 1.5-2.0 mg/dl. Blood samples were collected at the
end of each clearance period and inulin, PAH, Creatinine
(Cr), Urea, Na, K, Osmolality, Cy (polyclonal RIA) were
determined. Urinary samples were analysed for Inulin,
PAH, Na, K, creatinine. In addition, in NP quantitative
proteinuria was determined in all samples and protein
selectivity index ($C_{IgG}/C_{Transferrin}$) before and 3 hours
after Cy administration. Blood volume was measured by
Blue Evans method. Blood pressure and pulse rate were
checked every 20 min throughout the study.

RESULTS

Blood pressure and pulse rate did not change in both
groups. Mean blood volume was 56 ml/kg (SD 10) in NP.
In table 2 are summarized data of GFR, RPF and
Filtration fraction before and after 1, 2 and 3 hours
from Cy administration.

Table 2. Values of GFR, Renal Plasma Flow (RPF) and
         Filtration Fraction (FF) during the study.

	GFR		RPF		FF	
	C	NS	C	NS	C	NS
	ml/min/1.73 m^2		ml/min/1.73 m^2		%	
BASAL	118±16	90±25	564±210	383±135	21±3	27±8
I hour	93±15	70±19	305±47	300±135	26±4	27±12
II hour	88±18	68±22	361±121	232±100	24±5	34±15
III hour	98±21	63±13	323±296	247±137	26±8	30±13

The "nadir" percent changes of GFR after Cy was
significantly greater in nephrotics (-47% ± 14 vs -28% ±
15 of C, $p<0.05$). In NP, proteinuria decreased in all

during the 3 hours following Cy administration, from 19.8 ± 12.2 SD to a "nadir" value of 7.9 ± 6.5 SD (mg/min) (p<0.05); also protein excretion/GFR decreased from 24.34 ± 14.1 SD to 12.7 ± 9.38 SD (mg/min/GFR), but this difference was not significant. Proteinuria was non-selective in all NP in basal conditions and became highly selective (C_{IgG}/C_{Transf} < 0.10) in 5, near-selective (C_{IgG}/C_{Transf} 0.10-0.20) in 2, whilst remained non-selective in 2.

CONCLUSIONS

In conclusion, our data show that Cy acutely impairs renal function in nephrotics by reducing severely renal plasma flow; this reduction is greater of that observed in normal subjects. We have observed also a significant fall in urinary protein excretion: however, proteinuria/GFR, although lower, was not significantly different from basal values. This observation may partly (but not completely) account for the observed reduction of proteinuria, mainly due to the fall of GFR.
However, the effects of Cyclosporin are not purely haemo-dynamic: in fact, the observed improvement in the proteinuria selectivity index can not be explained by renal haemodynamic changes either by immunological effects induced by the drug. A possible explanation is that, since Cy has been demonstrated able to reduce acutely the ultrafiltration coefficient (Kf) in the rats (4), if a similar reduction occurs in humans, this could also account for the higher selectivity of proteinuria and, possibly, also for the observed trend to a reduction in "effective" proteinuria.

REFERENCES

1. Conte G, Sabbatini M, Napodano P, De Nicola L, Gigliotti G, Fuiano G, Testa A, Russo D, Esposito C, Libetta C, Dal Canton A, Andreucci VE, Transplant Proc 1988 (in press).

2. Myers BD, Sibley R, Newton L, Tomlanovich SJ, Boshkos
   C, Stinson E, Luetscher JA, Whitney DJ, Krashy D,
   Coplon NS, and Perlooth MG, Kidney Int, 1988,33:
   590-600.
3. Barros JG, Boim MA, Ajzen H, Ramos OL, Schor N, Kidney
   Int 1987, 32: 19-25.
4. Sabbatini M, Esposito C, Uccello F, De Nicola L, Alba
   MM, Conte G, Dal Canton A, Andreucci VE, Transplant
   Proc 1988 (in press).
5. Praga M, Martinez R, Lisazoain M, Arenas J Morales JM,
   Ortuno B, Prieto C, Ann Int Med, 1987,107: 786.

CYCLOSPORINE A THERAPY IN IDIOPATHIC NEPHROTIC SYNDROME

R.POVEDA, M.T.GONZALEZ, A.M.CASTELAO, J.M.MAURI and
J.ALSINA.
Department of Nephrology. Hospital de Bellvitge.
Barcelona. Spain.

INTRODUCTION

The resistence or dependence to steroids in Nephrotic
Syndrome (NS) is a frequent clinical situation. In these
cases, the persistence of NS after therapy or the appea-
rence of steroid toxicity after repeated courses of prednisone makes unsatisfactory this therapeutic modality.

Recently, remissions of NS have been reported after
treatment with Cyclosporine A (CsA) included some cases of
previous steroid resistences. Most described cases correspond to patients diagnosed of Minimal Changes Disease (MCD)
or Focal Segmental Glomerulosclerosis (FSGS) (1,2). In
other reports, Membranous Nephropaty (MN), or other glomerular disease, included the non immune Alport Disease
have shown decrease in proteinuria after CsA therapy (3).

Frequent NS relapses after CsA discontinuation and potential nephrotoxicity are the main problems due to this
drug.

We report the results of CsA therapy in four cases of
NS.

MATERIAL AND METHODS

The age of the patients, their histopathologic diag-
noses and previous therapy are:
  Case 1: Female aged 21. MCD. Steroid dependent.
  Case 2: Male aged 34. FSGS. Steroid resistant.
  Case 3: Male aged 14. FSGS. Steroid resistant.

Case 4: Male aged 59. Membranous N. Steroid resistant.

CsA therapy: CsA was given at dose of 3 mg/Kbwt/d and furtherly adjusted to reach a whole blood level of 100-200 ng/ml measured by polyclonal RIA. The mean time under CsA therapy was 8 month (6-12mo).

RESULTS

Three patients showed a significant proteinuria decrease during CsA therapy. Complete remission was produced in case No 1, in whom 15 mg/d of prednisone was added to CsA during the first month of therapy. In another patient (No 4), proteinuria decreased to less than 1 g/d from a level of 10 g/d. In both cases, hypercholesterolemia and hypoproteinemia returned to normal levels durin treatment and edema disappeared. The case No 2 showed proteinuria decrease (from 6 g/d to 2 g/d) with no other clinical benefit and finally, in the case No 3, a proteinuria of 8 g/d was not modified by the tratment.

In two cases beginning CsA therapy with minimal renal failure (Cases 2 and 4, plasma creatinin of 150 microMol/l) further impairement of GFR (Plasma creatinine of 250 microMol/l) was seen during therapeutic period.

FOLLOW UP AFTER CYCLOSPORIN A DISCONTINUATION (CsA Dis.)

Case 1: The NS relapsed three months after CsA Dis. Histologic renal control showed MCD. GFR: Remains in normal level 8 months after CsA Dis.

Case 2: Proteinuria returned to previous Csa therapy values. GFR: Increased creatinine remained unchanged until 5th month after CsA Dis. Furtherly, plasma creatinine reached to 500 microMol/l.

Case 3: Proteinuria not responsive to treatment, remained at same level after CsA Dis. GFR: Unchanged (Normal) until 3th month after CsA Dis. Furtherly, progressive impairement of renal function. Six months after CsA Dis., hemodialysis is needed. Histological renal control: advanced renal sclerosis (Previous renal biopsy one year before showed FSGS).

DISCUSSION

As reported by others in more extensive studies, our very short experience shows that CsA decrease proteinuria and improves clinical symptoms in nephrotic patients included some steroid resistant cases. The absence of steroid side effects is an important   advantage of this therapy.

Opposed to CsA therapy is, in our experience, the frequent impairement of GFR (three patients) in spite of low CsA blood levels. In two patients with minimal previous renal failure, increasing in plasma creatinine was seen during therapy and in the other one, rapid deterioration of renal function was seen few months after CsA discontinuation. To discard CsA induced nephrotoxicity is not easy in every case.

We think advisable to exclude of this therapeutic modality the patients with decreased GFR.

The association of low CsA and steroid doses given for a short time period could combine the therapeutic effects of both drugs minimizing its side effects.

REFERENCES
1. Meyrier,A. and Simon,P. In: Actualités Néphrologiques de l´Hôpital Necker (Ed. Flammarion), Paris 1987,pp.121-140.
2. Niaudet, P.,Habib, R., Gagnadoux,M.F., Tête,M.J.and Broyer, M. In: Actualités Nephrologiques de l´Hôpital Necker (Ed. Flammarion) Paris, 1987, pp. 142-160.
3. Weimar, W., Zietse, R., Wenting, G.J.and Kramer, P. In: Proceedings of the Second International Congress on Cyclosporine. Washington D.C. USA. November 1987.

CAPTOPRIL AS AN ANTIPROTEINURIC AGENT IN PATIENTS WITH CHRONIC GLOMERULONEPHRITIS

A. FABBRI, M. MANDREOLI, E. DEGLI ESPOSTI, A. LUCATELLO, R. COCCHI, M. FUSAROLI
Servizio di Nefrologia e Dialisi, Ospedale S. Maria delle Croci, Ravenna, Italia

In membranous nephropathy patients with nephrotic range proteinuria have a poor prognosis (1,2), while those with asymptomatic proteinuria show a more benigne course (1,3,4). Moreover, it has been reported (5) that patients with focal segmental glomerulosclerosis and massive proteinuria reached end stage renal failure in the first 6 years after renal biopsy. Since a positive correlation between the amount of proteinuria and the progression of renal damage emerges from these clinicl studies and from experimental data (6), any treatment aimed at decreasing the severity of proteinuria may have a protective role on renal function. Thus, we have wanted to check the efficacy of captopril in 14 patients with glomerulonephritis and persistent proteinuria, in accordance with some recent clinical observations (7,8) that show the antiproteinuric effect of the angiotensin converting enzyme inhibitors (ACE-I).

MATERIALS AND METHODS

In this work we consider 14 patients with various histological types of glomerulonephritis, all documented with renal biopsy, and persistent proteinuria. We used captopril on all the patients for a period of 6 months at a mean daily dose of 75 mg (range 50-100). In 8/14 patients renal function was normal (plasma creatinine <1.5 mg/dl). Six out of fourteen were hypertensive patients (mean arterial pressure ≥110 mm Hg). In 11/14 patients, proteinuria persisted in spite of the previous treatments with steroids, with or without cyclophosphamide. Of these 11 patients, 9 had already completed one or two cycles of therapy, while in 2 patients the steroids had been interrupted due to the presence of serious side effects. In 3/14 patients, however, captopril was used as a first choice drug. At every check, clinical parameters were taken (the presence/absence of edemas, arterial pressure, side effects) as well as laboratory ones (24 hours proteinuria, albuminemia, plasma creatinine). All the results are reported as mean ± SEM and the significance is calculated with Wilcoxon's test for paired data.

RESULTS

In table I we report the mean values of proteinuria, albuminemia and

plasma creatinine at 0, 1, 3, 6 months. After the first month of treat
ment we observed a reduction in proteinuria in all the 14 patients, with
a mean decrease of 40%. At the end of the 6 months average proteinuria
was significantly reduced. However,upon analyzing each behaviour, in 5
out of 14 patients proteinuria has a tendency to increase towards the
initial values after 3 months. Plasma creatinine remained constant for
all the 6 months of the treatment. The albuminemia showed a tendency to
increase even if this did not reach statistical significance. Mean arte
rial pressure was reduced during the therapy even if not in a statisti
cally significant way (from 108 ± 2 to 103 ± 2 mm Hg, p = NS).

Table I. Clinical and laboratory parameters evaluated during the 6
months period of observation. (* $p < 0.001$)

Time	months	0	1	3	6
Proteinuria	gr/day	3.1 ± 0.4	1.8 ± 0.3*	1.7 ± 0.3*	1.9 ± 0.3*
Albuminemia	gr|dl	2.7 ± 0.1	2.7 ± 0.1	2.9 ± 0.2	3.1 ± 0.2
P. creatinine	mg/dl	1.6 ± 0.2	1.6 ± 0.2	1.6 ± 0.2	1.6 ± 0.1

DISCUSSION

Considering all the works published up to now on the treatment of glomerulonephritis, beyond the differences in the therapeutic schedules
(3,9,10,11,12,13), we can notice a favourable effect of therapy, since
the long-term prognosis turned out to be significantly better in the
patients in whom the therapy induced prolonged remission of proteinuria
(2,10,11). Today, the idea seems to prevail, and we too are in agreement
with this, that if the pathogenetic therapy with steroids and other im
munodepressive drugs does not appear to be effective, then you need to
take an antiproteinuric symptomatic treatment into consideration (14,
15,16). An antiproteinuric effect of captopril was already reported in
the patients with glomerulonephritis, complicated by arterial hyperten
sion and by a various deficit in renal function (7,8). Our work, compa
red to the previous ones, is different in that it also includes normotensive and normofunctional patients. In our patients the reduction in
proteinuria was the same in all after the first month's therapy, which
suggested that the hemodynamic variation is experienced in all patients
in the same way, regardless of the underlying histological damage. In
9/14 patients that effect was maintained throughout the period of obser
vation, while in the other 5 patients we observed a tendency towards a
return to the initial levels in proteinuria after 3 months. In the patients of Taguma (17) there is a heterogeneous response to captopril
right from the beginning whereas the diversification of response of our
patients occurred after the third month. Moreover, also in the patient
series reported by Heeg (11) there are 3/13 patients in whom even from
the third month the same phenomenon of rise in proteinuria was evident.
We should however remember that beyond every relationship between intra

renal hemodynamics and proteinuria, we are faced with inflammatory and immunological lesions that cause proteinuria and recur. We believe that treatment with ACE-I should be considered every time we are faced with persistent proteinuria regardless of the conventional therapy. Recently Brenner and coll. (18) have demonstrated that in rats cortisone induces intracapillary hypertension and that ACE-I is able to counter-balance that effect. In view of this, ACE-I ought not to be viewed solely as a second-choice treatment in non responders but as a drug to be associated to steroids right from the beginning.

REFERENCES

1. Davison, A.M., Cameron, J.S., Kerr, D.N.S., Ogg, C.S., Wilkinson, R.W. Clin. Nephrol. 22: 61-67, 1984.
2. Ponticelli, C. Kidney Int. 29: 927-940, 1986.
3. Mallick, N.P., Short, C.D., Manos, S.G. Nephron 34: 206-219, 1983.
4. Honkanen, E. Clin. Nephrol. 25: 122-128, 1986.
5. Velosa, J.A., Holley, K.E., Torres, V.E., Offord, K.P. Mayo Clin. Proc. 58: 568-577, 1983.
6. Hostetter, T.H., Olson, J.L., Rennke, H.G., Venkatachalam, M.A., Brenner, B.M. Am. J. Physiol. 241: F85-F93, 1981.
7. Lagrue, G., Robeva, R., Laurent, J. Nephron 46: 99-100, 1987.
8. Heeg, J.E., De Jong, P.E.,Van der Hem, G.K., De Zeeuw, D. Kidney Int. 32: 78-83, 1987.
9. Collaborative study. N. Engl. J. Med. 301: 1301-1306, 1979.
10. Ponticelli, C., Zucchelli, P., Imbasciati, E., Cagnoli, L., Pozzi,C., Passerini, P., Grassi, C., Limido, D., Pasquali, S., Volpini,'T., Sasdelli, M., Locatelli, F. N. Engl. J. Med. 310: 946-950, 1984.
11. Tu, W.H., Petitti, D.B., Biava, C.G., Tulunay, O., Hopper, J. Nephron 36: 118-124, 1984.
12. West, M.L., Jindal, K.K., Bear, R.A., Goldstein, M.B. Kidney Int. 32: 579-584, 1987.
13. Suki, W.N., Chavez, A. Am. J. Nephrol. 1: 11-16, 1981.
14. Velosa, J.A., Torres, V.E., Donadio, J.L., Wagoner, R.D. Mayo Clin. Proc. 60: 586-592, 1985.
15. Vriesendorp, R., Donker, Ab.J.M., De Zeeuw, D., De Jong, P.E., Van der Hem, G.K., Brentijens, J.R.H. Am. J. Med. 81 (suppl. 2B): 84-94, 1986.
16. Laurent, J., Belghiti, D., Bruneau, C., Lagrue, G. Am. J. Nephrol. 7: 198-202, 1987.
17. Taguma, Y., Kitamoto, Y., Futaki, G., Ueda, H., Monma, H., Ishizaki, M., Takahashi, H., Sekino, H., Sasaki, Y. N. Engl. J. Med. 313: 1617-1620, 1985.
18. Garcia, D.L., Rennke, H.G., Brenner, B.M., Anderson, S. J. Clin. Invest. 80: 867-874, 1987.

STEROID-RESISTANT NEPHROTIC SYNDROME TREATED WITH CYCLOSPORIN A(CyA).

Riegler P.,Corradini R.,Eder P*,Valli A.**,Huber W.
Dept.of Nephrology,City Hospital,Bolzano,Trento**,
Dept of Intern.Med.,City Hospital,Brunico*,ITALY.

Introduction

Besides the important immunosoppressive functions
Cyclosporin A (CyA)showed also positive influences on
nephrotic syndromes(NS)of different origins
(1,2,3,4,5,6,7).
Therefore we treated eight patients affected by NS,
for whom we thought we had reached a therapeutic dead
end.

Patients and methods

Our patients were 6 males and 2 females(mean age 40.6
+/-18.8 years)and were treated with CyA over a period
ranging from 2 to 14 months(mean treatment time 8.2
+/- 3.5 months).
Two patients were affected by focal
glomerulosclerosis(FGS)and one by mesangial
proliferative glomerulonephritis(MPGN)with frequent
relapses ; each of them strongly
steroid-dependent.The one affected by MPGN was
treated with almost toxic dose of
cyclophosphamide.Three patients,one affected by
membranous glomerulonephritis(MGN)and two by
membranoproliferative glomerulonephritis(MemProlGN)
were steroid resistant.The two affected by
MemProlGN,when the disease began,had already a mild
renal failure.(serum creatinine 2.3 mg% and 1.9
mg%).In two more steroid resistant patients ,renal
biopsy was not performed because of
contraindications.
CyA was given orally in two equal doses each
day;serum blood through level,measured by
radioimmunoassay, was maintained between loo and 4oo
ng/ml.In one patient(FGS)the remission of NS relapse

was not obtained with CyA alone and so we administred methylprednisolone as a bolus intravenously(250mg/daily over three days)followed by methylprednisolone orally in decreasing dosage.Another one(MPGN)received prednisone orally at the same time.

Results.

Proteinuria improved initially in all patients;in fact five months after starting treatment,it came down in statistically significant measure from 13.2 +/- 8.3 g/d to 4.8 +/- 2.3 g/d(p< 0.05).Serum protein level rose to a near normal value in all patients at the 5th. month.Serum creatinine did not show increments in all patients but two affected by MemProlGN.In these two patients ,both hypertensive,after an initial improvement of their renal function,despite Cya blood through levels below 400 ng/ml,their renal function worsened.This compelled us to stop the treatment respectively in the 7th and 10th month.Now they are on regular hemodialysis treatment.One of these patients suffered a hypertensive encephalopathy during CyA treatment. Arterial hypertension was a mayor problem in the two affected by MemProlGN;two more patients (FGS and 1 undefined case)during the CyA treatment needed hypotensive medications;theyr renal function. was normal. Side effects like gum hypertrophy and hypertrichosis,tremor and nausea were mild and four patients didn't show any.One patient(MemProlGN)developed a severe hypertrichosis associated with combined CyA and minoxidil therapy . Two patients out of 8(MemProlGN)showing renal failure at the start of their renal disease,are now on dialysis,three are still on treatment and three more worsened their proteinuria after stopping treatment to a maximum af 5 g/d without clinical edema.

Conclusions

The results of our investigation indicate,that CyA is effective in the treatment of patients affected by steroid resistant or dependent NS.Further investigations should be performed to establish the duration of treatment with CyA.

References
1.H.C.Gunn,B.Ryffel,P.C.Hiestand and J.F.Borel .
 In:Cyclosporin in autoimmune disease ,pag.334
 (Ed.R.Schidler)Springer Verlag,1985
2.A.R.Watzon,Clin.Nephrol:25,5,273-274,1986

3.D.C.Cattran,J.Dossetor,P.Keown,C.Stiller,P.Halloran
  W.F.Clark.Kidney Int.29,82,1986
4.A.Meyrier,P.Simon,G.Perret & M.C.Condamin.Kidney
  Int.,29,197,1986
5.A.Tejani,K.Butt,R.Khawar,M.Suthanthiran,C.J.Rosen-
  thal,H.Trachtman and M.Fusi.Kidney
  Int.29,206,1986
6.K.N.Lai,F.M.Lai,P.K.T.Li,J.Vallance-Owen.Br.Med.J.
  295,165-168,1987.
7.Schulz W.,Rebstoeck W..2.Dec.1985.Faculte Saint
  Louis Lariboisiere,Paris

Miscellany

INTRAVASCULAR VOLUME EXPANSION AS THERAPEUTIC APPROACH TO THE UNDERFILL STATE OF PREECLAMPSIA

P. Stratta, C. Canavese, L. Gurioli, M. Porcu, M. Dogliani, T. Todros, G.C. Mattone, O. Fianchino, L. Gagliardi, A. Vercellone.

Department of Nephrology and Ostetric Pathology, University of Turin, Italy.

INTRODUCTION

Plasma volume expansion is a central physiological adjustment of normal pregnancy, and inadequate plasma volume expansion has been associated with specific complications of pregnancy, in particular preeclampsia (PE). In view of the important role of atrial natriuretic peptide (ANP) in volume homeostasis, ANP kinetics might help to understand plasma volume changes in different conditions (1). Nevertheless a direct relationship between ANP and plasma volume is evident only in physiological conditions, while in some pathological conditions such as PE, it is possible to observe a dissociation betxeen plasma volume contraction and high ANP level (2 - 5).

The aim of this study was to evaluate volume homeostasis in normal and complicated pregnancy, by using the ratio between Aldosterone and ANP instead of ANP alone. We assumed the first to be the symbol of the water-sodium saving forces, and the second as symbol of the water-sodium wasting forces.

PATIENTS AND METHODS

The study was undertaken in 34 normal pregnances, monitored monthly from the first trimester, and 15 PE, monitored from arrival to our unit until the birth.

We evaluated: plasma ANP (RIA-Peninsula) and Aldosterone, total sodium excretion, uteroplacental and fetoplacental flow (continuous wave ultrasound Doppler, DOPTEK 9021) and fetal ouctome (weight, APGAR).

RESULTS

In normal pregnancy Aldosterone sharply increases in the first weeks (431 $\pm$ 232 pg/ml) and again in the final weeks until birth (845 $\pm$ 449 pg/ml). Conversely ANP falls below normal values (21.7 $\pm$ 5.7 pg/ml) in the first trimester, reaches slightly above normal values at the beginning of the third trimester (35 $\pm$ 7 pg/ml), and after slowly decreases, though always within normal ranges (29 $\pm$ 5.8 pg/ml). The ratio between Aldosterone and ANP in normal pregnancy shows that the higher values in favour of the water-sodium retaining factors are in early (20.5 $\pm$ 5) and late (28.7 $\pm$ 8) pregnancy.

In preeclamptic patients, while Aldosterone is always in lower ranges, ANP levels range from the lowest to the highest values of the normal range. The ratio Aldosterone/ANP is significantly lower (8 $\pm$ 4) than that of normal pregnancy at the same gestational age, and total (80 $\pm$ 20 mEq/24) sodium excretion is significantly reduced. A comparison between the two subgroups with Aldosterone/ANP ratio (6 and 6) shows that the group with lower ratio has some significant differences: a greater number of cases with pathological uterine and placental flow (8/8 vs 2/7), and more cases of newborn small for their gestational ages (8/8 vs 3/7). After hyperoncotic albumin infusion (0.3-0.7 g/body weight), we observed variable changes in ANP (+5 to 100%), Aldosterone (-1 to 75%), BCrC (-20 to +50%) and Na excretion (-50 to +300%). Both

BCrC and sodium did not increase in patients with a lower pre-albumin Aldosterone/ANP ratio.

CONCLUSION

In conclusion, the ratio Aldosterone/ANP seems to be a better index than ANP alone in evaluating volume changes in normal pregnancy and in PE. In normal pregnancy this ratio shows that the maximum effort in order to gain and maintain adequate volumes is in the first and final weeks, at a time when, however, intravascular volume is "sensed" as underfill or bordeline owing to the vasodilation (6).

In PE, a significantly lower Aldosterone/ANP ratio is in accordance with a failure of water-sodium retaining factors to expand adequate maternal volume. In PE, a particularly low Aldosterone/ANP ratio due to inappropriately high ANP levels produced for unknown stimuli (perhaps more severe myocardial involvement) is associated with a poorer fetal outcome. Furthemore, a particularly low Aldosterone/ANP ratio may identify the "non responders" to albumin infusion, this non response being due to an exceptionally contracted intravascular volume.

BIBLIOGRAFIA
1. Weidmann P., Saxenhofer H., Ferrier C., Shaw SG. - Am. J. Nephrol. 8, 1-14, 1988.
2. Thomsen J.W., Stort T.L., Tham Sborg G., De Nully M., Bdker B., Skovby S. - Br. Med. J. 294, 1508-1510, 1987.
3. Rutherford A.J., Anderson J.V., Elder M.G., Bloom S.R. - Lancet 1, 928-929, 1987.
4. Cusson J.R, Gutkowska J., Rey E., Michon N., Boucher N., Larochelle P. - N. Engl. J. Med. 313, 19, 1230-1231, 1985.
5. Gant N.F., Whalley P.J., Everet R.B., Wolvery R.J., Macdonald P.C.- Am. J. Kidney Dis. 9, 4, 303-307, 1987.
6. Schrier R.W., Dür J.A.- Am J. Kidney Dis. 9, 4, 248-289, 1987.

A PROSPECTIVE RANDOMIZED THERAPEUTIC TRIAL FOR SCHISTOSOMAL SPECIFIC
NEPHROPATHY

Mohamed A. Sobh, Fatma E. Moustafa, Samir M. Sally, Mohamed Ashraf

Foda, Ander M. Deelder, Mohamed A. Ghoniem.

Urology & Nephrology Center, University of Mansoura, Egypt.

We have previously reported the existance in clinical settings

of schistosomal specific nephropathy and that this disease may

progress to end stage renal failure (1). Furthermore, we described

the histopathology and immunopathology of this disease in its early

and late stages (1,2).

The objective of this work was to study the effect of three

therapeutic modalities on schistosomal nephropathy.

MATERIAL AND METHODS

Patients with schistosomal specific nephropathy were randomly

distributed among three groups. Group I cases were given anti-

schistosomal treatment (Oxamniquine&Praziquantel), group II were

given anti-schistosomal treatment and prednisolone. Group III were

given anti-schistosomal treatment and ciclosporin.

Schistosomal specificity of kidney lesions were assessed as pre-

viously discribed (2,3).

Oxamniquine was given in a total dose of 40-60mg/kg, given on three

successive days, praziquantel was given as a single oral dose of

15mg/kg.

Prednisolone was given in a dose of 60 mg/d for 12 weeks, then gra-

dually withdrawn within 24 weeks.

Ciclosporin was given orally in a dose of 5mgkg/d, this was given in two divided doses and readjusted so as to have a whole blood trough level of 200-300 ng/ml. Ciclosporin was given for 12 weeks. Patients were evaluated before treatment and every other week for 12 months.

Special stress was directed towards degree of oedema, blood pressure, S. creatinine, albumin, cholesterol, 24h. urinary protein and kidney biopsy was performed before and 12 months after initiation of treatment.

RESULTS

24 patients fullfiled the criteria for admission to the study. There was no difference between the three groups regarding the main age, sex, clinical presentation, kidney function or histopathologic nature of the kidney lesions. The main age of the whole group was 23.5±0.5 years, 20 were male and 4 were female, 20 were nephrotic and 4 were presenting with non-nephrotic proteinuria, serum createnine was normal in 20 patients and mildly high in 4 cases. Mesangiocapillary glomerulonephritis was detected in 6 cases, FSGS in 6, mesangioproliferative glomerulonephritis in 7, membranous glomerulonephritis in 2 and no changes were detected in 3.

Following treatment, complete clinical and laboratory remission was documented in two cases in group II, the duration of remission was 4,8 months. Partial remission was reported in 3 cases in group II & in group III, there was no response to treatment in 8 cases in group I, 3 cases in group II and in 4 cases in group III. Ciclosporin was stopped in one case due to significant acute nephrotoxicity.

116

In no cases there was toxicity related to intake of antischistosomal drugs. In those received prednisolone, one developed osteoporosis and another suffered from steroid diabetes and gastro intestinal haemorrhage. In those received ciclosporin two & suffered from nephrotoxicity and one suffered from hepatotoxicity. Histopathologic reevaluation showed no regression of the lesion in any of the three groups. Progression of kidney lesion was observed in 2 in group I, 1 in group II and 2 cases in group III.

CONCLUSION

We have concluded that within the observation period, in patients with established schistosmal nephropathy, non of the tried therapeutic regimens will induce regression of the disease or prolonged remission.

REFERENCES

1. M. Sobh, F. Moustafa, M. Basta, A. Deelder, M. Ghoniem. Kidney Int. 31 : 1006-1011, 1987.

2. M. Sobh, F. Moustafa, S. Sally, A. Deelder, M. Ghoniem. Nephrol Dial Transpl. (in press).

3. M. Sobh, F. Moustafa, S. Sally, A. Deelder, M. Ghoniem. Nephrol Dial Transpl. (in press).

IMMUNOTACTOID GLOMERULOPATHY: WHAT ABOUT THERAPY?

C. ROLLINO, R. COPPO, G. BELTRAME, R. NOVARA, D. ROCCATELLO, B. BASOLO, A. AMORE, G. MARTINA, G. PICCOLI

Nefrologia Medica e Dipartimento di Scienze Biomediche e Oncologia Umana. Università di Torino. Divisione di Nefrologia e Dialisi. Ospedale Nuova Astanteria Martini. Torino.

INTRODUCTION

Immunotactoid glomerulopathy (ITGP) was identified in 1985 by Korbet (1). Its histologic characteristic is the presence on electron microscopy of mesangial and/or parietal structured deposits with fibrillar or microtubular configuration, while light microscopy and immunofluorescence aspects are non specific. No reports about therapeutic approaches are found in the literature; only one case (2), suffering from ITGP and vasculitis, was treated by steroids but nor the posology nor the response are mentioned. We are herein presenting a clinical study of 8 patients who were given different therapeutic schedules.

MATERIALS AND METHODS

In a recent review of the renal biopsies performed in our town and examined by the Pathology Department of the University of Turin among the cases which had been considered "non classified" or "atypical", 8 cases of ITGP were identified. They all presented the typical structured deposits. Mean age of patients, 5 males and 3 females, was 26.5 ± 13.8 years. Follow-up ranged from 31 to 156 months (mean 79.6 ± 51.6 months). At the onset mean proteinuria was 3.7 ± 2.6 g/day. 6/8 patients underwent renal biopsy because of a nephrotic range proteinuria, 1 (FP) because of an acute nephritic syndrome, 1 (VB) because of minor urinary abnormalities and symptoms of systemic disease. Hematuria was present in 6/8 patients but in only one (FP) it was important. Renal function was normal in 5/8 patients, modestly compromised in 2 (BM, CM), and severely in 1 (FP). Mean creatinine was 1.5 ± 1.3 mg%. Hypertension was present in 4 patients. Immunologic investigations were negative or normal in most patients. Only 1 patient (CA) had a sporadic positivity for ANA. Two patients (MB, VB) were given no therapy, the former, with nephrotic range proteinuria, on his own will, the latter because of the too modest urinary abnormalities. Three patients were treated by indomethacin: CA 150 mg daily for 8 years, CM 200 mg daily for 3 years; MF 100 mg daily for a few months.

One patient (BM), because of his diabetes secondary to pancreatectomy, was not given prednisone but chlorambucil alone 10 mg daily for a test period of one month. He had a carcinoma of the pancreas head 8 years before which was treated by removal of pancreas and spleen. One patient (LM) was started on prednisone 100 mg/day, cyclophosphamide 100 mg/day. The last patient (FP) had an acute nephritic syndrome with a rapidly progressive renal failure. An IgGK monoclonal gammopathy of unidentified significance (MGUS), but no Bence Jones proteinuria, was detected. We performed a treatment with 3x1 g methilprednisolone pulses, followed by 50 mg prednisone daily and cyclophosphamide 100 mg daily in association to 8 plasma exchanges. During the following year, 6 cycles were performed of prednisone 50 mg/day plus cyclophosphamide 100 mg/day for 6 days. Two relapses occurred afterwards and an analogous treatment was applied. After the last one the patient was maintained on a therapy of low dose steroids (deflazacort 30 mg every other day) and monthly cyclophosphamide cycles (100 mg daily for 5 days).

RESULTS

LM was lost from follow-up after few months. Renal situation of MB and VB, who received no treatment, was stable after 31 and 87 months. Of the 3 patients treated by indomethacin only one (CA) had a good reduction of proteinuria (from 5 to 0.5 g/day). Two attempts to discontinue the drug were followed by immediate relapses of proteinuria (from 0.2 to 4 g/day and from 0.6 to 7 g/day). Renal function modestly worsened in these years. CM had a poor response: proteinuria was stable around 4 g/day. Renal failure slowly progressed over 10 years. Of the last patient (MF) we observed no response over the few months of treatment as of the patient treated by the test period of chlorambucil (BM). The response in FP was good: few days after the starting of therapy we observed a rapid improvement of the renal parameters. At each relapse the response was satisfactory again. At the end of follow-up (35 months) cyclophosphamide cycles permitted to maintain stable renal function.

DISCUSSION

As the pathogenesis of ITGP is still unknown the rational basis for these therapeutic approaches were provided mostly by the analysis of histologic and clinical data of each patient and from some general considerations.

Case FP had a very peculiar clinical presentation. Extracapillary proliferation and inflammatory aspects other than rapidly progressive renal failure made the rational for the initial therapy whih was repeated at the relapses. The combined treatments permitted to obtain quick improvements in renal parameters. However we are aware that this good response might be referred to a good effect on the extracapillary proliferation rather than on the typical immunotactoid lesions. However the repeated positive outcome of therapy would suggest a direct effect on the ITGP itself. Moreover it can not be excluded that a superimposed nephritis was associated. Besides, the presence of structured deposits made from proteic material suggested a correlation between monoclonal gammopathy and glomerular disease. We can suppose that the paraprotein, precipitating itself, or determining the precipitation of other serum proteins into the kidney, had contributed to the formation of the immunotactoid deposits. The benefic effect of PE might likely be due to the removal of unknown factors modulating the precipitation of these proteins and hence the expression of the disease. In this sense we applied also chemiotherapic cycles similar to those performed in myeloma which permitted to maintain a quite long stabilization of the disease. Of the 2 patients treated by indomethacin for long time only one showed a good response. As in other nephropathies, the antiproteinuric effect might be related to hemodynamic mechanisms or to other unexplained effects on blood flow intrarenal distribution which could modify the glomerular response to an immunologic aggression (3). This patient progressed very slowly towards renal failure. Since Korbet identified in proteinuria a negative prognostic factor, this good clinical course may be referred to a better control of proteinuria or to a good direct effect of indomethacin on the progression of the disease. The data reported are only anecdoctic; hence it seems difficult to draw definitive conclusions. Anyhow it would seem that when signs of striking activity of the disease are present an aggressive treatment may be successful.

REFERENCES
1. Korbet, S.M., Melvin, M.S., Rosenberg, BF., Sibley R.K. and Lewis E.J. Medicine 64: 228-243, 1985.
2. Schifferli, J.A., Merot, Y. and Chatelanat, F. Clin. Nephrol. 27: 151-155, 1987.
3. Michielsen, P. In: Advances in Nephrourology (Ed. Plenum Press), New York, 1981, pp. 153-157.

RENAL PRESENTATION IS NOT A RELEVANT FACTOR IN PREDICTING RENAL OUTCOME IN PATIENTS WITH SYSTEMIC LUPUS

G. FUIANO, P. STANZIALE, M. VISCIONE, V. SEPE, B. GUIDA, G. MARINELLI, G. COLUCCI, D. SABELLA, M. BALLETTA

Department of Nephrology II Faculty of Medicine Naples Italy

INTRODUCTION

Lupus nephritis is the most important cause of death in patients with systemic lupus erythematous (1-4). For this reason, an early biologic and clinic evaluation could be of great prognostic rilevance.

To verify if any correlation exists between the functional renal involvement at presentation and the evolution of lupus nephritis, we analyzed data from 20 patients with different degrees of renal involvement.

PATIENTS AND METHODS

Twenty patients with lupus nephritis (18 F, 2 M) were divided in two groups according to renal function and proteinuria. Group 1 (n = 5, mean age 27.7 yrs ± 9.2 SD): patients with serum creatinine < 1.5 mg/dl and proteinuria < 3 g/24 hr. Group 2 (n = 15, mean age 23.9 yrs ± 6.6 SD): patients with serum creatinine > 1.5 mg/dl and/or proteinuria > 3 g/24 hr. Sexteen patients underwent renal biopsy. Specimens were processed for optical microscopy using conventional technique immunohistological studies were performed using a direct immunofluorescence method on frozen tissue. Renal histology was reviewed by three of us (GF, PS, MB). Morphologic diagnosis was made according to W.H.O. classification. The employed immunosuppressive therapy is shown in table 1.

Table 1.   Histological findings and immunosuppressive
                  therapy

| Category (WHO class) | | Methylprednisolone (MP) | | | MP + Azathioprine |
		Pat. (n)	Mean dos. (mg)	SD	Pat. (n)
I	Normal LM/EM/IF	Ø	Ø	Ø	Ø
II	Mesangial changes				
	II A	Ø	Ø	Ø	Ø
	II B	3	70	26.4	Ø
III	Foc. and seg. prol. GN	4	61.7	13.6	Ø
IV	Diffuse prol GN	3	158.3	123.3	4
V	Membr. Lupus Nephritis	1	25	Ø	1

Mean follow up was 36 months; clinical laboratory tests
were determined by standard laboratory procedures. Seven
patients were on antihypertensive therapy. Differences
between the two groups were analyzed by Student's t test.

RESULTS

        Table 2 and table 3 show the main laboratory
findings at presentation and at last control
in both groups, respectively.

Table 2.   Laboratory findings at presentation

| | Group 1 | | Group 2 | |
	mean	SD	mean	SD
Serum cret. mg/dl	0.87	0.23	1.22	0.62
Creat. clear. ml/min	72.75	20.24	74.5	36.47
Serum alb. g/dl	3.30	0.35	1.92	0.79
ESR mm/hour	33.25	24.89	76.9	31.86
Blood hemog. g/dl	13	1.8	10.5	1.53
White cells x 1000	6.45	2.6	6.9	3.7
Plateles x 1000	233		182	753
% PAT. WITH C3% < 66	50		62.5	
% pat. with C4% < 67	67		66.7	
% pat. Ab anti-DNA pos.	20		73.3	
Proteinuria g/24 h	1.13	0.64	6.04	3.58

Table 3.   Laboratory findings at the last control

	Group 1		Group 2	
	mean	SD	mean	SD
Serum cret. mg/dl	1.12	0.28	1.66	1.41
Cret. clear. mL/min	53.1	1.6	78.76	57.5
Serum alb. g/dl	3.15	0.75	3.07	1.35
ESR mm/hour	43.5	11.5	13.0	2.0
Blood hemogl. g/dl	13.8	2.9	14.3	1.1
White cells x 1000	11.7	5.9	12.1	6.5
Platelets x 1000	210	57	183	63
Proteinuria g/24 h	4.17	2.02	3.61	1.54

A rapid and steady normalization of both serum albumine and blood hemoglobin was observed in group 2 (1.92 ± 0.8 vs 3.07 g/dl and 10.5 ± 1.53 vs 14.3 ± 1.1 g/dl, $p < 0.05$). Renal function remained unchanged in both groups. Twenty-four hours proteinuria significantly increased (1.13 ± 0.64 vs 4.17 ± 2.02 g/24 hr, $p < 0.05$) in patients of group 1, while decreased (6.0 ± 3.58 vs 3.61 ± 1.54 , $p < 0.05$) in patients of group 2. Blood pressure was kept within normal values in both groups; clinical symptoms ameliorated in 5 patients. One patient developed end stage renal failure and underwent a regular dialysis treatment 12 months after the first control.

DISCUSSION

A prognostic evaluation of lupus nephritis on the basis of the sole histology is impossible as its course is variable and glomerular changes are often multiform and susceptible of spontaneus modifications (5). It is also possible that severe glomerular changes are present without a clinical renal involvement (6). For this reason in this study we tried to perform a prognostic evaluation on the basis of the degree of functional renal involvement at presentation. At the end of follow-up, no difference in renal function and daily proteinuria was observed between the two groups. Therefore we conclude that a worse renal functional involvement at presentation

does not indicate a poor prognosis, provided that blood
pressure and relapses of acute episodes are properly
treated.

REFERENCES
1. Cameron, J.S., Turner, D.R., Ogg, C.S., Williams,
    D.G., Lessof, M.H., Chantler, C., Leibowitz, S.
    Quart. J. Med. 189-1, 1979.
2. Estes, D., Christian, C.L. Medicine 50:85, 1971.
3. Urowitz, M.M., Bookman, A.M., Koehler, B.E., Gordon,
    D.A., Ogrylo, M.A. Am. J. Med. 60:221, 1976.
4. Wallace, D.J., Podell, T.E., Weiner, J.M., Cox, M.B.,
    Klinemberg, J.R., Forouzesh, S., Dubois, E.L. Am. J.
    Med: 72:209, 1982
5. Hill, G.S. In: Pathology of the kidney (Eds. R.H.
    Heptinstall) Little Brown, Boston, 1983, pp. 839-906.
6. Hecht, B., Siegel, N., Kashgarian, M., Hayslett, J.P.
    Medicine, Baltimore 55.163, 1976.

IS TUBULOINTERSTITIAL DAMAGE A RELIABLE INDEX FOR PREDICTING RENAL OUTCOME IN PRIMARY MEMBRANOUS NEPHROPATHY ?

P. Stanziale, V. Sepe, M.M. Balletta, A. Esposito, G. Colucci, P. Cianfrone, N. Comi, G. Fuiano
Dept. of Nephrology, 2nd Faculty of Medicine, University of Naples, Italy

INTRODUCTION

Interstitial changes are often observed in primary glomerular disease. However, the severity of these changes is not always mirrored by the glomerular involvement. Aim of this study is to evaluate if the presence of tubular, interstitial and vascular changes can predict the renal outcome of primary membranous glomerulonephritis (MGN).

PATIENTS AND METHODS

The analysis was performed on 65 patients with primary MGN. The patients were grouped on the basis of renal function in Group 1 (creatinine clearance, Ccr, $\geq$ 80 ml/min; Gr1) and Group 2 (Ccr < 80 ml/min; Gr2). All biopsies were reviewed by 4 of the authors without knowing the identity of the patients and were scored for glomerular stage, tubulo-interstitial and vascular changes: in particular, the following lesions were sought and evaluated: interstitial infiltrates, fibrosis, tubular dilations and atrophy and vascular sclerosis and intimal hyperplasia. All patients were followed for at least 26 months and clinical and laboratory controls were performed at least every three months, although the majority of them were checked monthly, particularly during the first 6 months after histological diagnosis and during steroid treatment.

The main clinical and laboratory features of patients are reported in Table I.

Table I. Clinical and laboratory features of patients
         at the time of histological diagnosis (M±SD)

	N	Age **	Males **	Time to onset Pr NS ns *			Protein uria	Serum Crea **	Follow-up **
		yrs	%	mts			g/day	mg/dL	mts
Gr 1	37	39±16	55	15	75	10	6.2±3.0	0.9±0.2	47±32
Gr 2	28	53±14	71	29	71	-	7.3±4.2	1.4±1.5	26±33

*Pr=proteinuria; NS=nephrotic syndrome; ns=nephritic
syndrome; **p<0.05

HISTOLOGICAL STAGE

Group 1: 10 had stage 1, 26 stage 2 and 1 stage 3;
Group 2: 3 had stage 1, 21 stage 2 and 4 stage 3.

STATISTICAL ANALYSIS

Paired and unpaired t-test, Fisher's exact test and
analysis of variance with repeated measures were used.

RESULTS

No difference was found between the two groups as
regard to interstitial infiltrates and tubular or
vascular changes: interstitial infiltrates were in fact
present in 6 of Gr1 and in 12 of Gr2; tubular atrophy in
17 of Gr 1 and in 16 of Gr 2; arteriolar degenerative
changes (mainly hyalinosis) were present in 8 of Gr1 and
in 10 of Gr2. By contrast, patients of Group 2 presented
a higher incidence and severity of interstitial fibrosis:
moderate to severe interstitial fibrosis was in fact
found in 2 patients of Gr1 (5%) and in 7 (25%) of Gr2 (p
< 0.05). The incidence of obsolete glomeruli was not
different between the two groups and in no case was
greater than 10% of the total number (Table II).

The observations of creatinine, creatinine clearance,
blood pressure and proteinuria are shown in Table III.
Gr2 patients were significantly older than patients

of Gr1 (p<0.02); this was particularly evident for patients of Gr2 with second stage MGN. At the last follow-up (i.e. after 47±32 and 26±33 months in Gr1 and Gr2 respectively) creatinine clearance was greater in Gr1 than Gr2 (84±31 vs 49±24 mL/min respectively; p<0.01). Renal function, as assesed by creatinine clearance, decreased in a different way (p<0.01) in both groups.

Table II. Histological findings

	absent Gr1 Gr2		mild Gr1 Gr2		moderate Gr1 Gr2		severe Gr1 Gr2	
	%		%		%		%	
Int. infiltrates	84	57	11	32	5	11	–	–
Int. fibrosis	49	21	46	54	5	18	–	7
Tub. atrophy	54	43	43	39	3	14	–	4
Tub. dilation	100	89	–	11	–	–	–	–
Art. changes	78	64	22	32	–	4	–	–
Obsolete glo.	81	61	19	35	–	4	–	–

Int.=interstitial; Tub.=tubular; Art.=arteriolar; glo.=glomeruli

Table III. Laboratory findings (M±SD)

	Time to onset Gr1	Gr2	After 6 months Gr1	Gr2	At the last follow-up Gr1	Gr2
Crea	0.9±0.2*	1.4±1.5	0.9±0.2*	1.5±1.0	1.4±1.1	2.4±2.6
Pro.u	6.2±3.0	7.3±4.2	4.5±3.9	4.9±4.6	5.2±5.4	3.2±4.2
Ccr	108±17 *	56±17	101±25 *	60±23	84±31 *	49±24
PAs	133±19	145±29	135±20	146±29	138±25	150±25
PAd	81±11	84±13	81±16	86±13	82±13	90±13

*p<0.01; Crea=serum creatinine mg/dL; Ccr= creatinine clearance mL/min;Pro.u=proteinuria g/day; PAs=systolic blood pressure mmHg; PAd=diastolic blood pressure mmHg

CONCLUSIONS

Patients of Gr2, with more severe renal functional impairment at the last follow-up, showed a more severe tubulointerstitial damage (1,2).

Age of Gr2 patients was significantly greater than Gr1, this may be responsible of the tubulointerstitial findings. Nevertheless, the different degree of renal functional impairment in the two groups, suggests that tubulointerstitial damage at the onset of MGN may be a reliable index for predicting renal outcome of MGN.

REFERENCES
1. Braden G, Rastegar A, Hession J, Garb J, Siegel N, Fitzgibbons J, Kashgarian M, Kidney Int, 1988,33: 183
2. Macrae J, Beyer MM, Nicastri AD, Chen CK, Friedman EA, Kidney Int, 1988,33: 200
3. Honkanen E, Clinical Nephrolgy, 1986,25: 122
4. Darenady EM, Offer J, Woodhouse MS, J Pathology, 1975,109: 195

SERUM IgA IN CHILDREN WITH ACUTE POST-INFECTIOUS GLOMERULONEPHRITIS

S. MARINGHINI, L. BELVEDERE, F. LUNETTA, I. CUTAJA, P. CARMINA, D. NATOLI.

Servizio Nefrologia e Dialisi, Laboratorio Analisi, Ospedale dei Bambini "G. Di Cristina", Piazza Montalto, 90134 Palermo, Italy

INTRODUCTION

Elevated serum IgA levels have been reported in a variable percentage of patients affected by IgA nephropathy (1) but also in other glomerulopathies (2). Reports on IgA levels in patients affected by acute post-infectious glomerulonephritis (AGN) are scanty (3). We therefore undertook a retrospective study on serum levels of IgA in children with AGN admitted to our Service.

MATERIALS AND METHODS

During the last seven years 186 children have been admitted for AGN. In order to exclude other glomerular diseases the analysis of data was restricted to those patients who had a low serum C3 on admission which rose to the normal range within 8 weeks. Serum levels of immunoglobulins (Ig) were determined on admission and at any subsequent visit in most patients and in a control group of 114 children who had no apparent renal, gastrointestinal or respiratory disease. Behring nephelometer and antisera were used for the measurements. Serum IgA were considered elevated when above two standard deviations from the mean of the control group of the same age. Statistical analysis included the Student's and the chi-square tests.

RESULTS

Table 1. Serum Ig levels in children of the contol group.

Age (yrs)	1-3	3-5	5-7	7-9	9-11	11
No	29	28	20	21	10	6
IgA (m±SD)	65±27	94±39	116±36	140±41	140±44	117±26
IgM ▪	160±59	155±69	159±62	175±70	150±40	152±66
IgG ▪	976±229	1100±296	1303±221	1406±210	1374±204	1160±112

Serum Ig were available on admission in 131 patients (88 males and 43 females) affected by AGN; age ranged from 1 to 13 years (mean ± SD = 6.0 ± 2.3). IgA were elevated in 44 (34%), IgG in 49 (37%) and IgM in 9 (7%) patients. Thirteen patients had high IgA and normal IgG and IgM. Only 2 patients had significantly low levels of IgA. Age, sex, serum creatinine were not significantly different in patients with high serum IgA levels. No significant correlation has been observed between serum levels of IgA or IgG and antistreptolysin-O titles. Serum Ig levels during the follow-up (23 ± 15 months) in 68 patients showed a decrease with time (Fig. 1). Sixty-eight patients have been followed for a minimum of one year and had at least 3 measurements of Ig; 13 (9%) had serum IgA consistently elevated. Clinical and laboratory data were not different in these patients when compared with the others. Hematuria was still present after one year of follow-up in 17 of 68 patients; only 4 had high serum IgA on admission and in none of these persisted elevated.

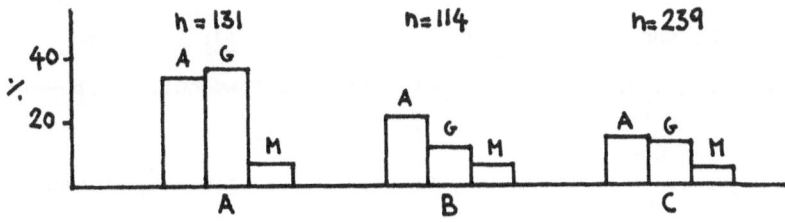

Fig. 1. Percentage of Ig values above 2 SD from the mean of controls (Table 1) in children with AGN on admission (A), after 3 months (B) and after 3 to 65 months (C).

DISCUSSION

IgA is the predominant immunoglobulin in the external secretions of humans, but the physiological role of IgA in blood is poorly understood (4). Serum IgA are elevated in patients affected by IgA nephropathy and other glomerular diseases (2). Some authors have noticed a strict correlation between serum IgA levels and IgA deposition in the glomeruli (2). Post-streptococcal acute glomerulonephritis is still a common disease in Sicily (5). IgA nephropathy in the context of a previous acute glomerulonephritis has been recently described (6). Elevated serum concentrations of IgG and IgM but not IgA have been reported in AGN (3); children were included in this study but normal values of serum IgA were questionable. Our data show that serum IgA levels may be elevated in AGN in children at the onset of the disease but also after recovery. Children with high levels of IgA are not different from the others as far as clinical and laboratory data or prognosis are concerned.

REFERENCES

1. D'Amico, G. Q. J. Med. 64:709-727, 1987

2. Withworth, J.A., Leibowitz, S., Kennedy, M.C., Cameron, J.S. and Chantler, C. Clin. Nephrol. 5: 33-36, 1976

3. Rodriguez-Iturbe, B., Carr, R.I., Garcia, R., Rabidau, D., Rubio, L. and McIntosh, R.M. Clin. Nephrol. 13: 1-4, 1980

4. Underdown, B.J. and Schiff, J.M. Ann. Rev. Immunol. 4: 389-417, 1986

5. Maringhini, S., Cutaja, I., Natoli, D., Cutaia, A., Lo Cascio, A., Savio, C., Bosco, A. Eur. J. Ped. 140: 209, 1983

6. Yoshizawa, N., McClung, J.A., Ohshima, S., Takahashi, K., Treser, G. Nephron 44: 167-173, 1986

EPIDEMIOLOGY OF IDIOPATHIC GLOMERULAR DISEASE IN A FRENCH AREA : A PROSPECTIVE STUDY

P.SIMON, MP.RAMEE, KS.ANG, G.CAM

Department of néphrology, La Beauchée Hopital 22000 SAINT-BRIEUC, FRANCE

INTRODUCTION

For the diagnosis of idiopathic glomerular disease (IGD),renal biopsy is required. Indications for renal biopsy may varie from country to country (1) and these geographic variations in the incidence and prevalence of IGD may, at least in part, reflect differences in the indications for renal biopsy. On the other hand, these observed differences may be also influenced by screening procedures for detecting asymptomatic patients. This data would be particularly true to explain incidence rates of IgA nephropathy found much lower in United States and United Kingdom than in France or Japan where young people and workers undergo routine screenings for renal disease (1) (2). In this prospective study, the incidence of IGD in a adult population over 15 years of age was determined by means of renal biopsies taken for a period of twelve years (1976-1987). Because a close cooperation with public health institutions for detecting renal diseases we were able to approach the real incidence of IGD in a French area.

PATIENTS AND METHODS

Patients The study was conducted between January 1976 and December 1987. Renal biopsy was indicated in 786 patients over 15 years of age who were born and lived in the studied area. Indications for renal biopsy were: 1) recent onset uremia, 2) recent onset nephroctic syndrome, 3) hematuria and significant proteinuria (24 H proteinuria $> 0,2$ g but < 3 g), 4) chronic microscopic hematuria (> 50000 cells/ml) or recurrent macroscopic hematuria in the presence of a normal urologic workup, 5) chronic idiopathic proteinuria with or without hypertension. Contra-indications for renal biopsy included the absence of one kidney, coagulation disorders, urinary tract infections and urogical abnormalities. Excluded from the study were glomerulonephritis secondary to systemic diseases (inclusive diabete mellitus, cirrhosis of the liver, Schönlein-Henoch purpura) and familial hematuria.

Analysis of renal biopsy All renal biopsies were processed and stained for light microscopy and immunohistochemistry using polyclonal antisera against human IgG, IgM, IgA, C3, C1q. Electron microscopy study of biopsy specimens was done only in patients with familial hematuria and those deriving from known Alport families (excluded from the study). All specimens were analysed by the same pathologist (MPR). Biopsies had to contain more than 5 glomeruli. The number of biopsies classified as technical failure was less than 1,5 % (n=12)

Method for the estimation of incidence of PGD In this area, the two census of population taken in 1977 and 1982 showed population growth of minor importance (less than 1 %). This area had the criteria to qualify as a "statistical area" (3) : 1) a large population nucleus with one city with 80 000 residents, 2) a total population of about 400 000 inhabitants, 3) adjacent communities that were well-integrated socially and economically with the major population nucleus. Finally, this area had a homogeneous and stable population in terms of migratory behaviour. Biopsies were taken in the single hospital nephrology unit that served the population of this area. Comparisons of incidence were made between for 4 years periods : period A 1976-79 ; period B, 1980-83 ; period C, 1984-87 for which the number of renal biopsies was 246, 294 and 241 respectively.

RESULTS

IGD was diagnosed in 401 patients (51,3%) corresponding to a prevalence for 12 years of 1/1000 about. As shown in Fig. 1, the incidence of IGD decreased during the period C (7,2 per 10^5) compared to periods A and B (8,6 and 9,2 per 10^5). IgA nephropathy (IgAN) was the commonest of IGD (34,2%) and its incidence remained stable for the period under review : 2,6 (A), 3,2 (B) and 2,8 (C) per 10^5. For membranous nephropathy (MN), crescentic idiopathic glomerulonephritis (IGN), mesangial proliferative glomerulonephritis (mes PGN) and focal glomerulosclerosis (FGS), annual incidence did not change significantly. In contrast, a significant decrease of incidence was observed for lipoid nephrosis (MC) : 1 (A), 1 (B) and 0,35 (C) per 10^5, membranoproliferative GN (MPGN) : 1,2 (A), 0,25 (B) and 0,3 (C) per 10^5 and post-streptococcal acute GN (AGN) : 0,6 (A), 0,12 (B) and 0 (C) per 10^5. Among 278 patients who were starting dialysis for the period under review, 82 (29,5%) had IGD and 80,2% of those had undergone renal biopsy. IgAN was the first cause of end stage renal failure (ESRF) (15%, incidence 0,85 per 10^5) before diabete (12%, 0,79 per 10^5). This study confirms the decrease of the incidence of MPGN, AGN and MN, and demonstrates that IgAN is not only the commonest of IGD but also among the most frequent causes of ESRF.

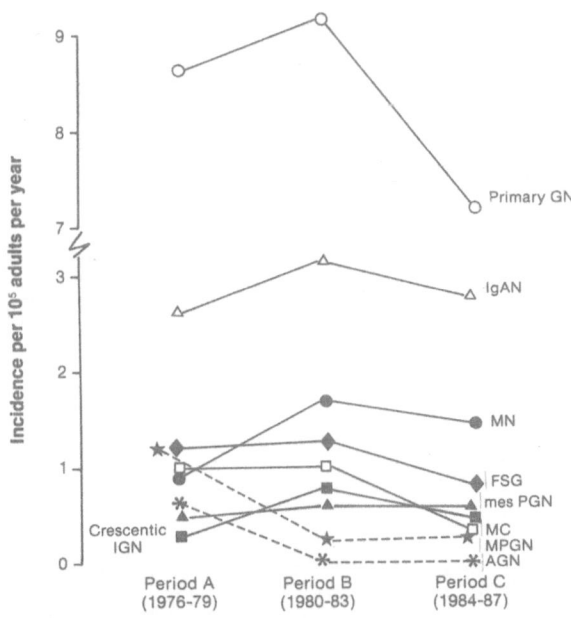

Fig. 1 Incidence of idiopathic glomerular disease and histological forms diagnosed by renal biopsy.

REFERENCES

1. D'Amico, G. The commonest glomerulonephritis in the world : IgA nephropathy. Q. J. Med. 64 : 709-727, 1987.
2. Tiebosch, AT., Wolters, J., Frederik, PF., Vander Wiel, TW., Zeppenfeldt, E., Van Breda Vriesman, PJ. Epidemiology od idiopathic glomerular disease : a prospective study. Kidney Int. 32 : 112-116, 1987.

II. THERAPY IN RENAL FAILURE

Plasma Exchange in Acute Renal Failure

Clinical course of rapidly progressive glomerulonephritis during immunosuppressive therapy, plasmaexchange and without specific therapy

Metz-Kurschel, U., Daul, A., Graben, N.
Department of Renal and Hypertensive diseases, University of Essen,
Hufelandstr. 55, D 4300 Essen, FRG.

Introduction

Rapidly progressive glomerulonephritis is an entity of glomerulonephritis with a fulminant progressively downhill course accompanied by oliguria or anuria.
In 1925 Theodor Fahr used the term subacute glomerulonephritis to emphazise the protracted course and to contrast it with the ordinarily self-limited course of acute glomerulonephritis.
In strict sence the "term rapidly progressive" describes the clinical course of the glomerulonephritis. Conversely today the term is used to describe the biopsy picture of this glomerulonephritis.
Histologically the most striking feature is the accumulation of cells within the Bowman´s space, so called crescents. Since patients with the clinical picture of rapid progressively glomerulonephritis (RPGN) may be found on biopsy to have endocappillary proliferative or necrotizing glomerulonephritis with crescentic lesions, it would seem preferable to avoid the use of a clinical term to describe pathological appearances (1).
It is generally accepted that the prognosis of RPGN is poor and that in absence of hemodialysis patients will die within several weeks or months.
Furthermore there are some prognostic criterions basing upon several findings in renal biopsies and upon the clinical course underlying the poor prognosis.
A poor prognosis is indicated when 70 % or more of the glomeruli are affected or when the biopsy picture shows severe tubular atrophy and interstitial fibrosis or extensive glomerular fibrosis (1).
To prevent progression of RPGN several therapies were initiated during the last 20 years. Besides glucosteroids even in high doses of 1000 mg/day, trials with cytotoxic agents such as cyclophosphamide and / or azathioprine in some patients combined with plasmaexchange were investigated (2,3,4).
Fibrinrelated antigenes in the glomerular lesions lead to the use of anticoagulants. All studies using heparin or warfarin in conventional doses showed no benefit refering to renal function (4,6,7).
In our study we investigated whether there is a positive effect in regard to renal function in patients treated with glucosteroids combined with cytotoxic agents with or without plasmaexchange in contrast to patients without specific therapy.

Patients and methods

Retrospectively we investigated the data of 31 patients.

Since 1971 we observed 31 patients , 18 males and 13 females with histologically proven rapidly progressive glomerulonephritis. The age ranged between 24 and 69 years.

In 17 patients there was no hint of an underlying disease. In these patients RPGN is called primary or idiopathic RPGN or idiopathic diffuse crescentic glomerulonephritis. In 5 patients RPGN occured in association with various infectious diseases. In 7 patients RPGN occured in association with Wegener's granulomatosis, in 2 patients with systemic lupus erythematodes.

We divided our patients into 3 groups. Patients of group **IS** received combined immunsuppressive therapy, consisting of prednisone, azathioprine and /or cyclophosphamide. Patients of group **PS** received plasmaexchange , additionally. Patients of group **WT** received no specific therapy.

At the onset of therapy 16 patients presented with end stage renal failure, 5 of group IS, 5 of group PS and 6 of group WTthe others with impaired renal function.

The histological picture showed in all 31 patients in more than 70 % crescents. Additionally in 4 patients the glomerular tuft showed areas of fibrinoid necrosis. In the majoritiy of patients RPGN was accompanied by acute renal failure.

As I said patients of group IS and PS were treated with cytotoxic agents. 11 patients were treated with a threefold combined chemotherapy consisting of prednisone, cyclophosphamide and azathioprine. 5 patients received prednisone in a dose of 1,5 mg/kg b.w. and cyclophosphamide, and 5 other patients received a combination of these 2 agents, but prednisone in a dose of 1000 mg.

Therapy was given at least 8 weeks, in responders up to 1 year.

8 patients of group PS were treated with plasmaexchange (5 l, 3 times the week), additionally.

10 patients of group WT received never immunsuppressive therapy nor plasmapheresis.

One year after initiation of therapy 5 patients of group IS were still on hemodialysis, 5 had impaired renal function and 3 had died following infectious diseases during chemotherapy. After 5 years renal function had worsened in 2 patients. By that time 7 patients were on hemodialysis, 3 had impaired renal function and 3 were dead (Fig. 1).

In group PS during the first year 3 patients had temporarily improvement of renal function, 2 patients died following infectious diseases and 2 patients remained still on hemodialysis. After 5 years 3 patients are on hemodialysis, only 1 of 8 patients had impaired renal function and 2 patients had died additionally due to progression of underlying diseases (Fig. 1).

Only in group WT 4 patients had normal renal function after 5 years, 3 are on hemodialysis and 3 had died. The reason of death was independent of RPGN (Fig. 1).

In all 4 patients, having normal renal function after 5 years, RPGN occured after various bacterial infectious. All these patients did not received cytotoxic chemotherapy or plasmaexchange at any time. The only therapeutic agents given to them were antimicrobial agents. If neccessary they reveived antihypertensive drugs and hemodialysis.

| | RPGN n = 31 | | | | | | | | | |
| | IS 13 | | | PS 8 | | | WT 10 | | | |
	IRF	HD	+	IRF	HD	+	NRF	IRF	HD	+
before therapy	8	5	—	3	5	—	—	4	6	—
after initiat. therapy 0-1 year	5	5	3	4	2	2	4	2	4	—
1-4 years	5	5	3	2	4	2	4	2	2	2
5 years	3	7	3	1	3	4	4	0	3	3

IS = immunsuppressive therapy, PS = Plasmaexchange, WT = without specific therapy
IRF = impaired renal function, NRF=normal renal function, HD = Hemodialysis

Fig. 1: Clinical course of RPGN in 31 patients during immunosuppressive therapy (IS), plasmaseperation (PS) and without specific therapy (WT).

Discussion

In general the outlook for recovery in patients with RPGN is poor. Our data show that the prognosis of RPGN depended on the assumed pathogenetic pathway. RPGN in connection with infectious diseases needs no other specific therapy than antibiotics and had a very good prognosis concerning renal function if the infection is eliminated. Glucosteroids and / or cytotoxic agents or plasmaexchange may be hazardous in these patients because of septic complications. For this reason it is necesarry to exclude an underlying infectious disease before starting immunsuppressive chemotherapy.

Besides the patients with RPGN and infectious diseases there were no other patients with normal renal function after 5 years. All other patients had only temporarily improvement of renal function or they remained on hemodialysis or they died.

In patients with primary RPGN without infections there was no additional positive effect in the group treated with membrane plasmaexchange compared with patients treated only immunsuppressive. Only patients with Wegener's granulomatosis or lupus erythematodes and secondary RPGN benefit from plasmapheresis with regard to their renal function and the symptoms of the underlying diseases. These data are in accordance to the literature. In 1988 a german multicenter study showed that patients treated with immunosuppressive therapy and plasmasperation had no better prognosis than patients treated only with immunosuppressive therapy (8). To avoid septic complications it is necessary to exclude underlying infectious diseases before starting therapy. Patients with primary RPGN without infections are to be treated only with immunosuppressive therapy. Only patients with secondary RPGN should be treated with immunosuppressive therapy and plasmaseperation.

Literature

1. Glassock R J, Adler S G, Ward H J, Cohen A H (1986): Primary glomerular diseases. In: Brenner B M, Rector F C (eds): The Kidney, Bd. 1, third edition. W B Saunders Company, 929 - 1013.
2. Nakamoto S, Dunea D, Kolff W J , McCormack L J (1965): Treatment of ologuric glomerulonephritis with dialysis and steroids. Ann. Int. Med., Vol. 63, No 3, 359 - 368.
3. Schulz W, Gessler U (1977): Diagnostik, Therapie und Verlauf der rasch progressiven gloermulären Insuffizienz. Therapiewoche 27, 7441 - 7462.
4. Oredugba O, Debesh C, Mazumdar M B Meyer J S , Lubowitz H (1980): Pulse Methylpredinsolone therapy in idiopathic, rapidly progressive glomerulonephritis. Ann. Int. Med., Vol . 92, No 4, 504 - 506.
5. Suc J.M, Durand D, Conte J, Mignon-Conte M, ORFILA C, Ton That H, Duchet J P (1976): The use of heparin in the treatment of idiopathic rapidly progressive glomerulonephritis. Clin. Nephr., Vol. 6, No 1,9 - 13.
6. Pinggera W F, Djawan S, Singer F, Stummvoll H K, Wolf A (1973): Heparintherapie bei perakuter glomerulonephritis. Wien. Z. inn. Med. 54 ,8/9, 417 - 421.
7. Arieff A I, Pinggera W F (1972): Rapidly progressive glomerulonephritis treated with anticoagulans. Arch Intern Med, Vol 129, 77 - 84.
8. Glöckner W M, Siebert H.-G, Wichmann H E et al (1988): Plasmaexchange and immunsuppression in rapidly progressive glomerulonephritis: a controlled, multi - center study. Clinical Nephrology, 29, No. 1, 1 - 8.

PLASMA EXCHANGE IN TREATMENT OF ACUTE VASCULAR REJECTION

G.SAKELLARIOU, M.DANIILIDIS, E.ALEXOPOULOS, E.KOKOLINA, P.KOUKOUDIS, D.GAKIS, M.PAPADIMITRIOU.

Departement of Nepthrology, Hippokration General Hospiotal, Aristotelian University of Thessaloniki-Greece.

INTRODUCTION

Renal transplant rejection may occur as a result of both cellular and humoral immunologic injury. Recently, plasma exchange has been used as an adjunct to immunosuppressive therapy in order to reverse humoral rejecrtion episodes in the early posttransplant period [1-5].

In this paper we report our experience with the use of plasma exchange therapy in renal transplant recipients with proven histologic evidence of acute vascular rejection and who were unresponsive to conventional immunosuppressive treatment.

PATIENTS AND METHODS

From 1980 to December 1987 a total of 153 kidney transplants were performed in 150 patients (114 LRD, 39CD) with chronic renal failure.

Twelve of 17 pts underwent percutaneous needle biopsy of the allograft to obtain histological confirmation of the diagnosis of rejection before P.E. was performed. The characteristic histologic findings consisted of arterular intimal damage characterized by endothelial cell proliferation with or without fibrinoid necrosis of the glomerular cap. A total of 17 pts (9 males) who were unresponsive to conventional treatment were subjected to plasmapheresis. The mean age of the pts was 31 yrs (range 18-47 yrs) All were first graft recipients (15 from a LRD, 2 from a CD). In 11 pts the initial standard immunosuppressive regiment consisted of azathioprine 1mg/kg/day, MP 0.15 mg/kg/day and CyA 4-5mg/kg/day. In 6 cases immunosuppressive therapy consisted of azathioprine 1.5-2.5 mg/kg/day and MP 0.30-0.40 mg/kg/day.

PE treatment was performed with a flat plate membrane plasma separator (TPE System Cobe). During each treatment a total of 3 to 4L of plasma were removed and simultaneously replaced with 4% albumin and Ringer's Lactate solution.

Before, during and after each PE treatment we studied the following immunologic parameters:serum immunoglobulin levels, C_3, C_4 and factor B, were measured by radioimmunodiffusion. Cytotoxic antibodies (anti HLA-A or B) were detected by utilizing microlymphocytotoxicity test. T-cell subsets were studied by monoclonal antibodies using OKT3, OKT4, OKT8 monoclonal antibodies (Ortho Pharmaceutical Corp Raritan NJ).

Biochemical, hematological and radionuclide evaluations of renal transplant function (99^m Tc DTPA) were performed in all cases.

RESULTS

Nine of 17 pts (53%) showed an excellent response with complete reversal of the rejection episode. Four of 17 pts (23,5%) demonstrated a partial response and 4 pts (23,5%) showed no response. The changes in immunoglobulin levels were significant but varied from patient to patient. We observed a 10-48% decrease in IgG, up to 60% in IgA and up to 28% in IgM, serum levels. However, immunoglobulin levels returned to pretreatment levels within ten to 16 days after discontinuation of P.E. A significant decrease in the level of cytotoxic antibodies (CA) was observed. Before initation of P.E. the mean levels were $31.1 \pm 36.6\%$ and decreased to $4.8 \pm 10.5\%$ ($p < 0.001$). Following therapy similar changes were observed in the serum complement (C_3, C_4, Bf). The OKT4/OKT8 ratio was normal in 10 patients and low in 7 patients.

DISCUSSION

The validity of plasmapheresis in renal transplant rejection remains one of the most controversial issues in the whole field of therapeutic application of this procedure. The results reported in the literature are extremely conflicting with improvement reported to occur from 30% to more than 90% of cases[2,6].
Renal transplant rejection may result from both cellular and humoral mechanisms of injury. When humoral mechanisms predominate the rejection is usually characterized by vascular lesions in the graft with poor response to conventional treatment. The humoral factors involved in acute vascular rejection includes:1. Antibodies (anti T-cells, anti B-cells, anti vascular endothelial cells, anti GBM, anti TBM etc) 2) Immune complexes (CIC), 3) Cytokines (interleukin 1,2, macrophage stimulating factors, interferon, B-cell growth factor etc) 4) Acute phase proteins (C reactive protein, fibrinogen) 5) other factors (Complement, congulation factors, kinins) [5]. It has been

postulated that some of the aforementioned humoral factors are removed by PE and that this leads to improvement in graft function[4,7]. On the other hand AVR is not satisfactorily controlled by high doses of steroids, ALG, ATG, and monoclonal antibodies. For this reason, PE may be used to reverse AVR in a proportion of such cases without producing adverse side effects. In the present study initial improvement of transplant function was observed in 9 of 17 patients. Four patients showed only a partial response in as much as recurring rejection episodes were observed ten to 60 days after discontinuation of PE treatment. In the remaing patients no response was observed. Other investigators have reported variable results[6,8]. In two controlled studies plasmapheresis failed to reverse AVR[3,6,8]. On the other hand , results similar to ours were reported by Frasca et al[3] Vangelista A et al [5] and Fassbinder W [2]. It has been demonstrated that when an anti-HLA antibody of restricted specificity directed against the graft is present at the time of AVR, its removal by PE is associated with an improvement, in graft function[5]. In all of our patients a significant decrease in titer of the cytotoxic antibodies was observed following PE and this was more prominent in six patients who improved after PE. The ratio of OKT4/OKT8 was normal or low. Nevertheless the analysis of lymphocyte subpopulations revealed reduced levels of OKT3, OKT4, and OKT11, while the levels of OKT8 were significantly higher as compared to other types of rejection. In conclusion, PE treatment should be considered as the treatment of choice in patients with proven AVR, especially since these patients show a poor response to other treatment modalities. Plasmapheresis should be considered especially in recipients of a first transplant and in particular in those with serum creatinine concentrations balow 5,0 mg/dl.

REFERENCES
1. Rifle, F. Chalopin, J.M. Turc, J.M. et al: Transplant Proc. 11:20-22, 1979
2. Fassbinder, W. Erust, W. Stutte, H.J. et al: Int J Artif Organs 6:61-63, 1983
3. Frasca, G. Vangelista, A. Sermasi, G. et al: Int J Artif Organs 6:57-60, 1983
4. Fassbinder, W. : Life Sup Systeme 3:336-339, 1986.
5. Vangelista, A. Frasca, G.M. Bonomini: Clin Nephrol 26(1):564-567, 1986
6. Kirublakaran, M.G. Disney, APS. Norman, J. et al: Transplantation 32:164-166, 1981.
7. Vangelista, A. Frasca. G.M. Nanni-Costa, A. et al: Trans ASAIO 28:599-602, 1982.
8. Cardella, C.J. Suffen, D M. Falk, J.A. et al: Transplant Proc 10:617-619, 1978
9. Sakellariou, G. Paschalidou, E. Tsobanelis, et al: Transplant Proc 6:2779-2781, 1985

EVALUATION OF PLASMA EXCHANGE EFFECT IN PATIENTS WITH LUNG HEMORRHAGE AND RAPIDLY PROGRESSIVE GLOMERULONEPHRITIS EITHER IDIOPATHIC OR VASCULITIS ASSOCIATED.

Mauri J.M., González M.T., Poveda R., Romero M., Gabas J., Sarrias X., Carreras J., Andres E., Díaz C., Ferrer P.

Hospital de Girona (Girona).
Hospital de Bellvitge (Hospitalet de Ll. Barcelona).

INTRODUCTION

We comment here our experience on 19 patients presenting 23 episodes of pulmonary hemorrhage (PH) and 21 nephritic crises. Patients started conventional immunosuppression or immunosuppression plus plasma exchanges (PEX) by applying random criteria.

PATIENTS AND METHODS

Ninenteen patients, 10 males and 9 females, aged 21-73 y.o., are reported. In all of them the following criteria were found: 1) Lack of evidence of congestive heart failure, valvulopathy, pulmonary infection or embolism, tuberculosis, bronchiectasia or pulmonary neoplasm, 2) Absence of collagen disease, 3) Negative anti-GBM detection in both serum and glomeruli, 4) Lack of coagulation disorders, 5) Hemoptysis with pulmonary opacities on X-ray chest films, 6) Acute nephritic syndrome and rapid loss of renal function in patients in whom a crescentic nephritis -epithelial proliferation in 60% or more of the observed glomeruli- was documented.

In these 19 patients 23 episodes of PH were noticed and treated by means of either Prednisone (P) and Cyclophosphamide (CY) or P, CY plus PEX by applying random selection criteria.

Pharmacological treatment was the same for both groups. Therapy in the first month included P (1 mg/k.b.w.) and CY (2 mg/k.b.w.).

Data were analyzed in an HP 3000 computer by means of the

SPSS package program.

RESULTS

On admittance all patients were found seriously ill and restless. Out of 23 episodes of PH, hemoptysis weakness, shortness
of breath -in 17 cases associated to severe hypoxemia- fever
and malaise were the complaints more currently found.

X-ray pulmonary involvement ocurred in all 23 episodes. In
almost all of cases an alveolo-interstitial diffuse bilateral
pattern was observed.

Improvement and subsequent resolution period of pulmonary involvement as evaluated by X-ray chest films were significantly
reduced in the PEX treated cases.

In 8 cases conventional immunosuppression was applied. Only
one out of 4 with hemodialysis (HD) requirements improved, and
two out of four cases with starting serum creatinine levels lower than 800 micro.mol/l. worsened, without significative changes in the other two patients. Improvement of pretreatment serum creatinine values were seen in 12 out of 13 PEX treated cases. Three out of 4 cases with HD requirements and all 9 pa -
tients without HD needs improved.

A bifactorial analysis for all patients showed significative
the improvement in the serum creatinine values observed in the
PEX treated patients ($p = 0.009$). A multivariate desing showed
that serum creatinine values improved significantly in both
PEX treated cases, those with and those without HD requirements,
($0.0001 > p < 0.05$).

DISCUSSION

Pulmonary hemorrhage and RPGN anti-GBM unrelated constitues
a rather unfrequent clinical association.

Previous reports have suggested that on such a patients better therapeutic results might be obtained by associating an intensive PEX regime to the conventional steroid and CY treatment.
Though the short number of cases studied, our results would
strongly confirm previous experiences when considering the sig-

nificative shortening of the ventilatory impairment and X-ray pulmonary abnormalities observed in the PEX treated patients.

The significative serum creatinine improvement observed in PEX treated patients with HD requirements would be in a good agreement with previous studies. In this report, however, a benefitial effect of PEX when applied to patients without HD requirements could be appreciated too. Whereby it seems important to remark the significative renal function improvement observed in PEX treated patients when compared with the analog untreated group.

From our results we may conclude suggesting that: a) Plasma exchanges may be useful for controlling the X-ray pulmonar abnormalities in patients with idyopathic pulmonary hemorrhage and that, b) Plasma exchanges might be an interesting therapeutic tool for improving renal function in patients with RPGN.

CURRENT TREATMENT OF ACUTE RENAL FAILURE(ARF) FROM LEPTOSPIROSIS

PECCHINI F.,ARISI M.°,BERTOLI G.°°,BORGHI M.,CAVALLI P.°°°,CROTTI M.°°°,GRUTTAD'AURIA C.,ROMANINI G.°°°

Division of Nephrology,Health Physics Service°,Pathological Anatomy°° and Blood Bank°°° - Hospital of Cremona, Italy.

INTRODUCTION

Leptospirosis occurs through the world and have multiple clinical presentations: firstly,cases have to be distinguished when jaundice and ARF developed;secondarily European and U.S.A. cases seem partially different from East(Philippine,Thailand) ones. Treatment,traditionally based on penicillin and fluid replacement,get advantage from hemodialysis(HD)and plasma-exchange(PEx) (1). Recently the type of dialysis,PEx itself(2) and use of corticoids and/or continuous positive airway pressure (CPAP)have been discussed(3). During thirteen years,41 patients have been treated in our center: we have studied their clinical course and their outcome in order to obtain some therapeutic advantage.

MATERIALS AND METHODS

41 pts treated(3,2/year),whom illness' gravity based on the presence of at least two of the following conditions:a)Arterial hypotension: < 90 mm/Hg

b)Total bilirubin: >15 mg/dl

c)Blood urea nitrogen: >100 mg/dl

d)Platelets(plts): < 70.000 and/or hemorrhage.

While during the 70th yrs,peritoneal dialysis was used (15 cases),since 1980 PEx(fresh plasma replaced) was introduced at the same time with extracorporeal intensive dialysis(also twice a day)(26 cases). Both series had also penicillin(6 g/day)and plts infusions(3 to 6 bags, each containing 0,7 x $10^9/1$ plts)in the first hours. Besides the other clinical signs as conjunctival suffusion and lymphadenopathy(rare) our pts presented Herpes Labialis frequently(38%). Farmworkers and fishermen are strongly prevailing in the series. Other laboratory and anamnestic data are summarized in Table I.

TABLE I

	1975-80 (15)	1980-87 (26)	t Student test (p)
Highest BUN (mg/dl)	180,2±53,4	118,0±29,6	< 0,001
Platelets (x 10⁹/1)	94,1±101	40,2±27,2	< 0,01
Highest T.Bil (mg/dl)	15,9±7,0	23,2±7,7	< 0,005
Pre-PEx (days)	6,8±1,0	6,2±1,7	N.S.
Age (years)	52,5±11,7	49,8±14,9	N.S.
I.Hemorrh. (I.H.)	66%	n.v.	

Patients of the 80th yrs had also valued fibrin degradation products(FDP)as 62,4±82,4 mg/dl(n.v.< 8),fibrinogen
as 835,2±322,9 mg/dl(n.v.350-550)and CPK as 1362,2±1629,2
(n.v.< 170 mU)during the first day. Direct(before and after)effect of PEx(42,5±25,9/61,6±35,2)and PEx+HD(26,0±6,9
/42,2±21,2)on plts was not significative.

RESULTS

During 70th yrs,deaths were 8 from 15(53%): necropsy
revealed 3 shock lung,1 pneumonitic and 4 hemorrhagic
causes. Six of the 8 dead had received corticoid. From
1980,3 only pts dead(11%),2 of them,suffering of hepatic
cirrhosis,for shock lung and 1 for bilateral pneumonia
from Aspergillus Fumigatus(the man had falled with his
tractor in a filthy channel with water entrance in upper
respiratory tract;he was already well when pneumonitis
developed)(4). In table II the exit in many a series.

TABLE II

British Isles	Cases	Deaths	%
Brit.Med.J.287:1365-1983	9	4	44
U.S.A.(5)	-	-	15-40
Padova(3)	18	5	28
Cremona	26	3	11
Treviso(2)	70	6	9

DISCUSSION

Weil's syndrome,defined as severe leptospirosis with
jaundice and azotemia usually accompanied by anemia,
hemorrhages and disturbances in consciousness is mostly
due to the I.H. type. Our cases had prevalence of I.H.

and we think it so on,also if in the last years confirmation was difficult for testing serum lack and PEx interference. Conditions for entry in treatment schedule distinguish our cases from East ones without even plts
count(6)where mortality is almost negligible(7)or from
ones(2)with more plts(72.600),lesser CPK(1009)and no data
about azotemia. Efficacy of intensive HD appear from the
different exit in our series,with perit.dialysis used(not
rarely together with corticoids)only before 1980.With the
exception of BUN(higher in previous series),pts forward
from 1980 seem more serious: but they had a better cour_
se. Some focused the additional uremic risk of bleeding
and hypercatabolism of the illness. However no direct effect was found on plts,PEx is recommended in hyperbiliru-
binemic ARF(7)and to obtain rapid reduction of vasoactive
substances and fibrinogen(9).Similarity to thrombotic
thrombocytopenic purpura might request plasma(and not albumin)as replacement and might explain worse outcome(3).
Acute respiratory distress syndrome(ARDS)seems today almost the only cause of death: quick restoration of body
fluids and sympathomimetic drugs(dopamine)to oppose hypotension claimed.Early CPAP failed to prevent ARDS(10).
Our experience in two cases was complicated by cirrhosis:
we don't used CPAP. Today conflict persists between sup-
porters(6)and opposites(5)to penicillin: we think it useful for collateral symptoms.

REFERENCES
1)Pecchini F.Borghi M.,Bodini U.,Copercini B.,Gruttad'Auria C.,Romanini G.,Romano C. Clin.Nephr. 18:164,1982
2)Teodori T.,Gatti P.L.,Da Porto A.,Bocci C.,Amici G.
   G.Clin.Med. 67:159-164,1986
3)Bonadonna A. et al. Giorn.It.Nefr. 3:117-122,1986
4)Pecchini F.,Bertoli G. Min.Electr.Metab. pg.269,1986
5)Sanford J.P. New Engl.J.Med. 310:524-525,1984
6)Watt G.,Padre L.P.,Tuazon M.L.,Calubaquib C.,Santiago E
   Ranoa CP,Laughlin L.W. The Lancet pg.433,Feb.27,1988
7)Sitprija V. Acute Renal Failure,M.Nijhoff,pg.319,1984
8)Kennedy N.D.,Pusey C.D.,Rainford D.J.,Higginson A.
   Postgr.Med.J. 55:176-179,1979
9)Borghi M.,Bertoli G.,Bodini U.,Copercini B.,Forzani F.
   Gruttad'Auria C.,Pecchini F.,Romanini G.,Scaravonati P.
   Therapeutic Apheresis:a critical look.Nosè,Malchesky
   and Smith,Cleveland,1984,pg.57-60.
10)Pepe P.E.,Hudson L.D.,Carrico C.M.,New Engl.J.Med.
   311: 281-286,1984

PLASMAEXCHANGE INDUCED IMPROVEMENT ON EXTRA-RENAL MANIFESTATIONS OF SYSTEMIC LUPUS ERYTHEMATOSUS

L. FURCI, A. BARALDI, M. LEONELLI, E. LUSVARGHI

Cattedra e Divisione di Nefrologia e Servizio di Emodialisi Università di Modena, Italy

INTRODUCTION

Recent observations suggest that plasmaexchange (PE) may be determinant in controlling extra renal manifestations of Systemic Lupus Erythematosus (SLE) (1, 5).
Cerebral lupus, vasculitis, thrombocytopenia and skin lesions may, in some instances, be resistent to conventional therapy with steroid and cytostatics. Also lupic interstitial pneumopathy in our experience may be controlled with PE after failure of methyl-prednisolone pulses and cyclophosphamide treatment.

CASE REPORT

In September 1986 a young man aged 21, affected by SLE, on treatment with low doses of prednisone (0.2 mg/Kg) was admitted to our Hospital with evident signs of lupus activity: fever, mild hypertension, arthropathy and dyspnoea. Serological examination confirmed: ANA 1:1280, double strain DNA antibodies 100 (normal range < 20) C3 = 36 mg/dl, C4 = 3 mg/dl, IgG 2150 mg/dl, IgA 225 mg/dl, IgM 157 mg/dl. Renal function was within normal range.
A chest Roentgengraphy showed bilateral basal opacity, mild pleural effusions, bilateral elevation of diaphragms and biventricular enlargement. No pericardial effusion was found at ecocardiography. Blood and sputum were repeatedly cultured and were free of pathogens. Gas-analysis, functional respiratory tests, single breath DLCO confirmed the presence of severe restrictive respiratory failure expressive of interstitial pneumopathy of lupus. Since active urinary sediment and

nephrotic proteinuria appeared, the patient was referred to our nephrological division.

Renal biopsy showed a mesangial diffuse proliferative GN (class IIB WHO). Methylprednisolone pulses and i.v. cyclophosphamide were given and subsequently pleural effusions disappeared, while proteinuria, urinary activity and serological indexes of SLE persisted. In spite of immunosuppressive full therapy, after a few months the patient was repeatedly hospitalized because of intermittent fever, dyspnoea and nephrotic proteinuria.

In June 1987 renal deterioration (serum creatinine 1.7 mg/dl), poorly controlled hypertension and impending respiratory failure induced us to repeat methylprednisolone pulses. Renal deterioration reversed but fever, dyspnoea and serological indexes of SLE activity persisted and after a few days generalized seizures, expressive of acute lupus encephalopathy, ensued. Intensive PE treatment (2.5 l three times a week for two weeks) with replacement with albumin, and gammaglobulin was started while continuing prednisone and cyclophosphamide; soon afterwards PE was tapered (one treatment weekly and then one treatment/month and withdrawn after 4 months. Serological indexes of SLE activity were negative and fever, arthropathy and dyspnoea disappeared within two weeks from the start of PE.

Today, after one year's follow-up, the patient is still free of clinical manifestations, non nephrotic proteinuria is present while the serological indexes of SLE activity remain low (ANA 1:80; anti-DNA antibodies:absents). Respiratory functional tests have improved but reduced vital capacity, total lung capacity and DLCO are still present as in chronic restrictive defect; diaphragmatic elevation is almost completely reduced.

DISCUSSION

Plasmatic levels of Circulating immuno-complexes (CIC), antibodies to DNA and nucleoprotein antigens are known to correlate with clinical manifestations of lupus activity

(6, 7). Removal of CIC and antibodies reduces. the burden on the mononuclear phagocyte system and provides a rational basis for PE treatment.

Chronic PE treatment alone or associated with immuno-suppressive therapy has been proposed in lupus nephropathy with good general conditions but its usefulness is still debated (1, 8).

Intensive PE is presented as resolutive in many anecdotal reports on critically ill SLE patients. In our case intensive immunosuppressive therapy failed to control either fever or lupus interstitial pneumopathy, and did not prevent encephalopathy ensuing, while intensive PE rapidly resolved acute lupus activity.

Actual estimate of fatalities during PE has been evaluated in 3/10,000 treatments in USA, 20/10,000 in France and none in U.K. (9). This variety of incidences may be related to different infusional replacement (plasma everywhere in France, plasma in some centres in USA, as against albumin in U.K. as in our Nephrology Unit). This relatively high rate of mortality should not constitute a reason for delaying PE when classical therapy fails to control most severe life-threatening SLE manifestations.

REFERENCES

1. Jones,J.V. Clinc. Rheum. Dis. 8: 243, 1982.
2. Lewis,E.J. Am. J. Kid. Dis. Suppl. 2: 182, 1982.
3. Fruchter,L., Gauthier,B., Marino,F. J. Rheum. 10: 341,1983.
4. Wall,B.A., Weinblatt,M.E., Agudelo,C.A. South. Med. J. 75: 1277, 1982.
5. Johannessen,A., Gutteberg,T., Husby,G. Acta Paed. Scand. 71: 347, 1982.
6. Clough,J.D., Calabrese,L.H. Plasma Ther. Transf. Tecn. 2: 73, 1981.
7. Notman,D.D., Kurata,N., Tan.,E.M. Ann. Int. Med. 83: 464,1975.
8. Wei,N., Klippel,J.H., Huston,D.P., Hall,R.P., Lawley,T.J., Balow,J.E., Steinberg,A.D., Decker,J.L. Lancet Vol. 1, No.8314/5 17, 1983.
9. Huestis,D.W. In: Therapeutic Hemapheresis (Eds. M. Valbonesi, A.A.Pineda, JC Biggs), Wichtig Ed., Milano 1986. pp. 179-186.

Medical Therapy in Chronic Renal Failure

FEASIBILITY OF AN INTEGRATED DIET-DIALYSIS PROGRAM (IDDP) AS A
TREATMENT OF ESRD.

Andrulli S. Di Filippo S, Pontoriero G, Ponti R, Citterio A, Tentori
F, La Milia V, Locatelli F.

Divisione di Nefrologia - Ospedale di Lecco - Lecco - Italy

INTRODUCTION

The aim of this study is to evaluate the clinical role of IDDP
among the strategies of ESRD substitutive treatment.

PATIENTS AND METHODS

84 patients (pts), 43 male and 4I female, aged 56.9±I7 years,
started the ESRD substitutive treatment between November I5th, I985
and April I5th, I988 (28 months) in our Department. 55 out of Them
(65%) entered the preliminary phase (PP) of IDDP. The IDDP consisted
of hypoproteic diet (0.4 g/kg/day), supplemented with essential aminoacids (E) or with a mixture of essential aminoacids and ketoanalogues (K), and hemodialysis once a week (28 acetate, 27 bicarbonate),
scheduled to maintain predialysis BUN < 90 mg/dl. The caloric intake
was ⩾ 35 Kcal/kg/day; 9.6 g/day of E or 0.I47 g/kg/day of K were administered. E and K composition is reported elsewere (I, 2). The pts
were given folic acid, vitamin BI, B6, BI2 and iron supplement, to
overcome the diet deficiency, as well as sodium bicarbonate, calcium
carbonate, vitamin D, antihypertensive drugs and diuretics as needed.
The length of hemodialysis session was less than 5.5 h; cuprophan
and polymethylmethacrylate dialysers with surface areas ranging from
I to 2 m^2 were used. Mean blood flow was 250 ml/min, dialysate flow
500 ml/min.

RESULTS

9 out of the 55 pts (16%) admitted to the PP of IDDP were excluded during the PP (lack of compliance 4, insufficient urine output 3,
E and K intolerance I, intercurrent surgery I) and 46 (84%) entered
the experimental phase (EP). 22 out of these 46 pts (48%) are still
on IDDP and 24 (52%) dropped out (lack of compliance 11, renal transplantation 2, insufficient daily urine output 2, brain sufferance I,
renal function recovery I, death 7; causes of death: cachexia 3, sepsis 2, pseudomembranous colitis I, myocardial infarction I).

The features of the pts before entering the PP of IDDP are shown
in Table I. No significant differences were found among subgroups
with regard to basal values of GFR, diuresis, serum creatinine and
BUN. The only significant difference was found between the age of pts
excluded and that of pts admitted to EP.

Table I. Basal features of the patients (Mean ± SD).

Pts	N.	age (years)	GFR (ml/min)	diuresis (ml/24 h)	sCreat. (mg/dl)	BUN (mg/dl)
all	55	60.8±14.2	2.3±0.9	1022±354	14.8±3.6	146±42
Ex	9	47.2±19.0 ★	2.0±1.1	874±393	15.2±1.7	141±31
EP	46	63.4±11.3	2.4±0.8	1051±338	14.7±3.8	147±44
On	22	65.4±10.9	2.4±0.7	1137±355	15.6±3.7	148±55
DO	24	61.6±11.3	2.4±0.9	973±302	13.9±3.7	146±30

sCreat. = serum creatinine; Ex = patients excluded during the PP;
EP = patients entered the experimental phase; On = patients still on
IDDP; DO = dropped out patients. ★ $p < 0.002$ vs EP (Student's T test)

The percent program survival in all pts and in subgroups by age,
at 3, 6, 9, 12 and 18 months is shown in Table II.

Table II. Percent program survival in pts entered EP (Mean ± SE).

	N.	3 months	6 months	9 months	I2 months	I8 months
all	46	98±2	85±5	63±8	59±8	35±I0
< 60 y	I7	-	93±6	68±I3	58±I5	I4±I3
> 60 y	29	96±3	8I±8	58±I0	-	47±I3

< 60 y, > 60 y = pts aged less or more than 60; Cox-Mantel Test: NS.

DISCUSSION

In our experience IDDP was applied to 55 out of 84 pts needing renal substitutive treatment (65%). It was feasible in 46 of these 55 pts (84%), that is at least 55% of pts starting substitutive treatment. Excluded pts were significantly younger than pts admitted to the experimental phase. The lack of compliance with the diet was the main cause of exclusion and drop out. The program survival rate was 59% at I2 months and 35% at I8 months, showing that IDDP is an actual, although temporary, alternative to standard hemodialysis or CAPD, especially for old pts.

CONCLUSIONS

IDDP is feasible in more than 55% of pts needing renal substitutive treatment. It better suits old pts and those strongly determined to accept heavy dietetic restrictions in order to get a two thirds cut in the frequency of the hemodialytic treatment. For them it represents an actual, although temporary, alternative to standard hemodialysis or CAPD. Its duration is variable and not foreseeable at the start of the treatment.

REFERENCES

I. Pontoriero G, Di Filippo S, Andrulli S, Tentori F, Citterio A, La Milia V, Ponti R, Locatelli F. Int J Artif Organs (in press).
2. Zimmermann E, Gretz N, Meisinger E, Huber W, Stranch M. Proc 2nd Intern Congress on Nutrition in Renal Disease, Bologna, 1979.

TREATMENT OF UREMIC ANEMIA WITH ETRETINATE: COMPARISON WITH
RECOMBINANT HUMAN ERYTHROPOIETIN (rHuEPO)

S.LAMPERI, S.CAROZZI, A.ICARDI, M.G.NASINI, G.B.TRAVERSO

Nephrology Department, St. Martin's Hospital, Genoa, Italy

INTRODUCTION

Cis-retinoic acid(CRA)and its metabolites have been shown
to increase,in vitro,the number of Burst Forming Units Erythroid
(BFU-e),the more immature erythroid precursors,in a dose-dependent
manner(1).Thus,besides EPO,also retinoids might be able to correct
the defective bone marrow(BM)erythroid proliferative activity in
uremics (2).

The aim of this study was,therefore,to evaluate the effects
of CRA derivative,etretinate (E) on the BM and peripheral blood
abnormalities in a group of anemic dialysis patients,compared to
a group of patients treated by rHuEPO.

PATIENTS AND METHODS

Of the patients studied,15 (7 in hemodialysis-HD- and 8 in
continuous ambulatory peritoneal dialysis-CAPD-) were treated for
28 weeks with E (25mg p.o.)and 10, in HD, with rHuEPO for 32 weeks
(IV bolus in progessively increasing doses). In vitro BM BFU-e and
Colony Forming Units Erythroid(CFU-e) growth was determined by
Iscove's method (3). Hemoglobin (Hb)levels and reticulocyte (Ret)
count were assessed by the standard techniques.

RESULTS

In HD patients,treatment with E induced a slow rise in Hb

values,from the 16th week,reaching a maximum (about 25% increase)
the 24th week. A noticeable increase(nearly 5-fold)in the Ret
count was also seen, from the 2nd through the 28th week. Before
E therapy, study of BM erythroid progenitor growth showed that
both BFU-e and CFU-e growth was significantly decreased compared
with controls. From the 2nd week, treatment induced significant
increases in the number of BFU-e. Contemporaneously, non-signifi-
cant modification of in vitro CFU-e growth was seen.

In HD patients treated for 12 weeks with increasing IV doses
of rHuEPO(1st phase), progressive rises in Hb values and Ret count
were observed from the 2nd week. In vitro evaluation of BM
erythroid proliferative capacity showed a marked improvement
of CFU-e growth from the 2nd week of therapy, reaching normal
levels the 12th week. During the 2nd phase of therapy, from the
12th to the 32nd week, the Hb values were stationary, while the
Ret count decreased. There was also a slight increase of the BFU-e,
although they never reached the normal range; and decrease of the
CFU-e which, however, remained within the normal range.

DISCUSSION

Our results with E show the possibility of obtaining positive
effects on the peripheral hematologic parameters of anemic uremics
consisting of a modest increase in the Hb levels,while significantly
greater is the increase in the Ret count. In the patients treated
with rHuEPO, there were more marked rises in these parameters.The
in vitro effects of E on BM erythroid proliferation also differed
from those of rHuEPO. E stimulated the proliferation and differentiation
of the more immature erythroid elements, the BFU-e, while in the
more mature CFU-e, considered the physiological target of EPO (4),
there was no significant change. This indicates that the mechanism
of action of retinoids on BM cells in anemic uremics is different

from that of EPO. As E stimulates only the more immature erythroid precursors (BFU-e), when EPO is lacking its is unable to affect the peripheral hematologic parameters, while EPO leads to their near normalization. However, our studies have shown that after prolonged therapy even with relatively high doses of rHuEPO there tends to be a decrease in the number of CFU-e in vitro,associated with a drop in the Ret count in vivo. This reduction of the effects of rHuEPO is probably due to a deficit of CFU-e, which is secondary to a lack of their precursors, the BFU-e. Since retinoids stimulate the proliferation of BFU-e, their addition to rHuEPO could help avoid this problem by providing more BFU-e to become CFU-e and be stimulated by EPO.

In conclusion, our results have shown that E and EPO act at different stages of erythropoiesis. Therefore, the addition of E could potentiate the effects of rHuEPO in the treatment of uremic anemia, as well as permit a reduction of its dosage.

REFERENCES

1. Douer, D., Koeffler, H.P. J. Clin. Invest 69: 1039-1041,1982.
2. Winearls, C.G., Pippard, M.J., Downing, M.R., Oliver, D.O., Reid, C. and Cotes P.M. The Lancet 22: 1175-1178, 1986.
3. Iscove, N.N. Cell. Tiss. Kinet. 10: 323-334, 1977.
4. Erslev, A.J. New England J. Med. 316: 101-103, 1987.

ACUTE EFFECTS OF CARNITINE ADDITION TO THE DIALYSIS FLUID DURING HEMODIALYSIS IN PATIENTS WITH CHRONIC RENAL FAILURE

G. TOIGO, L. CRAPESI, R. SITULIN, G. TAMARO, M.A. DEL BIANCO, M. CORSI, *P. LO GRECO, °A. VASILE, G. GUARNIERI

Institute of Patologia Medica, Trieste University; *Central Laboratory, Udine General Hospital; °Div. Nephrology, Palmanova Hospital (Italy)

L-Carnitine (C) is required for intramitochondrial transport of FFA to the sites of beta-oxidation: in muscle the oxidation of long chain fatty acids is mostly C dependent. It is also accepted that C may shuttle acetyl-groups from the mytochondrial matrix to the cytosol for FFA synthesis and, in liver, TG synthesis.

Plasma C fractions are often increased in chronically uremic patients on conservative treatment. In hemodialysis (HD) patients the percentage of free C is generally lower and that of short-chain acylcarnitine is higher (1). It is generally agreed that muscle C content is lowered by chronic hemodialysis treatment, but probably not all HD patients are C deficient.

After C administration in HD patients the clinical status and some neuromuscolar symptoms have been reported to improve. However, the multifactorial pathogenesis of this type of disturbances makes the interpretation of these therapeutic effects very difficult.

The effect of C supplementation on lipid metabolism in chronic uremic patients in HD treatment is still under investigation. Controversial effects have been found after C supplementation on hypertriglyceridemia and lipoprotein abnormalities of HD patients: these inconsistent results may depend on inadequate controls, on poor patient compliance, on variations in dietary intake, and on different C dosages or schedules.

Paradoxical responses, with increase of triglyceride plasma concentration after C supplement, have been sometimes reported and these results may be due to C dependent shuttling of acetyl group from mitochondria to the cytosol, where they can be utilized for fatty acid, triglycerides and VLDL synthesis.

Besides, some patients on maintenance HD show an "intolerance" to the acetate load used as alkalinizing salt during HD treatment.

In a previous study (2) we treated 9 hemodialysis patients for 6 weeks with a high dosage of i.v. C at the end of the dialysis and we unexpectedly found higher serum acetate and triglyceride and lower blood bicarbonate levels during the HD treatment. These paradoxical effects might depend on the large amount of C infused or on the acute i.v. bolus infusion following dialysis.

METHODS

In this new protocol we examined 9 patients during two hemodialysis treatments, without or with C addiction to the dialysis fluid.

During hemodialysis we measured the plasma concentration of C fractions, acetate, lactate, pyruvate, acetoacetate, 3-hydroxybutyrate, FFAs, triglycerides and the blood acid-base status, collecting blood from the arterial line before, 30', 60', 120', 150' after the beginning, at the end and 60' after the end of dialysis.

C fractions were determined by the method of Cederblad; serum acetate by gas-chromatographic method; lactate, pyruvate, acetoacetate and 3-hydroxybutyrate by enzymatic methods; FFAs by the kit "NEFA Quick BMY', triglycerides by the kit "Testomar triglycerides". The blood acid-base status was evaluated by standard methods. Mann-Whitney U test and ANOVA were obtained from SPSS.

RESULTS

The basal values of short chain acylcarnitine were significantly higher than in normal controls, whereas concentration of long chain acylcarnitines and the free to esterified and total C ratios were lower.

HD induced significant changes in serum free C, free to esterified and to total C ratios, FFAs, 3-hydroxybutyrate, acetoacetate, 3-hydroxybutyrate/acetoacetate and lactate/pyruvate ratios and in blood pH, pCO_2 and HCO_3^-.

Significant differences were observed after C addition to the dialysis fluid for serum free C, free to esterified and total C ratios, lactate to pyruvate ratio, and blood HCO_3^- and pCO_2 (Table 1).

TABLE 1. Effect of hemodialysis and carnitine in uremic patients.

	HD ($p<$)	CARNITINE ($p<$)
Free C	0.01	0.017
FC/EC	0.001	0.001
Acetate	0.001	N.S.
Triglycerides	N.S.	N.S.
3-OH-BUT/ACAC	0.002	N.S.
Lactate/Pyruvate	0.001	0.012
pCO_2	0.001	0.002
HCO_3^-	0.001	0.011

DISCUSSION

Short-chain acylcarnitine concentration was higher and long-chain acylcarnitine concentration was lower in our patients than in controls, and free to esterified and total C ratios were decreased: these data could suggest that FFAs oxidation is impaired in chronic uremia and C acts as a carrier of the excesso of short-chain acylcarnitines.

During HD with carnitine-enriched dialysate, free C and free to esterified and total C ratios were higher than before C addition (short-chain acylcarnitines, in fact, did not change), but, despite the high C concentration in the dialysate, they decreased during HD: these data suggest that the C flux from dialysate was not sufficient to counteract the free C consumption for acetate and FFA esterification. It is also possible a slower C diffusion due to a pH--dependent change of dissociation.

3-hydroxybutyrate/acetoacetate ratio and lactate/pyruvate ratio increased during HD, suggesting vascular instability and tissue hypoxia; the latter ratio significantly decrease after C, suggesting a better oxidative metabolism; however, no effect on the plasma levels of acetate and triglycerides was seen during C supplementation, and blood bicarbonate and pCO_2 (possibly derived from metabolized acetate) decreased during dialysis.

Further studies on acetate kinetics during HD with a C-enriched bath are necessary to optimize the dosage and to assess efficacy of the compound.

REFERENCES
1. Corsi, M. Secondary carnitine deficiency in renal disease. In: Clinical Aspects of Human Carnitine Deficiency (Ed. P.P. Borum), Pergamon Press, New York, 1986, pp. 194-212
2. Guarnieri, G., Toigo, G., Crapesi, L., Situlin, R., Del Bianco, M.A., Corsi, M., Lo Greco, P., Paviotti, G., Mioni, G. and Campanacci, L. Carnitine metabolism in chronic renal failure. I. Metabolic effects of carnitine supplementation during acetate hemodialysis. Kidney Int: 32(suppl.22): S116-S127, 1987

CLONIDINE IS EFFECTIVE IN THE TREATMENT OF
"RESTLESS LEGS" SYNDROME IN CHRONIC UREMIC PATIENTS

M. AUSSERWINKLER, P. SCHMIDT
1st Medical Department, Landeskrankenhaus
9026 Klagenfurt, AUSTRIA

INTRODUCTION

The "restless legs" syndrome is a disorder in witch
patients feel an irresistible urge to move the legs,
generally when sitting or lying down. Obove all patients
undergoing chronic hemodialysis treatment have an
unpleasant deep discomfort inside the calves, requiring
that the legs be moved.
A variety of medicaments have been used to treat this
syndrome. Such as L-dopa, bromocriptine, opoid drugs,
clonazepam or carbamazepine.
The first report on the efficancy of clonidine was
given by Handwerker et al (NEJM 313 (1985) 1228).
In order to evaluate this therapy 20 consecutive uremic
patients with restless legs syndrome were included into
a double-blind study.

PATIENTS AND METHODS

20 patients with chronic renal failure were included
into the trial. 11 patients were treated conservatively
9 were on chronic hemodialysis treatment. The mean age
was 50 years. All of them showed symptoms of restless
legs syndrome for at least 3 weeks.
The study was a double-blind comparison of placebo
and clonidine.

10 patients received 0,075 mg clonidine twice daily,
10 patients a placebo. The blood pressure was   measured
three times a day.
3 days after starting therapy, the patients were examined
to determine the effectiveness of the treatment.
Blood pressure was measured at least twice daily and
compaired with blood presure before treatment.

RESULTS

In the clonidine-treated group there was complete relief
of symptoms in 8 out of ten patients and in 1 patient a
striking improvement was noted, in 1 further patient
the symptoms remained unchanged.
In contrast only 1 out of 10 patients of the placebo
group showed some improvement of the symptoms.
(chi square = 12,8; p   0,001).
Blood pressure was not significantly different in the
two groups.

DISCUSSION

The beneficial effects of the antihypertensive drug
clonidine in the treatment of migraine, anxiety disorders,
vasomotor symptoms, spasticity in spinal cord injured
patients have been proved. Many authors have demonstrated
the analgesic effects of clonidine. The favourable effect
of clonidine in three nonuremic patients suffering from
symptoms of the restless legs syndrome was shown by
Handwerker et al. (NEJM 313, (1985) 1228).
Our data show that lowdose administration of the central
alpha 2-adrenergic agonist clonidine is a very effective
approach in the treatment of the restless legs syndroms
in chronic uremic patients.

REFERENCES

1. Akpinar, S.   Chlin. Neuropharm. 10 (1987)
   69 - 79

2. Callaghan N.,   Neurology 16 (1966) 359 - 361

3. Forssberg H.   Brain   Research 50 (1973) 184 - 186

4. Fox   G. N., Am. Fam. Physician 33 (1986) 147 - 152

5. Gold M. S., JAMA 243   (1980) 343 - 346

6. Handwerker J., Palmer R.,   NEJM 7 (1985) 1228 -29

7. Lugaresi E., Cirignotta F., Coggagna G.,
   Montagna P., Adv. Neurol. 43 (1986) 295 - 307

8. Missak S. S., Med. Hypoth., 24 (1987) 161 - 165

9. Scheele C.,   Lancet, 2   (1986) 426 - 427

HEMORHEOLOGY AND HYPERTENSION IN END-STAGE RENAL FAILURE PATIENTS TREATED WITH ERYTHROPOIETIN

R.M. SCHAEFER, M. LESCHKE*, B. KUERNER, M. ZECH, A. HEIDLAND

Department of Internal Medicine, Universities of Wuerzburg and *Duesseldorf, FRG

INTRODUCTION

With the advent of recombinant human erythropoietin (r-HuEPO) effective treatment of renal anemia has become possible (1-3). However, with the increase of hematocrit levels some of the patients treated developed hypertension. Since blood viscosity determines vascular resistance (4, 5) and thereby blood pressure (6, 7), we investigated blood pressure behaviour and blood viscosity in long-term dialysis patients during treatment with r-HuEPO.

PATIENTS AND METHODS

Fifteen long-term hemodialysis patients suffering from severe anemia were treated with r-HuEPO. The hormone was produced by recombinant DNA techniques (Amgen, Thousand Oaks, CA, USA) and obtained from Cilag GmbH, Alsbach-Hähnlein, FRG via Ortho Pharmaceuticals, Raritan, NJ, USA. All rheological determinations were performed with the ORCD device (Anton Paar Co., Graz, Austria) et 37°C using an oscillating viscosimeter.

RESULTS

After 4 months of therapy with r-HuEPO hematocrit rose from baseline values of 23.7 + 1.2 to 35.7 + 0.2 % (Table 1). With the correction of anemia mean predialytic blood pressure increased from 131/79 to 139/85 mm Hg. This was mainly due to the development of frank hypertension in 3 patients who had to be put on anti-hypertensive therapy.

Table 1. Hemorheology in healthy subjects and dialysis patients prior to and during treatment with r-HuEPO.

	r-HuEPO		healthy subjects
	0	16 weeks	
	n = 8	n = 8	n = 15
Hematocrit %	23.7 ± 1.2	35.7 ± 0.2^a	42.7 ± 3.5^b
Whole blood viscosity mPas			
gamma = $2s^{-1}$	3.58 ± 0.20	5.08 ± 0.37^a	6.85 ± 0.38^b
gamma = $100s^{-1}$	2.34 ± 0.13	3.11 ± 0.18^a	3.99 ± 0.23^b
Plasma viscosity mPas	1.38 ± 0.04	1.42 ± 0.02	1.27 ± 0.04^b

Data are given as means + SE. [a]p 0.05 for values during versus prior to treatment and [b]p 0.05 for healthy subjects versus hemodialysis patients (t_o).

Rising hematocrit levels in these patients caused whole blood viscosity to increase by 42 % at low shear rates and 32 % at high shear rates. Plasma viscosity was significantly higher in anemic dialysis patients as compared to healthy controls (Table 1). This increment in plasma viscosity was predominantly caused by enhanced levels of fibrinogen in hemodialysis patients as compared to normal controls (335+26 versus 230+21 mg/dl). During therapy with r-HuEPO, a small but insignificant increase in plasma viscosity was observed.

DISCUSSION

The present investigation clearly showed that during r-HuEPO therapy whole blood viscosity increased both at low and high shear rates. The increase at high shear rates is mainly due to higher hematocrit values which will give rise to a greater viscous resistance of blood to flow. The increment in whole blood viscosity at low shear rates will influence flow conditions in the microcirculation.

As whole blood viscosity is one of the factors that determine vascular resistance (4), it is conceivable that a rise in whole blood viscosity may contribute to high blood pressure under these circumstances. Neff et al. (8) made similar observations when they increased hematocrit levels in dialysis patients acutely from 20 to 40 % by transfusions of packed red cells. Peripheral resistance increased by 80 % with a concomitant increase in diastolic blood pressure of 20 mm Hg.

Besides this notion, a second hypothesis for the rise in blood pressure has been forwarded. Accordingly, it was suggested that severe anemia produces peripheral vasodilatation due to hypoexemia. Correction of this condition will therefore abolish hypoxic vasodilatation and increase arteriolar vasoconstriction and thus resistance and blood pressure (8).

REFERENCES
1. Winearls, C.G., Oliver, D.O., Pippard, M.J., Reid, C., Downing, M.R., and Cotes, P.M. Lancet 2: 1175-1178, 1986.
2. Zins, B., Drueke, T., Zingraff, J., Bererhi, L., Kreis, H., Naret, C., Delons, S., Castaigne, J.P., Peterlongo, F., Casadevall, N., and Varet, B. Lancet 2: 1329, 1986.
3. Eschbach, J.W., Egrie, J.C., Downing, M.R., Browne, J.K., and Adamson, J.W. N. Engl. J. Med. 316: 73-78, 1987.
4. Schmid-Schönbein, H., Rieger, H., and Fischer, T. Angiology 31: 301-319, 1980.
5. Harris, T., McLoughlin, G. Q. J. Med. 23: 451-464, 1930.
6. Letcher, R.L., Chien, S., Pickering, T.G., Sealey, J.E., and Laragh, J.H. Am. J. Med. 70: 1195-1202, 1981.
7. Leschke, M., Motz, W., Blanke, H., and Strauer, B.E. J. Cardiovasc. Pharm. 10 (Suppl. 6): 103-110, 1987.
8. Neff, M.S., Kim, K.E., Persoff, M., Onesti, G., and Swartz, C. Circulation 18: 876-883, 1971.

EFFECTS OF CHRONIC HYPERPROTEIC DIET ON RENAL FUNCTION AND ALBUMIN EXCRETION

F.J. GAINZA, M.J. DOMINGUEZ, R. MUÑIZ, I. LAMPREABE

Nephrology and Nuclear Medicine Services, Cruces Hospital, Bilbao, Spain

INTRODUCTION

An acute overload of protein intake produces glomerular hyper-filtration (1). Brenner et al. proposed that sustained hyperfiltration can produce glomerular sclerosis (2). It has been demostrated that "microalbuminuria" is a predictor of glomerulosclerosis (3). This study was undertaken to investigate the effects of chronic hyperproteic diet on renal function and if there is any evidence of microalbuminuria present.

SUBJECTS AND METHODS

We have evaluated 31 healthy male physicoculturists with an average age of 27 (ranging from 20 to 37). None had history of metabolic or nephrourologyc diseases. All of them presented normal urinalysis, blood pressure, glucemia and plasma lipids. They were divided into two groups in regard to dietary protein intake:

Control group (CG)

11 of the 31 males studied followed a normal protein diet.

Hyperproteic group (HG)

The other 20 remaining were following hyperproteic diet with oral powder protein supplements for at least 12 months before the study (an average 48 mo; ranging from 12 to 180).

There were no differences between two groups in age and body surface area.

Prtein intake (PI) estimation

$$PI = (\text{Non urea nitrogen} + \frac{\text{urinary urea nitrogen (UUN)}}{\text{body wt in kg}}) \times 6.25$$

PI expresed in g/Kg body wt and UUN in g/24-hr.

Glomerular filtration rate (GFR)

GFR was measured by endogenous creatinine clearance (CCr) with a 24-hr urine collection. The morning after the completion of the urine collection, plasma creatinine level was tested in the fasting state (AutoAnalyzer Astra 4).

Quantitative tests for proteinuria

We include sulfosalicylic acid method (nephelometer) and radioimmunoassay (RIA) for albumin excretion rate (AER) in a 24-hr urine collection.

Tubular function

Tubular reabsortion of phosphate (TRP), fractional excretion urate (FE urate) and beta-2 microglobulin excretion were calculated. And pH was measured in the first morning fresh urine.

RESULTS

In Table 1 are shown the results expresed as mean+1 sd.

Table 1.

Parameter	C GROUP	H GROUP	Statistic test
Plasma creatinine	$1.06^{\pm}0.14$	$1.03^{\pm}0.13$	NS t Student
CCr (ml/min/1.73m2)	$115^{\pm}22$	$156^{\pm}38$	p<0.01; Mann-Whtney
BUN (mg/dl)	$12.6^{\pm}3.3$	$19^{\pm}3.4$	p<0.001 t Student
Urea clearance	$67^{\pm}19$	$84^{\pm}15$	p<0.01; " "
UUN (g/24-hr)	$11.6^{\pm}1.7$	$23^{\pm}5.5$	p<0.001 Mann-Whitney
PI (g/Kg body wt)	$1.3^{\pm}0.1$	$2.2^{\pm}0.4$	p<0.001 " "
TRP (%)	$87.8^{\pm}4.7$	$84^{\pm}6.8$	NS t Student
FE urate (%)	$8.7^{\pm}2.3$	$10.9^{\pm}4.5$	NS " "
Proteinuria-sulfo-salicylic (g/24-hr)	$180^{\pm}40$	$270^{\pm}140$	p<0.05; " "
AER (mg/24-hr/1.73)	$5.8^{\pm}4.4$	$7.2^{\pm}7.1$	NS " "

None of them failed to obtain normal tubular function.

It was a positive correlation (Fig. 1) between 24-hr urinary urea nitrogen and creatinine clearance.

DISCUSSION

High oral protein intake was demostrated in HG who were eating oral protein powder supplements. And it was in lesser degree in CG.

Creatinine clearance is significantly greater in HG than in CG but plasma creatinine is similar in both of them. Other authors (1)

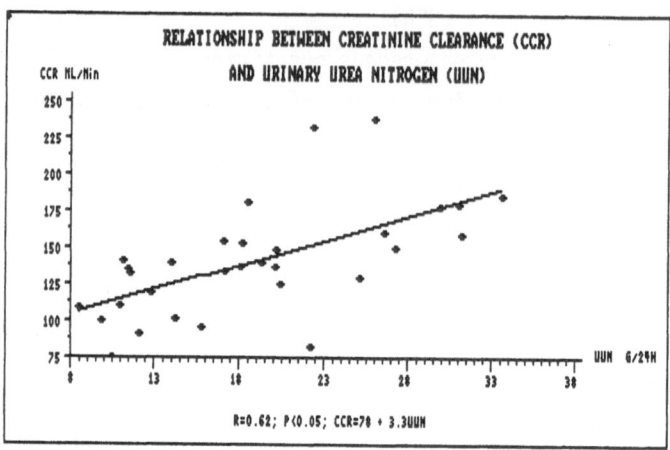

Fig. 1. Relationship between UUN and CCr.

had demostrated glomerular hyperfiltration with acute oral protein overload and they did not find differences between CCr and Cinulin.

When AER was greater than normal human excretion (30 mg/24-hr) is called microalbuminuria (4). Only one of the HG presented 32 mg and there were no differences between the two groups in average AER.

Chronic exercise training ameliorates progresive renal disease in rats with subtotal nephrectomy (5). It is also possible that this effect can act preserving renal injury in physicoculturists.

We have found that hyperproteic diet for at least 12 months produced sustained hyperfiltration without any other changes in renal function and no evidence of microalbuminuria has been found.

REFERENCES
1. Bosch J.P.,Saccaggi A.,Laver A.et al. Renal Functional Reserve in Humans. Am J Med; 75: 943-950, 1983.
2. Brenner B.M.,Meyer T.W.,Hosteter T.H. Dietary Protein Intake and the progressive nature of Kidney Disease.N Eng J Med 307;632, 1982.
3. Viberti G.C.,Hill R.D.Jarret R.et al.Microalbuminuria as a pretor of clinical nephropaty in ID diabetes.Lancet I:1430-32, 1982.
4. Mogensen C.E. and Christensen C.K.Predicting diabetic nephropaty in insulin-dependent patients.N Eng J Med 311:89-93, 1984.
5.Heifets M.,Davis T.A.,Tegtmeyer E.,Klahr S.Exercise training amelio rates progresive renal disease ...Kid Int 32:815-20, 1987.

This study was partially supported by a grant from The Health Dept. of the Basque Country Government.

ACE INHIBITION AND PROGRESSION OF RENAL INJURY IN MAN.

G. GRAZI, C. CIRAMI, V. PANICHI, A. BARONTI, E. MONTAGNANI, A.M. BIANCHI, M. PARRINI, R. COMINOTTO and R. PALLA.

2nd Medical Clinic, University of Pisa, 56100 Pisa, Italy.

INTRODUCTION

Enalapril maleate, an angiotensin Converting Enzyme Inhibitor (CEI), is an effective antihypertensive agent. It lowers peripheral and Renal Vascular Resistances (RVR), increases Renal Plasma Flow (RPF) and Blood Flow (RBF), whereas Glomerular Filtration Rate (GFR) is usually unchanged. Since Angiotensin II (AII) alters renal hemodynamics by increasing efferent arteriolar resistance, reduces GFR by decreasing ultrafiltration coefficient (LpA), the product of the glomerular capillary wall hydraulic conductivity (Lp) and the effective capillary surface area available for filtration (A), and produces proteinuria, CEI may have the potentiality to correct intraglomerular hypertension, to normalize GFR and to decrease proteinuria.

MATERIALS AND METHODS

Ten subjects with hypertension (recumbent diastolic Blood Pressure (BP) > 95 mmHg) and histological evidence of glomerulonephritis (4 IgA nephropaty, 3 chronic glomerulonephritis, 2 focal schlerosis, 1 lupus nephritis - WHO II class) were admitted to the study. They received 10 mg/day p.o. of Enalapril, in single dose, for 16 weeks. Serum and urine creatinine and electrolytes were assessed by Astra

Autoanalyzer. Daily Urinary Protein Excretion (UPE) was determined by Bradford's method (1). GFR was assessed by inulin plasmatic clearance (2) and RPF by I-131-Hippuran clearance (3). RVR (mean BP:RBF ratio), Filtration Fraction (FF) (GFR:RPF ratio) and Proteinuria Index (PI) (mg of UPE:mmol of urinary creatinine ratio) were calculated. Biochemical and functional parameters were evaluated before starting therapy and after 16 weeks. Results were expressed as mean $\pm$ SEM. Data were analyzed by Student's T paired test; a difference was considered statistically significant when p<0.05.

RESULTS

All patients showed a good BP response to Enalapril therapy (Table 1) and no evidence of tachycardia or postural hypotension; renal effects are showed in Table 2.

Table 1. Blood Pressure response

	Baseline	16th week	
Recumbent			
Systolic BP mmHg	141.2+3.8	122.1+3.7	p 0.01
Diastolic BP "	97.1+2.2	80.1+3.0	p 0.01
Upright			
Systolic BP mmHg	128.7+3.4	112.5+3.4	p 0.01
Diastolic BP "	92.8+2.3	77.9+2.9	p 0.01

Table 2. Functional and hemodynamic effects.

	Baseline	16th week	
Serum creat. (mg/dl)	1.3+ 0.2	1.3+0.1	
Creat. cl. (ml/min/1.73sqm)	92.7+10.5	89.8+9.9	
GFR (ml/min/1.73sqm)	77.4+13.1	77.2+11.5	
RPF (ml/min/1.73sqm)	513.4+69.8	615.6+74.4	p 0.01
FF	17.1 %	13.2 %	p 0.02
RVR	0.149+0.025	0.102+0.014	p 0.01
UPE (mg/day)	2,082+661	1,117+383	p 0.02
PI (mg/mmol)	1,458+461	849+107	p 0.05

DISCUSSION

The drop in UPE after Enalapril therapy reflects a blunting of AII effects on one or more parameters of the ultrafiltration rate for a single glomerulus: 1) Ultrafiltration Coefficient (LpA); 2) transcapillary hydraulic pressure gradient (ΔP); 3) colloid osmotic pressure gradient ($\Delta\pi$). CEI administration is associated with unchanged GFR, increased RPF and decreased FF, reflecting an efferent arteriolar dilation. The reduction in efferent arteriolar resistance decreases glomerular capillary hydrostatic pressure and results in a drop in ΔP, inhibiting transglomerular passage of proteins. A reduction in FF decreases plasma proteins concentration along the lenght of glomerular capillary and therefore $\Delta\pi$; this in turn reduces transglomerular passage of proteins, whereas the paired reduction in ΔP should not alter the ultrafiltration rate. Alternatively the reduction in Lp could account for the decrease in UPE. Since CEI increases A by mesangial cells relaxation and does not change GFR, it should decrease Lp.

In summary, Enalapril may reduce proteinuria by decreasing ΔP, glomerular plasma proteins concentration and Lp. In man, being impossible a direct evaluation of these parameters by glomerular micropuncture study, remains the doubt about their quantitative effects, but it seems very probable an interaction of these factors in regulating nephron adaptative changes to renal injury and producing secondary glomerular sclerosis and proteinuria.

REFERENCES

1) BRADFORD, M.M. Anal. Biochem. 72 :218-221, 1976.
2) COLE, B.R. et al. N. Engl. J. Med. 287 :1109-1114, 1972.
3) BLAUFOX, M.D. et al. Nephron 3 :274-281, 1966.

ONE YEAR EXPERIENCE WITH HYPOPROTEIC DIET AND ONCE A WEEK HEMODIALYSIS (LESS THAN 5 HOURS).

G. PONTORIERO, S. DI FILIPPO, S. ANDRULLI, F. TENTORI, A. CITTERIO, V. LA MILIA, R. PONTI, F. LOCATELLI.
Divisione di Nefrologia e Dialisi - Ospedale di Lecco - Lecco, Italy.

INTRODUCTION. The aim of this study is to evaluate the long term depurative and nutritional adequacy of an integrated diet-dialysis program (IDDP: low protein diet supplemented with essential amino acids (EAA) plus once a week hemodialysis).

PATIENTS AND METHODS. Patients (pts) with glomerular filtration rate (GFR, calculated as the mean of creatinine and urea clearances) (1) under 5 ml/min, and a residual diuresis sufficient to avoid sodium and water overload were eligible for the IDDP. The pts were dialyzed once weekly, receiving a total dose of dialysis therapy (dialyzer urea clearance x dialysis time) to keep the predialysis BUN under 90 mg/dl. They were presribed a protein intake of 0.4 g/kg/day, supplemented with 9.6 g/day of oral EAA, and a caloric intake of at least 35 Kcal/kg/day. Data are presented on 11 pts (8 males and 3 females; mean age 55.4±9.9 years) who have followed the IDDP for at least one year. Before entering the IDDP their mean GFR was 3.3±1.0 ml/min, BUN 170.5±64.4 mg/dl, serum creatinine (SCr) 15.5±5.0 mg/dl. After hypercatabolism was excluded, the depurative adequacy and nitrogen balance were evaluated: predialysis SCr (PSCr) and BUN (PBUN) levels were determined; for at least two days immediately preceding the dialysis treatment, the total nitrogen production was calculated by summing urinary urea nitrogen (UUN), non urea nitrogen (NUN, taken as 31 mg/kg/day (2)) and change in urea pool (ΔN). ΔN was calculated as (ΔBUN x V)+ (BUN x ΔBW), where V was the volume of urea distribution, ΔBUN the change in BUN levels and ΔBW the change in body weight. V was calculated according to Lowrie et al (3). The protein catabolic rate (PCR) was calculated as 6.25 x (UUN + NUN + ΔN) (4) and compared with the prescribed protein intake to assess dietary compliance. Nutritional adequacy was evaluated by anthropometric indexes: body weight (BW), tricipital skinfold thickness (TSF), mid arm muscle circumference (MAMC) (5). GFR was evaluated in at least two 24 hour samples collected before the dialysis day. Statistical analyses were performed using the ANOVA.

RESULTS. PBUN remained within the preset range of adequacy whereas PSCr increased significantly. The difference between the PCR observed (PCRo) and the PCR expected according to dietary prescription (PCRe) was not statistically significant throughout the study. UUN and GFR showed a significant progressive reduction. ΔN tend to increase but the changes were not significant. All the anthropometric indexes, but MAMC, improved significantly (Table 1).

Table 1. Nitrogen metabolism, GFR and anthropometric indexes.

months	basal	6	12	P
PBUN (mg/dl)	84.9±18.2	88.2±13.0	88.1±26.3	NS
PSCr (mg/dl)	13.3±4.2	16.3±5.0	16.4±5.2	<0.001
PCRo (g/day)	37.5±8.7	37.7±9.2	34.5±9.2	NS
PCRe (g/day)	33.5±3.3	33.6±3.2	33.6±3.2	NS
ΔN (g/day)	1.9±1.2	2.7±1.3	1.8±0.9	NS
UUN (g/day)	2.1±1.0	1.3±0.7	1.6±0.8	<0.01
GFR (ml/min)	2.9±1.0	1.8±0.5	1.7±0.4	<0.001
BW (Kg)	65.0±10.8	68.3±9.8	68.9±9.9	<0.001
TSF (mm)	7.2±4.1	9.1±4.8	8.9±4.4	<0.001
MAMC (cm)	24.4±2.3	24.9±2.2	24.8±2.9	NS

DISCUSSION. As already reported (6), we chose a predialysis BUN < 90 mg/dl as index of adequate depuration. The observed mean values of predialysis BUN remained stable within the range of adequacy, whereas predialysis SCr increased significantly. This is possibly explained by the different performances of natural and artificial kidneys in removing the two solutes. In fact, whereas urea clearance by the human kidney is about 60% of creatinine clearance at the same level of renal function, urea clearance with the artificial membranes commonly used is about 30% higher than creatinine clearance. Thus replacement therapy can result in increased predialysis creatinine values, even in the presence of unchanged BUN values, muscle mass and total (renal and dialytic) urea clearance. This trend warrants careful evaluation, possibly requiring an increase in dialysis efficiency for this molecule. UUN decreased significantly (parallel with the reduction of GFR) and thus ΔN tended to increase. As a consequence, to maintain a stable predialysis BUN the dose of dialysis therapy increased progressively. Nevertheless the time of dialysis never exceeded 5.5 hours. It is widely recognized that malnutrition is the main risk of dietary protein restriction. In our study all the anthropometric indexes, but MAMC, improved significantly. This resul warrants further study to exclude the influence of an overhydration clinically not evident in our pts.

In conclusion satisfactory depurative and nutritional indexes can be maintained by IDDP with very short weekly dialysis treatment not only in the short term (4, 6) but also after one year.

REFERENCES.
1 Milutinovic J., Cutler R.E., Hoover P., Meiysen B., Scribner B.H. Kidney Int 8: 185-90, 1975.
2 Maroni B.J., Steinman T.I., Mitch W.E. Kidney Int 27: 58-65, 1985.
3 Lowrie E.G., Teshan B.P. Kidney Int 23 (suppl 13): 113-22, 1983.
4 Mitch W.E., Sapir D.G. Kidney Int 20: 122-6, 1981.
5 Lucas P.A., Meadows J.H., Roberts D.E., Coles G.A., Kidney Int 29: 995-1030, 1986.
6 Pontoriero G., Di Filippo S., Andrulli S., Tentori F., Citterio A., La Milia V., Ponti R., Locatelli F. Int J Artif Organs (in press).

CALCITRIOL AND RENAL FAILURE

M. BERTOLI, G. LUISETTO* A. RUFFATTI, P. GALUPPO* M. URSO
G.F. ROMAGNOLI.
Department of Nephrology - *Institute of Semeiotica Medi
ca, University - Hospital, Padova, Italy.

INTRODUCTION

Uremic patients have calcitriol deficiency, due to
reduced renal synthesis. Treatment with calcitriol in
these patients, however, reportedly worsens renal func
tion (1). The aim of our study is to verify this hypothe
sis.

MATERIALS AND METHODS

Seven patients (3 males and 4 females), ranging in
age from 32 to 68 years (mean 50.72 ± 10.40) with stable re
nal insufficiency (serum creatinine range, 2 to 8 mg/dl;
mean 5.07 ± 2.19 mg/dl) were administered 0.5 μg of
$1,25(OH)_2D_3$ (Rocaltrol - Roche) for a period of 4 months.
The following parameters were measured at the beginning
of therapy, and then every 15 days during the entire tre
atment period, and the first 2 months following suspen
sion of the drug: serum creatinine (cr), calcium (Ca),
phosphate, alkaline phosphatase, parathyroid hormone(PTH)
and calcitonin (CT). At the beginning and at the end of
treatment, the glomerular filtration rate (GFR) was eva
luated by inulin clearance and cr clearance following

ureteral catheterism.

RESULTS

The results are reported in the Table 1.

	Start	End	60 days after
SERUM CR μmol/l	448.18±193.59°	610.84±273.1°	494.15±238.6
SERUM CA mmol/l	2.32±0.17*	2.51±0.11*	2.31±0.125
PTH (MM) pmol/l	305.83±263.42*	173.17±115.9*	306.25±227.1
CT pg/ml	64.33±30.62	49.80±17.31	54.50±35.05
CR CLEARANCE ml/min	22.77±9.63^	17.87±12.51^	
INULIN CLEARANCE ml/min	11.80±9.53	12.05±7.31	

$°p < 0.005$
$*p < 0.002$
$^p < 0.04$

Calcitriol therapy: variations observed in some parameters.

DISCUSSION

In agreement with most workers (1), we observed an increase in serum cr and a decrease in cr clearance during therapy with calcitriol, but these findings don't seem related to a worsening in renal function. In fact during calcitriol treatment, GFR measured by inulin clearance, the most reliable and precise method to evaluate this parameter (2), did not show any significant change. Furthermore serum cr returns to basal levels 60 days after drug suspension.

We suggest that the cr increase is due to a cr release

181

from muscle. In fact, uremic patients present myopathy,
mostly secondary to a vitamin D deficiency. Replacement
therapy with calcitriol may improve the abnormal muscle
condition and increase the release of cr from the muscle.
Similar findings have been reported in vegetarian osteo
malacic men (3); these subjects have a low dietary intake
of vitamin D and show lower than normal serum cr levels.
However, serum cr increases to normal values when vitamin
D is added to their diet.

The reduction in cr clearance at the end of therapy ob
served in our series seems in contrast with this explana
tion. However, it is possible that such apparent deterio
ration in renal function might be due to a reduced tubu
lar reserve. In fact, renal cr excretion is partly due
to a reduced tubular secretion, and in advanced renal
failure cr secretion falls quickly, due to the severity
of tubular injury; under these conditions, even a slight
increase of cr in blood can readily saturate the system.

REFERENCES

1. Christiansen, C., Rodbro, P., Christiansen, M.S.,
   Hortnach, B. and Transbol, I. Lancet ii: 700-703,
   1978.
2. Rehling, M., Moller, M.L., Thamdrup, B., Lund, J.O.
   and Trap-Jensen, J. Clin. Sci. 66: 613-619, 1984.
3. Fonseca, V., Mohiuddin, J., Weerakoon, J., Boss, M.,
   Mikhailidis, D.P. and Dandona, P. Lancet i: 1093-1095,
   1984.

TORASEMIDE, A LOOP DIURETIC, USEFUL IN CORRECTING ECF VOLUME EXPANSION IN PATIENTS WITH CHRONIC RENAL FAILURE.

D. RUSSO, A. TESTA, R.M. GAZZOTTI, P. MAZZONE, F. SAVINO, V.E. ANDREUCCI.

Department of Nephrology, II Faculty of Medicine, Naples, Italy;

INTRODUCTION

In patients with chronic renal failure (CRF) the reduced nephron mass causes salt and water retention and consequently ECF volume expansion; thus diuretic drugs have to be administered. The efficacy of diuretics, however, is hampered by the loss of functioning nephrons; furthermore residual nephrons are already in intensive diuresis due to both ECF volume expansion and increased osmotic load per nephron. Under such circumstances only high doses of loop diuretics may induce an adequate increase in salt and water excretion.

Torasemide (T) is a new loop diuretic with no structural similarity to the other available diuretic drugs. This study has been carried out to evaluate the diuretic efficacy of T in patients with CRF.

MATERIALS AND METHODS

T has been administered in 11 patients with CRF requiring diuretic treatment for both hypertension and peripheral oedemas. Serum concentration of sodium (Na), potassium (K), urea (U), creatinine (C) were measured before T and then on 4th, 7th, 9th day of the study; 24 hours urinary excretion of water (V), sodium (UNaV), potassium (UKV), were measured daily, starting on the 2nd day before untill the 2nd day after T administration. Body weight and blood pressure were recorded daily throughout the study.

The doses administered of T, chosen empirically, since the drug had never been used before in patients with CRF, was 0.77 mg/Kg/die.

RESULTS

Na, C and U were significantly increased by T. UNaV, UKV and V were significantly increased; this increase, however, was present only in the first three days of treatment with T. The reduction was significant already on the first day of treatment and was maintaned even after drug withdrawal.

DISCUSSION

T is a new high-ceiling loop diuretic claimed to have a longer duration of action than other loop diuretics; clinical studies, however, have been performed only in healthy volunteers or in patients with cardiac diseases. This study has been carried out in chronic uremia to investigate the natriuretic and diuretic effects of T. In CRF the natriuretic activity of a diuretic drug is hamperedby the reduced nephron mass and by the osmotic overload of the residual nephrons which are already in an intensive diuresis. In our study T significantly increase V and UNaV despite the severe impairement of renal function. This natriuretic effect allowed the correction of ECF volume expansion, as mirrored by normalization of blood pressure and reduction of body weight; during treatment with T both C and U increased in relation to the correction of ECF volume expansion. T significantly increased UKV leading to significant decrease in K; this kaliuretic effect, however, is not troublesome since uremic patients have serum potassium at high limit of normal values.

These results show that T is an high-ceiling loop diuretic useful in treating ECF volume expansion in patients with advanced CRF.

Table 1. Effects of T on serum sodium (Na), potassium (K), creatinine (C), urea (U), 24 hours urinary excretion of water (V), sodium (UNaV), potassium (UKV), body weight (BW) and blood pressure (BP). Numbers are means values $\pm$SEM.

	basal	4th	7th	9th	days after T
Serum					
Na	141.3	136.7°	134.9*	135.8*	
mEq/L	$\pm$1.0	$\pm$1.2	$\pm$1.4	$\pm$1.2	
K	4.4	3.9*	3.7*	3.8*	
mEq/L	$\pm$0.2	$\pm$0.2	$\pm$0.1	$\pm$0.1	
C	4.1	5.3*	5.1*	4.9*	
mg%	$\pm$0.5	$\pm$0.6	$\pm$0.6	$\pm$0.6	
U	1.1	1.5°	1.8*	1.9*	
g/L	$\pm$0.1	$\pm$0.1	$\pm$0.1	$\pm$0.1	
Urine					
V	1.5	1.7	1.7	1.3	
L/24 hr	$\pm$0.1	$\pm$0.1	$\pm$0.1	$\pm$0.1	
UNaV	66.1	72.8	59.7	21.6*	
mEq/24 hr	$\pm$6.9	$\pm$14.5	$\pm$17.5	$\pm$5.1	
UKV	33.2	48.2	41.1	32.0	
mEq/24 hr	$\pm$3.2	$\pm$3.3	$\pm$3.3	$\pm$3.0	
BW	68.4	66.7*	66.6*	66.8*	
Kg	$\pm$1.6	$\pm$1.0	$\pm$2.0	$\pm$1.7	
BP mean	126.6	110.0*	100.0*	106.6*	
mmHg	$\pm$5.8	$\pm$3.7	$\pm$4.3	$\pm$2.6	

° = p 0.05

* = p 0.01

1. Lesne, M., Clerckx-Braun, F., Dohoux, P., Uan Ypersele de Strihou, CH. Int. J. Clin. Pharm. Ther. Toxic. 20:382-397, 1982
2. Ambroes, Y., Ronflette, I., Dodion, L. Eur. J. Clin. Pharm. 31: s1-s7, 1986.
3. Lambe, R., Kennedy, O., Kenny, M., Darragh, A. Eur. J. Clin. Pharm. 31: s9-s14, 1986.
4. Broekhuysen, J., Deger, F., Douchamps, J., Ducarne, H., Hercauelz, A. Eur. J. Clin. Pharm. 31: s29-s34, 1986.

Miscellany

TREATMENT OF RAPIDLY PROGRESSIVE LUPUS GLOMERULONEPHRITIS

M.KOSELJ, J.DRINOVEC, S.KAPLAN, A.LIČINA, R.PONIKVAR
University Medical Center, Department of Nephrology, Ljubljana
Yugoslavia

INTRODUCTION

Rapidly progressive lupus glomerulonephritis (RPLGN) is a
severe and unfavorable complication of systemic lupus erythematosus.
(SLE). Progress in supportive and aggressive therapy in recent
years has considerably improved the prognosis. Since there is no
agreement about the most efficient therapy, the treatment of RPLGN
remains a highly controversial topic in clinical medicine (1,2).
In this paper, we report a follow-up of 11 patients with RPLGN,
monitored for 2-64 months. All patients were treated with prednisone
cyclophosphamide or azathioprine and plasma exchange.

PATIENTS AND METHODS

Patients who fulfilled at least 4 preliminary criteria of the
American Rheumatism Association and who showed a histological and
clinical picture of diffuse proliferative glomerulonephritis and
rapidly deteriorating renal function were included. 4 men and 7
women, aged from 20 to 49 years, were followed from 2-64 months.
Our treatment protocol consisted of prednisone 40-60 mg/day,
cyclophosphamide or azathioprine 1-2 mg/kg and plasmapheresis:
namely membrane plasma exchange at 2,3,7 and 14 day intervals for
2 months was performed. The exchanged volume was 4 % body weight;
the substitution solution was 5 % human albumin. Before the
therapy, infections were excluded and secondary hypertension
controlled.

RESULTS

Of 11 RPLGN patients treated, 7 completed the therapy while 4 died during therapy.

As shown in Table 1 the improvement in renal function, proteinuria and serologic parameters was observed in 7 patients at the end of therapy.

Table 1. Laboratory data of 7 RPLGN patients before and after therapy

Patient	S-creatinine (umol/L)		Proteinuria (g/24h)		Anti DNA (%)	
1	471	340	14.0	4.4	45	0
2	350	140	10.2	6.6	96	66
3	530	156	12.0	8.6	43	35
4	590	300	3.6	1.3	96	12
5	246	160	4.0	0.5	40	2
6	206	176	2.1	1.2	78	36
7	309	160	2.9	1.8	45	11

4 patients remained stable over a period of 2-64 months.

3 patients progressed to terminal renal failure in 12-36 months after treatment (Table 2).

Table 2. Outcome in RPLGN patients (n=7)

Patient	Follow up months	S-creatinine, umol/L		
		before th.	after th.	final value
1	12	471	340	HD
2	36	350	140	HD
3	64	530	156	260
4	24	590	300	HD
5	16	246	160	N
6	2	206	176	N
7	48	309	160	180

COMPLICATIONS

4 patients died before the end of therapy. All received cyclophosphamide orally. Their data are shown in Table 3.

Table 3. Complications of treatment in RPLGN patients

Patient	Age (yr)	Sex	Duration of SLE	S-creatinine (umol/L)	Side effects	Death
1	30	F	7 months	310	tbc sepsis	day 59
2	29	F	12 months	420	ARDS	day 7
3	24	M	4 months	390	pneumonia	day 29
4	30	M	1 month	240	ARDS	day 10

DISCUSSION

The improved prognosis of diffuse lupus glomerulonephritis is related to a more efficient management of arterial hypertension, infections and aggressive treatment of renal disease.
Encouraging results have been reported recently for intermittent cyclophosphamide pulses (3) or short course of metilprednisolone pulses (4).
Our treatment with immunosuppressive durgs and plasmapheresis was effective in the preservation of renal function, but the side effects of aggressive therapy were frequent and fatal.

REFERENCES

1. Donadio,J.V. N.Engl. J. Med. 311, 528-529, 1984.
2. Williams,D.G. Contr. Nephrol. 43, 25-35, 1984.
3. Austin,H.A., Klippel, J.H., Ballow, J.E. et al. N.Engl. J. Med. 314, 614-619, 1986.
4. Ponticelli,C., Zucchelli,P., Moroni,G.,et al. Clin. Nephrol. 28, 263-271, 1987.

THE EFFECT OF A SINGLE PERINATAL TREATMENT WITH CAPTOPRIL ON CYTOTOXICITY IN RATS

S. SONKODI AND Y. MÁNDI

1st Department of Internal Medicine and Department of
Microbiology, Albert Szent-Györgyi Medical University,
Szeged, Hungary

INTRODUCTION

Captopril, the first orally active inhibitor of
angiotensin-converting enzyme, is one of the most useful
medicines in the therapy of hypertension. Since a
suppressive effect of captopril has been found in the
cellular immune system (1), we have investigated the
cytotoxicity of this agent in rats treated perinatally.

MATERIALS AND METHODS

The experiments were performed on Wistar rats.
Pregnant animals were used 4-5 days before, the birth.

Group 1: through an abdominal incision (sterile)
0.1 ml captopril (Tensiomin; EGIS) or D-penicillamine
(Sigma) solution was injected into each amniotic
compartment space of the embryos (1 mg/ml concentration).

Group 2: the same procedure was followed, but only
the solvent was injected. Work-up was carried out 8,
16 and 32 weeks after the birth.

The natural killer (NK) cell activity (cytotoxicity)
of splenic lymphocytes was investigated with a ^{51}Cr
release assay (2). The results were expressed for 25:1,
50:1, 100:1 and 200:1 effector:target (E/T) cell ratios.

Statistical significance was calculated by
Student's two-tailed t-test.

RESULTS

Figure 1a shows that in 16-week-old captorpil-trea-
ted rats the cytotoxicity was significantly lower at each
E/T ratio than in the control animals.

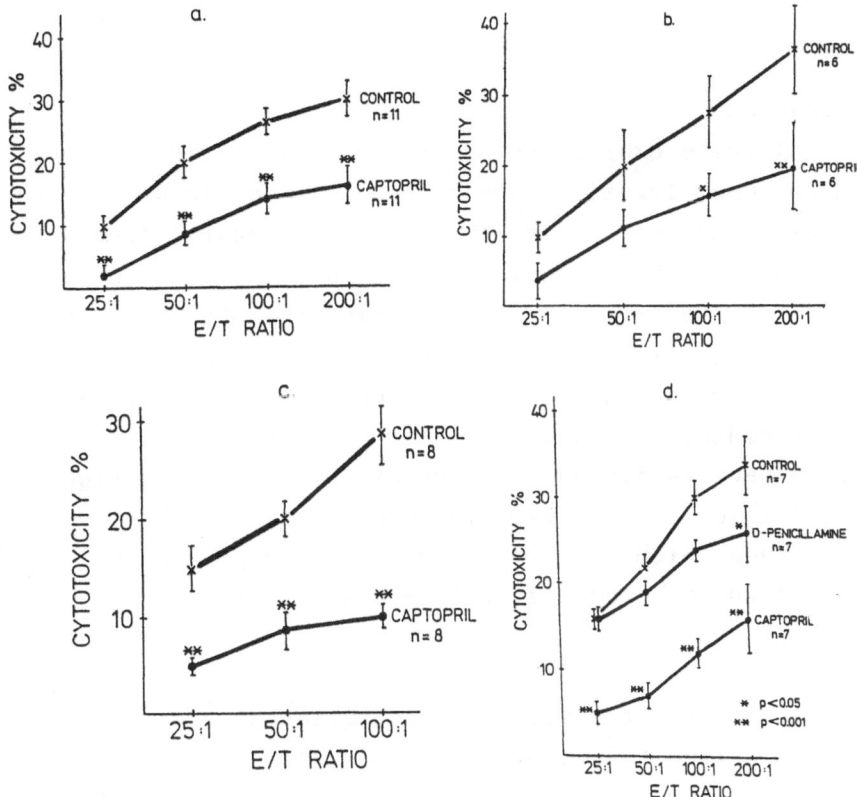

Fig.1. Effect of perinatal captorpil treatment on NK
activity of rat splenic lymphocytes. Spleen cells of
16-week-old (a), 8-week-old (b),32-week-old (c) animals
were isolated on Ficoll-Uromiro gradient (1.080), and
the cytotoxicity was then, determined by using ^{51}Cr-
-labelled YAC-1 target cells in a 4hr cytotoxic assay.
(d) Comparison of effects of captorpil and D-penicillamine on NK activity.

Similar results were obtained with 8-week-old (Fig. 1b) and 32-week-old (Fig. 1a) treated animals, but the difference was less pronounced in the younger rats.

The effect of D-penicillamine in the same experimental set up hardly differed from that of the solvent (Fig. 1d).

DISCUSSION

NK cells exhibit cytotoxicity against virus-infected or tumor targets among others (3). Our results demonstrated that a single perinatal captopril treatment caused a long-lasting effect in decreasing the cellular cytotoxic reaction in rats after birth. This effect appears to be fairly specific, as D-penicillamine, which has a similar chemical structure and is a useful medicine in the treatment of some immunological and connective tissue diseases,did not display a significant effect. These results suggest the possibility that drugs which enter the embryo during pregnancy might lead to chronic immune defets after birth.

SUMMARY

A single perinatal treatment with captorpil caused a long-lasting effect by decreasing the, cellular cytotoxic reaction in rats.

REFERENCES
1. Delfraissy, J-F.,Galanaud, P., Balavoine, J-F., Wallon, C. and Dormont, J.: Kidney Int. 25, 925-929, 1984.
2. Böyum, A.: Scand.J.Clin. Lab. Invest. 21, Suppl. 97, 77-89, 1979.
3. Hong, L.: Immun, Invest. 16, 453-499, 1987.

NEW EVIDENCE FOR THE NEUROTOXICITY OF PTH IN UREMIA

P.M.J.M. DE VRIES, M.G.G. CORTENRAAD, R.L.M. STRIJERS, P.L. OE and
S.L. VISSER

Departments of Hemodialysis and Clinical Neurophysiology, Free
University Hospital, Amsterdam, The Netherlands

INTRODUCTION

Peripheral neuropathy is recognised as a complication of uremia
in 60-65 % of the patients. There is still much discussion about its
pathophysiology and the best way to diagnose it. As neurotoxic agents
myoinositol, middle molecules and parathyroid hormone (PTH) were mentioned. Regarding diagnosis, no relation could be found between the
peripheral nerve conduction velocity and the prevalence and severity
of clinical neuropathy (1). It has been shown that H-M interval (late
response) can be delayed while motor and sensory nerve conduction ve-
locities are normal (2). The H-M interval has a very narrow normal
range and is easy to obtain.

The aims of this study were to (I) establish the prevalence of
impaired nerve conduction in patients with chronic renal failure on
maintenance hemodialysis; (II) investigate the course of nerve function during a period of maintenance hemodialysis and (III) correlate
electrophysiological changes and blood parameters that reflect the
adequacy of treatment.

PATIENTS AND METHODS

71 patients (36 women and 35 men) were followed during a mean
period of 32 months beginning at their first dialysis. All were dialysed five hours twice a week. The following parameters were studied:
* laboratory (once a month):
  - parathyroid hormone
  - urea, creatinine, uric acid
  - sodium, potassium, chloride, calcium, phosphate, alkal.phosphatase

* neurophysiology (every 6 months):
  - maximal motor nerve conduction velocity (MNCV) of the peroneal
  and ulnar nerves (m/sec). Skin temperature was measured and MNCV
  was corrected to 33 degrees C.
  - H-M interval (msec). This is the latency between the maximal
  H-response and the maximal M-response of the posterior tibial
  nerve. These values were normalised for age and body length.

Three groups of patients were formed according to the course of
their MNCV and H-M interval during the study: (I) Improvement, (II)
Deterioration and (III) No Changes. The values of MNCV and H-M interval were plotted against time. The linear regression lines were calculated. If the slope was significantly positive for MNCV and significantly negative for H-M interval, the patient was put in group I.
If the slope was significantly negative for MNCV and positive for
H-M interval, the patient was put in group II. All other patients
were put in group III.

RESULTS

At the start of the study 43 patients (60 %) showed neurophysiological signs of polyneuropathy whereas only 2 patients had clinical
signs (see table I).

Table 1. Electrophysiological abnormalities at the start of the study

Neurophysiological parameter	% abnormal
H-M interval	28 %
Motor Nerve Conduction Velocity (MNCV)	2 %
H-M interval and MNCV	30 %
total	60 %

At the end of the study 67 patients could be statistically evaluated. According to the changes of the neurophysiological parameters
they could be divided in the three considered groups:

I.   Improvement   n = 7   (10 %)
II. Deterioration n = 22   (33 %)
III. No Changes   n = 38   (57 %)

Some differences between these groups are shown in table 2.

Table 2. Some characteristics of the three groups.

Group	H-M interval (msec)	PTH (pmol/1)	age (years)	follow-up (months)
Improvement	28.2 + 0.5	28.3 + 8.3	32.0 + 4.6	17.0 + 1.6
Deterioration	30.7 + 0.7	52.8 +10.7	45.8 + 3.7	42.3 + 5.2
No changes	29.4 + 0.5	29.6 + 4.2	50.1 + 2.1	33.7 + 3.5

The start H-M intervals and MNCV values were not significantly different. The same accounted for the mean MNCV during the follow-up period. However mean H-M interval during the 32 months was significantly higher in the Deterioration group. PTH level was the only biochemical parameter that was different between the groups. The Improvement group showed a lower mean age and a shorter follow-up period. Because it seemed that a shorter dialysis period gave a better chance for improvement, the first 24 months of follow-up in each patient were investigated separately. The division into groups then was: Improvement 17 %, Deterioration 23 % and No Changes 60 %. Again the Deterioration group showed a longer H-M interval and higher PTH.

CONCLUSIONS

1. H-M interval is a more sensible test for polyneuropathy during chronic renal failure than MNCV.
2. the course of nerve function during a period of maintenance hemodialysis is 10 % improvement, 33 % deterioration and 57 % unchanged.
3. only PTH concentration correlated with neurophysiological parameters.
4. during the first 24 months of hemodialysis the chance for improvement is slightly higher than afterwards.

REFERENCES

1. Nielsen, V.K. Acta. Med. Scand. 194: 455, 1973.
2. Lachman, T., Shahani, B.T. and Young, R.R. J. Neurol. Neurosurg. Psychiat. 43: 156-162, 1980.

CONNECTION BETWEEN CHRONIC RENAL INSUFFICIENCY AND ALLUVIAL SOILS IN
CENTRAL GREECE.

TH. GALEAS, D. MYLONAS, P. FOUNTA.
General Hospital of Trikala, Artificial Kidney Department, Greece.

INTRODUCTION

Central Greece is available for the study of the influence of
soil on health for two reasons. First because it consists of   two
kinds of soils clearly separated between each other and secondly
because there hasnót been any significant moving of the population
in the recent years. (1,2). These two kinds of soils are   the
alluvial soils and non-alluvial soils. (Fig. 1).
In this work it is examined whether the constitution of the soil has
any influence on the frequency of appearance of chronic renal insufficiency. (3).

MATERIAL AND METHOD

We recorded the 224 patients who have been in the programme of
chronic hemodialysis since 1981. On the basis of the geochemical
constitution of the soil (1,4) we clasified them, bearing   in
mind their place of birth or residence for the last 20 years, in
two categories: a) patients living on alluvial soils and b)patients
living on non-alluvial soils. Using the X^2 method we considered
whether the increased number of nephropathies has any connection
with the constitution of the soil.

RESULTS

We observed a) 188 patients from the 224 were born   or were
residents in the last 20 years in areas with alluvial soils.(Fig.II)
b) 36 patients were born or lived on non-alluvial soils.

It is noticed that frequency of nephropathies was significantly higher on alluvial soils than on non-alluvial soils ($P < 0,05$).

DISCUSSION

In our attempt to estimate the distance the patients had to travel to receive their regular hemodialysis at the artificial kidney departments of the area we experienced an unexpected finding which led us to make a chartography study of the places in which these patients were born or lived.

In a smaller scale study of Galeas et al. (5) it had been shown that there is a close interconnection between the geochemical environment and the geographical distribution as it concerns chronic renal insufficiency. Extending our study in Central Greece we examined the relation of alluvial and non-alluvial soils with chronic renal insufficiency.

Alluvial soils are soils with the highest capacity in the exchange or cations. (4). Cation-exchange processes are known to exist in the smallest molecules of the soil (4). It is also known that plants take up the nessacery elements for their feeding, in the form of ions, from the territorial solution and from the colloidal components.

We assume that in the areas with alluvia soils where concentration of nephropathies was observed the following might happen:1. Essential metals nessacery for life (Fe, Zn, Co) are exchanged with heavy, toxic metals (Ca, Bi, Mn, Ni, Pb) (4) non essential for life.

To explain this we refer to law of masses (4) or to the theory that some cations have greater exchange capacity compared with others (cation exchange) (4) 2. There might be a deficiency of bioessential trace elements (Se, Zn, Cr, Ni, Si, F) in the endemic areas (3,6).

CONCLUSION

According to our study part of the nephropathies in this area might have a connection with the chemical constitution of the soil. Although international bibliography (7,8,9) has not come to definite conclusions we believe that geographical distribution shows that the whole investigation should be re-examined.

REFERENCES

1. Territorial chart of Greece by Dr. S. Katakouzinos.
2. Census 1981. National Statistic Service.
3. Maksimovic Z. 2nd Symposium on Geochemistry and Health,
   Royal Society London. 20-23.4.1987.
4. Katakouzinos S. Vol I, II. 1958.
5. Galeas Th., Mylonas D., Mavrikakis M., Sdrakas L. 43rd Panhellenic
   Meeting of the Iatrosurgical Society.
6. Klaws Schwarz. Med. Cl. N. Am. 60:981-997, 1976.
7. Fitzgerald Pr., Peterson J., Lue-Hing C. Am. J. Vet. Res.46 (3)
   703-7. 1985.
8. Baars Aj., Van Beek H., De Graaf Gj., Spierenburg Tj.,Beeftink Wg.,
   Nieuwenhuize J. Arch Toxicol (suppl), 9: 410-3. 1986.
9. Stoewsand Gs et al. J. Toxic.Env.Health.18 (3) 369-76. 1986.

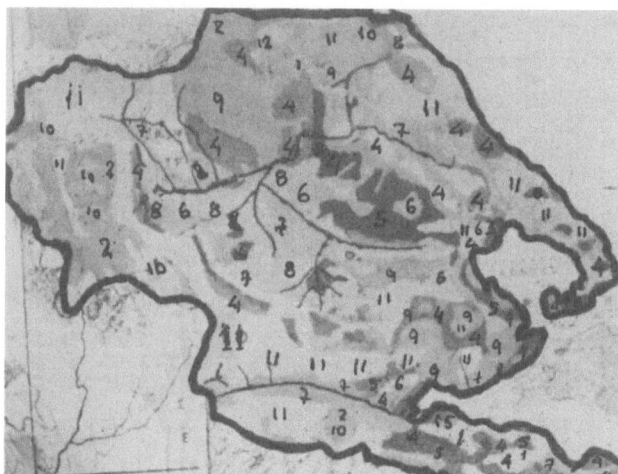

Fig. 1. 1-9 alluvial soils. 10-14 non-alluvial soils.

Fig. 2. We can clearly see the concentration of nephropathies in certain areas.

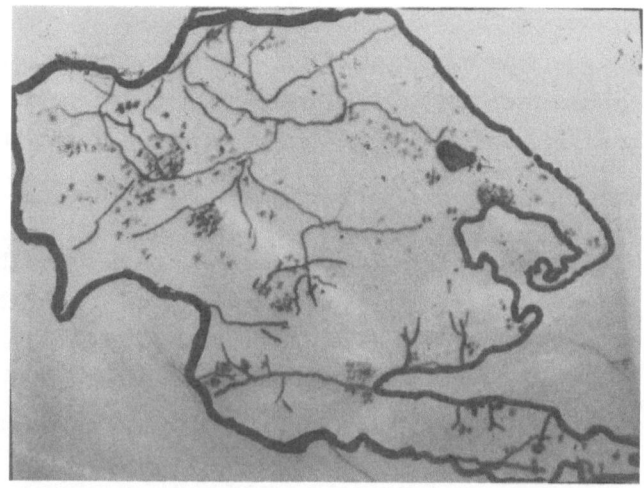

III. DIALYSIS

New Techniques

CLEARANCES OF SMALL SOLUTES IN HEMODIAFILTRATION AND PAIRED FILTRATION DIALYSIS.

B. Memoli, R.M. Gazzotti, T. Rampino, C. Libetta, G. Iorio°, E. Drioli° and V.E. Andreucci.
Dept. of Nephrology, II Faculty of Medicine and °Dept. of Chem. Eng., University of Naples, Italy.

INTRODUCTION.

Hemodiafiltration (HDF) can be performed both in one single hemofilter in which the two processes, dialysis and hemofiltration, are simultaneously carried out, or in two separated devices (Paired Filtration Dialysis, PFD) one of which works in ultrafiltration and the other one as a traditional dialyzer. Aim of this study was to compare the performances of HDF and PFD treatments on the basis of "in vivo" clearance tests.

MATERIALS AND METHODS.

The study was performed on 2 patients treated with HDF and 2 patients treated with PFD.   Blood axial flow rate was in both treatments 300 ml/min. "In vivo" clearance tests of urea, creatinine, phosphate and uric acid, were performed in both treatments by collecting simultaneously two blood samples at the hemofilter inlet and outlet. The clearances (total (diffusive + convective), diffusive and convective) were calculated referring to plasma solute concentrations and plasma volumetric flow rates.

RESULTS.

Table I shows ultrafiltration flow rates and total, diffusive and convective clearances of urea, creatinine, phosphate and uric acid in HDF and PFD treatments.

Paired measurements of diffusive and convective clearances in HDF, obtained at different ultrafiltration flow rates (range 33.75 - 82.5 ml/min), showed an inverse relationship for urea ($r = -0.7422$, <p 0.01) (Fig.1), creatinine ($r = -0.7797$, $p < 0.01$), phosphate ($r = -0.8368$, $p < 0.01$) and uric acid ($r = -0.9212$, $p < 0.01$).

TABLE I.

Comparison of ultrafiltration flow rates (Uf) and Total, Diffusive and Convective clearances of urea, creatinine, phosphate and uric acid in HDF and PFD.

	Total	Diffusive	Convective	Uf
Urea clearances				
HDF	176.9±12.2	128.8±16.7	48.1±6.0	71.5±5
PFD	210.2±17.3	170.2±17.4	40	40
p	<0.001	<0.001	<0.005	<0.001
Creatinine clearances				
HDF	156.5±7.4	99.7±10.8	53.2±5.2	71.5±5
PFD	153.1±13.5	113.1±13.5	40	40
p	ns	<0.001	<0.001	<0.001
Phosphate clearances				
HDF	150.3±9.6	96.3±14.2	54.0±6.3	71.5±5
PFD	141.7±8.3	101.7±8.3	40	40
p	ns	ns	<0.001	<0.001
Uric acid clearances				
HDF	142.7±11.2	87.2±15.2	55.4±6.2	71.5±5
PFD	135.9±11.6	95.9±11.6	40	40
p	ns	ns	<0.001	<0.001

DISCUSSION.

The results of clearance tests indicate a greater efficacy of PFD in which diffusive and convective mass transfer mechanisms are completely separated, as compared with HDF where these mechanisms mutually interfere. In particular we observed that: a) in HDF convective clearance is always lower than ultrafiltrate flow rate, unlike in PFD where they coincide; b) diffusive clearances, specially

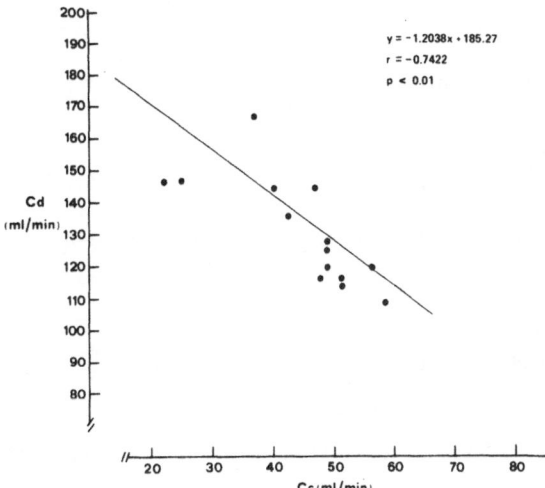

Fig.1. Relationship between diffusive (Cd) and convective (Cc) urea clearance in postdilutional HDF.

for highly diffusible solutes like urea and creatinine, are higher in PFD than in HDF; c) urea total clearance is greater in PFD than in HDF although ultrafiltration flow rate is higher in HDF than in PFD.

The diffusive clearance decrease observed in HDF may be accounted for by: 1) reduction of axial flow rate along the filter due to ultrafiltration and 2) accumulation of plasma proteins on the pressurized side of the membrane leading to the formation of a macromolecular gel that may affect diffusive transport (concentration polarization) (1).

REFERENCES.

1) Drioli E, Luchini P, Pozzi A, Memoli B, Calderaro V, Terracciano V, Andreucci VE, Salvatore M, Bazzicalupo L and Alfano B. ASAIO Journal, 5:16-21, 1982.

L-CARNITINE ADDITION IN THE DIALYSIS FLUID: A NEW THERAPEUTICAL
APPROACH FOR HEMODIALYSIS PATIENTS.

G.M. VACHA, G. GIORCELLI, S. D'IDDIO, G. VALENTINI, E. BAGIELLA,
A. PROCOPIO, S. DI DONATO and M. CORSI

Department of Nephrology and Dialysis, Ospedale Mauriziano
Umberto I, Turin, Italy

INTRODUCTION

In a previous study (1) we postulated that the long-term i.v.
administration of L-carnitine in hemodialysis patients is inadequate
since it induces an excessive accumulation of carnitine (free and esters)
in blood and muscle. In order to further elucidate the appropriate dosage
regimen and route of administration the present study has been carried out.

MATERIALS AND METHODS

A group of 22 stable hemodialysis patients of either sex who had
been on L-carnitine therapy (2 g/i.v./each dialysis) for a minimum of 12
months were selected. Dietary intake was standardized. Following baseline
evaluations intravenous L-carnitine therapy was discontinued for 4 months.
Then the patients received L-carnitine i.v. (1 g/end dialysis) for 1 month.
Finally the patients were divided into two subgroups of 11 patients each
and L-carnitine was added to the dialysate for 3 months (Group 1: 75 μml/l;
Group 2: 150 μmol/l). Pre-dialysis blood samples (carnitine and lipid
determination) were obtained at the enrollment and at the end of each
of the eight months of the study. Muscle biopsies (carnitine determination)
were obtained at the baseline, after 4 and 8 months.

RESULTS

All the patients exhibited marked elevations in serum total carnitine
(875 $\pm$ 292 μM; normal value: 53 $\pm$ 18 μM) and in muscle total carnitine (45

± 17 μmol/gNCP, normal value: 19 ± 5 μmol/gNCP). Following the 4 months wash-out period the muscle values were comparable with dose of normal subjects and did not significantly change during the second treatment. Also the serum concentrations showed a decrease and a new steady-state reflecting the concentration of L-carnitine added in the dialysate. Serum lipid pattern (Fig. 1) showed significant changes during the study.

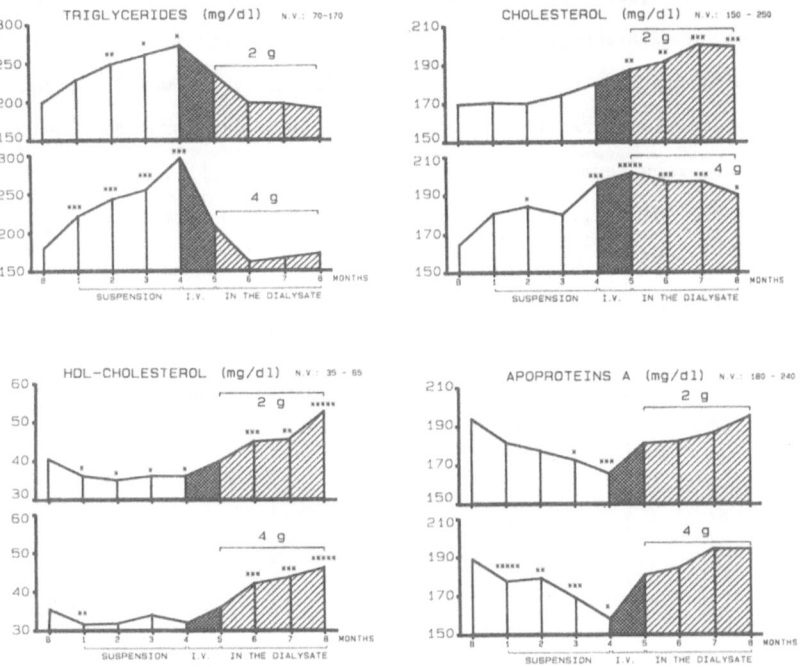

Fig. 1 Serum lipid profile during the study. In the figure the symbols (*) indicate the p value of paired Student's "t" test versus the baseline (B) - *p < 0.05; **p < 0.02; ***p < 0.01; ****p < 0.001. ANOVA analysis showed the following results: Triglycerides p < 0.005; Cholesterol p < 0.025; HDL-Cholesterol p < 0.001: Apoproteins A p < 0.025. No significant differences between the groups were observed.

DISCUSSION

The present results suggest that serum carnitine concentrations of 100 to 200 μmol/l may be appropriate as a target range to achieve the desired results. If we accept the proposed level as being optimal, then the task becomes one of finding the most efficient and cost effective method of achieving that level. In the present study we have demonstrated positive lipid effects with the addition of either 2 or 4 g of L-carnitine to the dialysate. Although the data are not conclusive, it is our opinion that the addition of 2 g of L-carnitine to the dialysate would adequately meet therapeutic requirements. In patients in whom carnitine deficiency is suspected, long-term hemodialysis patients for example, priming with an initial period of i.v. therapy may be desirable to restore muscle carnitine stores to normal levels.

REFERENCES

1. Vacha, G.M., Corsi, M., Giorcelli, G., D'Iddio, S. and Maccari, F. Curr. Ther. Res. 37(3): 505-516, 1985

BIDIRECTIONAL BLOOD-PUMP WITH A BIDIRECTIONAL BLOOD-PASSAGE THROUGH THE ARTIFICIAL KIDNEY.

R. HOMBROUCKX, R. BEELEN, L.LARNO, F. VAN WETTER, J.Y. DE VOS.
Dialysis Unit, Kliniek Hogerlucht, Ronse, Belgium.

INTRODUCTION

Inspired by the very efficient respiratory system of the pigeon, a new single-needle dialysis system has been developed, whereby a double passage of the blood through the exchange organ (this being the artificial kidney-AK) was contemplated.

We tested a bidirectional blood-pump,(BDP)(Fig.1) which through one needle and one blood-line pumps the blood from the bloodvessel, then guides it through the AK (first passage) (Fig. 2) to an expansion chamber (EC), located above the AK; the pressure is monitored in that EC, and upon attaining a preset max. pressure, the pump changes direction, empties the arterial chamber through the AK (second passage) (Fig.3) and directs the blood back into the patient's blood-vessel. The pump is controlled by a min. and max. manometer setting, the pressures being recorded in the EC.

EQUIPMENT AND METHODS

The system consists of a bipuncture needle, a modified blood-line, the BDP, this being a compact peristaltic blood-pump, modified for bidirectional functioning by us. Further, there is the AK that may be of any type, on condition that it has a low blood-priming volume, a low dialysate priming volume and a rigid membrane structure (thus for preference a capillary kidney). There also is the EC, which should consist of a tubular structure of about 5 cm diameter and about 15 cm in height, with a rigid wall, ending conically below in the blood-line towards the kidney,and above provided with a pressure line with a bacterial-filter.

Finally, we would mention the incorporation in the pressure line of a large <u>compliance chamber(CC)</u> with a capacity of 2000 ml of air. That large air chamber is necessary as a buffer for preventing large pressure fluctuations on the manometer (and in the AK).

Thet BDP is controlled by way of min. and max. pressure adjustment on a manometer with min. and max. settings in the positive and/or negative areas ; these settings are determining the <u>ultrafiltration</u>.

RESULTS

The overall dialysis ratio's for most molecules are comparable with the double head-pump (DHP) results (Fig. 4); however, the bidirectional AK passage results in a better extraction pattern for phosphate, especially when the direction of the dialysate flow is changed (Fig. 5).

DISCUSSION

The greatest disadvantage of the system is the <u>recirculation</u> of the dead-volume blood, (content of bloodline and pumpsegment) which reduces the overall efficiency of the system.

However, as soon as the <u>stroke volume</u> becomes three to four times greater than the dead volume, this recirculation has an almost negligible effect on the ultimate efficiency. To avoid excessive stroke volumes, we naturally miniaturise the system as much as possible.

The <u>ultrafiltration control</u> is easily obtained by the min. and max. pressure setting of the manometer.

P.S. <u>It is the only single-needle system wherein the high peak flows that pass through the needle, also effectively pass through the kidney and this in both directions per cycle.</u>

CONCLUSION

1* Simple system, which renders it suitable for home- and low-care dialysis (can be carried out by a patient without a partner), but just as suitable for routine dialysis or haemofiltration.

2* The high effective bidirectional flow through the artificial kidney renders the system, according to the direction of the dialysate flow, suitable for a more selective clearing of either small molecules or for phosphorus and middle molecules.

3* Easy ultrafiltration monitoring, independent of the bloodflow.

4* Low priming volume, which reduces periods of hypotension during the dialysis and which also makes a rinse-back with a minimal quantity of physiological solution possible.

5* By the lower number of pumphead switchings, also less haemolysis than in other tidal single-needle systems.

6* Very economical system, as concerns both the disposables and the hardware.

PRINCIPLE

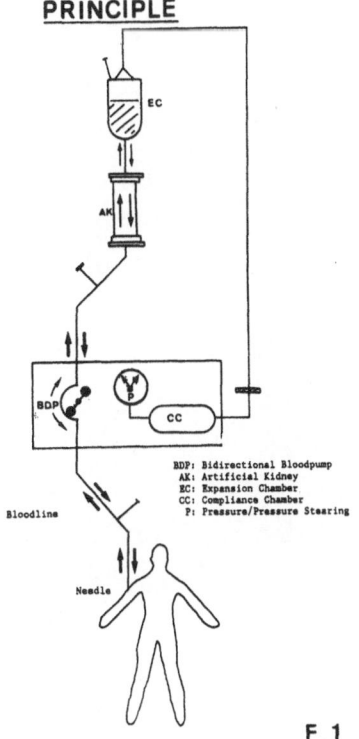

BDP: Bidirectional Bloodpump
AK: Artificial Kidney
EC: Expansion Chamber
CC: Compliance Chamber
P: Pressure/Pressure Steering

F.1

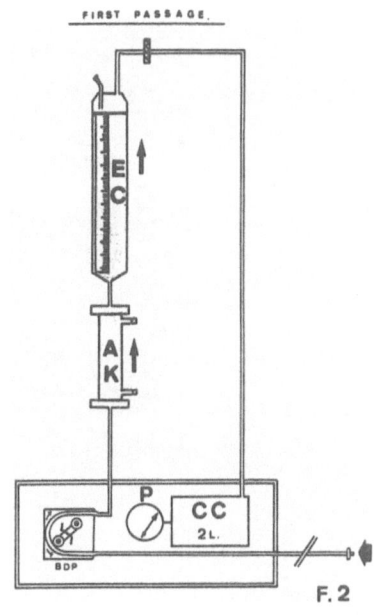

FIRST PASSAGE

F.2

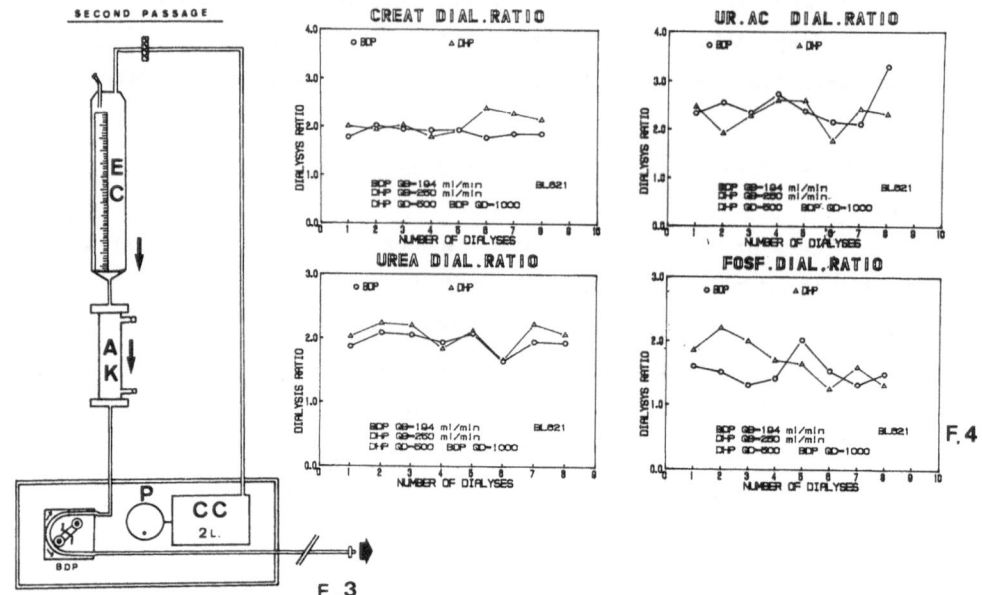

F.3

F.4

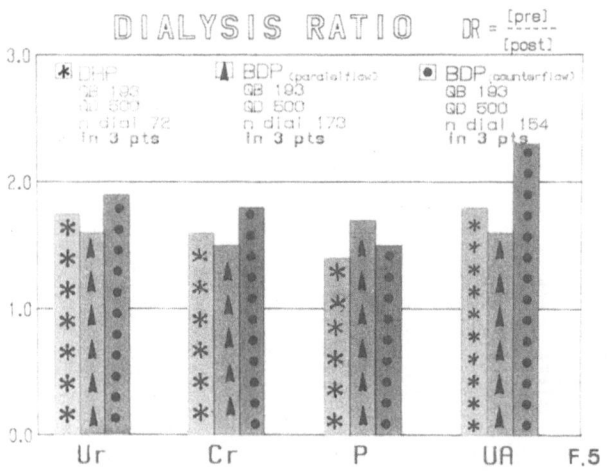

F.5

HEMODIALYSIS WITH LOW FLOW OF STERILE DIALYSATE (LSDH). EXPERIENCE OF TWO YEARS

BRIGNON P., FALLER Bernadette, MARICHAL J.F. - Service de Néphrologie - Hôpital Pasteur - 68021 COLMAR - FRANCE ; RICHALLEY G., HOSPAL, BASEL, CH.

Over the past several years the strategy of renal replacement therapy in seriously ill and hemodynamic unstable patients with acute renal failure (ARF) changed. First a continuous technique was proposed : CAVH (3). But, in order to increase the clearances to the level required by hypercatabolic patients diffusion was added in CAVHD (2).

We report our experience of an intermittent technique which combines low flow rates in order to achieve maximum diffusion of the solutes : low flow sterile dialysate hemodialysis : LSDH. We have extended this treatment to patients with chronic renal failure (CRF).

PATIENTS

With ARF

138 sessions of LSDH were performed in 32 patients (18 males, 14 females) aged 69 $\pm$ 12 years. Each patient underwent an average of 4.8 $\pm$ 3.2 sessions. Beside ARF, the patients presented congestive heart failure (5), cancer (8) and unstable cardiovascular state (16).

With CRF

8 patients (5 males, 3 females) aged 67 $\pm$ 9 years, have been treated with LSDH during a cumulative period of 71 patients-months. That is 128 $\pm$ 107 sessions during 8.9 $\pm$ 8.6 months for each patient. All patients were with congestive heart failure or poor general condition. For 2 patients, LSDH represents the first renal replacement therapy, 3 were transferred from conventional hemodialysis because of hemodynamic intolerance, 3 from CAPD after persistent peritonitis. 2 patients are still in treatment. LSDH was stopped in 6 patients, for inadequate dialysis (1 case), technical reasons (4) and because of death (1).

METHOD

Description of the technique

The hemofilter is an AN-69 SCU-CAVH flat plate of 0.43 m2. Both the blood and dialysate circulation are monitored by an BSM 22*. The blood flow provided by either an internal jugular vein catheter (ARF) or an arterio-veinous fistula (CRF) averages 150 ml/mn. The sterile dialysate is conditionned in 5 1-plastic bags. The composition (m-mol/1) is : Na 140, K 0 to 4, Cl 109.5, lactate 40, Ca 2. It is administered at a flow rate of 83 ml/mn (1 bag/h). The outlet line remains open so that the dialysate with the additional ultrafiltrate is collected in a container. The 6-hour sessions are repeated every other day.

Evaluation of the adequacy of dialysis

The urea generation rate is obtained by measuring the concentration of urea in the dialysate and additional ultrafiltrate.

The evaluation of protein catabolic rate (PCR) is based on the urea generation rate (1).

RESULTS

The excellent hemodynamic tolerance dramatically improves the quality of life of the patients with CRF. This result makes the patient accept the duration and the frequency of the sessions. We did'nt observe clinical or electric symptoms of neuropathy after 2 years of treatment.

The biological results are summarized in Table I and II.

BIOLOGICAL RESULTS

	BEFORE SESSION					CLEARANCE		
	UREA mmol/1	CREATININE umol/1	PHOSPHORUS mmol/1	HEMATOCRITE %		UREA ml/mn	CREATININE ml/mn	PHOSPHORUS ml/mn
C R F	30 +/- 9.02	928 +/- 238.68	1.56 +/- 0.58	26.91 +/- 5.56	C R F	54.40 +/- 5.09	48.19 +/- 2.90	39.30 +/- 2.97
A R F	40.58 +/- 6.01	805.35 +/- 231.60	-	28.88 +/- 2.49	A R F	59.69 +/- 6.36	47.73 +/- 3.61	-

* HOSPAL, Basel, CH.

The adequacy of dialysis is regularly followed by the evaluation of PCR. The patients still on treatment show a stable PCR after 1 and 2 years.

CONCLUSION

LSDH is simple, easy to handle technique. It does'nt require complicated devices, any water treatment or dialysis fluid delivery system. It is usuable anywhere, especially in Intensive Care Unit by nurses not trained in hemodialysis. The disavantages of the technique include the lenght of the sessions and the cost of the bags of dialysate.

Because of the good hemodynamic tolerance LSDH may be considered as a modality of renal replacement therapy in ARF. The procedure realizes biocompatible conditions by the combined use of sterile dialysate and AN-69 hemofilter.

Nevertheless, in the treatment of CRF, LSDH still is of interest from the hemodynamic tolerance point of view, but, as shown by the biological results, its use is limited to elderly patients with low catabolic rate.

REFERENCES

1. Farrel, P.C., Gotch, F.A. - Dialysis therapy guided by kinetic modelling : applications of a variable-volume simple-pool model for urea kinetics - Second Austral-Asian Conference on Heat and Mass Transfer, Sydney, 77, 29-37.

2. Geronimus, R., Schneider, N. - Continuous arterioveinous hemodialysis : a new modality for treatment of acute renal failure - TRANS AM SOC ARTIFICIAL INTERN ORGANS, 1984, XXX, 610.

3. Kramer, P., Wigger, W., Rieger, J., Mathali, D., Scheler, F. - Arterioveinous hemofiltration : a new and simple method for treatment of overhydrated patients resistant to diuretics - Klin WSCHR, 1977, 55, 1121

CONTINUOUS VENO-VENOUS HEMOFILTRATION (CVVH) FOR HEMODYNAMIC STABILIZATION BY BLOOD COOLING IN SEPTIC SHOCK

K. SODEMANN, G.E. SCHÄFER

Med. Klinik III, Städtische Kliniken, D-6050 Offenbach/M, FRG

INTRODUCTION

Despite all the endeavors of intensive-care medicine, septic shock is still a clinical picture with a high lethality. When multiple organ failure is present in addition, the survival rate is at best 10% to 20%. Here, acute renal failure is a feared complication in which the necessary detoxication and dehydration measures can contribute to further destabilization of the disease course. We therefore investigated the influence of continous veno-venous hemofiltration (CVVH) in patients in septic shock.

In general, a distinction is made today between early hyperdynamic and the late hypodynamic phase. In this stage, an acute oligo-anuric renal failure is to be expected almost regularly.

As an alternative to conventional renal replacement therapy (RRT) by means of hemodialysis, the method of continous arterio-venous hemofiltration (CAVH) developed by CRAMER (1) in 1977 has been used with increasing frequency in recent years in critically ill patients.

We used a pump-supported CVVH which was presented for the first time in this form by BISCHOFF (2) in 1982.

MATERIALS AND METHODS

Besides an especially developed blood pump (NFG 05, Dialysetechnik), we use two commercially available devices to balance the input and output (Intramat 1000, MSB). Here, a continous excess of filtrate is produced by the polysulfone filter used, which has a surface of 1.35 m² (AV 600, Fresenius) with a low rate of blood pumping of 120 to 150 ml/min, so that no suction of filtrate is produced by the infusion pumps used. The influence on hemodynamic parameters was measured by Swan-Ganz-thermodilution catheter.

All the patients we investigated were in the hypodynamic phase of septic shock and displayed an acute oligo-anuric renal failure without hyperhydration syndrome. Besides the catecholamine-refractory hypotension, there was in addition respiratory insufficiency requiring artificial ventilation in all patients.

RESULTS

	BT	MAP	HR	RA	CO	SV	SO₂PA	TPR
before	41.2±1.0	46±17	149±14	5±2	4.7±1.1	32±8	52±11	685±112
during	36.8±1.0*	98±10**	101±9*	7±2	6.8±1.5*	68±2*	65±8*	1091±144*

* p<0.01, ** p<0.001   RA=right atrial pressure

Within an average of 16±9.5 hours, the mean body temperature (BT) fell from 41.2°C to 36.8°C by extracorporeal cooling of the blood as well as input of cooled substitution solution. The mean heart rate (HR) also fell from 149 to 101 beats/minute. In connection with the lowering of temperature, the mean arterial blood pressure (MAP) rose from 46 mmHg to 98 mmHg, and the total peripheral resistance (TPR) rose from 685 to 1091 dyn.sec.cm^{-5}. We observed an improvement of the other hemodynamic parameters: the cardiac output (CO) rose from 4.7 l/min to 6.8 l/min, the stroke volume (SV) from 32 ml to 68 ml. The mixed venous oxygen saturation (SO₂PA) rose from 52% to 65%.

DISCUSSION

We were able to record an astonishing improvement in findings in connection with the lowering of the BT by CVVH. It is known from the results of hemodynamic follow-up that a significant increase of the CO as well as an elevation of metabolic rates with increased oxygen consumption occur in patients with cancer diseases who were subjected to extracorporal hyperthermia up to 42°C by CAVH (3). We interpret our results in the following terms: the reverse effect contributes to cardiac relief of the insufficient heart by reduction of the metabolic rates. In addition, WELTER and THAUER (4) already proved in 1943 that a lowering of the BT by 2°C leads to pronounced rise of total peripheral resistance. This is likely to be the second major effect contributing to hemodynamic stabilization.

It is possible that the elimination of mediators by means of hemofiltration is significant in anuric patients in septic shock (5).

The present results are the more remarkable since existing circulatory instabilty is additionally intensified by most methods of renal replacement therapy.

MAURITZ (6) has presented the largest-scale study showing the favorable effect of CVVH compared to acetate dialysis with regard to survival rate. From our own observations, but also in evaluation of the literature, the advantages of continous treatment methods appear to predominate compared to the intermittent forms of RRT. We also expect advantages from CVVH compared to CAVH: the large amount of filtrate always enables adequate detoxication. This is also a precondition for an adequate cooling of the blood in highly febrile progress forms.

CONCLUSIONS

In septic shock, CVVH can contribute to hemodynamic stabilization by lowering of BT. It is possible that the elimination of toxins plays an additional role. In the developement of an acute renal failure, CVVH should be used at an early stage.

REFERENCES:

(1) KRAMER, P. et al. : Arterio-venous hemofiltration, Klin. Wschr. 55, 1121, 1977
(2) BISCHOFF, K., M. DOEHN : Kontinuierliche Pumpen-getriebene Ultrafiltration bei Nierenversagen, in: KRAMER, P.(Ed.): Arterio-venöse Hämofiltration, Göttingen, 226-242, 1982
(3) MAETA, M. et al. : Effect of extracorporeally induced total body hyperthermia for cancer on cardiovascular function., Jpn Heart J, 25 (6) 993-1000, 1984
(4) WELTER, K., THAUER, R., Der Kreislauf im Dienste der Wärmeregulation., Ges Exptl Med 112: 345-379, 1943
(5) CORAIM, F.J., Acute respiratory failure after cardiac surgery: Clinical experience with the application of continous arteriovenous hemofiltration, Critical Care Medicine Vol.14 No.6, 714-718, 8.1986
(6) MAURITZ, W., Akutes Nierenversagen bei abdomineller Sepsis, Anästh. Intensivther. Notfallmed. 21, 212-217, 1986

BLOOD VOLUME CHANGES DURING HEMODIALYSIS DETECTED BY CONDUCTIVITY
MEASUREMENTS

P.M.J.M. DE VRIES, P.M. KOUW, J.H. MEIJER, V. VISSER,
P.L. OE, H. SCHNEIDER AND A.J.M. DONKER

Departments of Hemodialysis and Medical Physics,
Free University, Amsterdam, The Netherlands

INTRODUCTION

Hypotension is one of the most frequently observed complications
during hemodialysis. It is partly due to a decrease of blood volume
by ultrafiltration. Refilling of the blood compartment with fluid
from the overhydrated interstitium is not rapid enough to compensate
this ultrafiltration. A continuous on-line monitoring system to detect variations in blood volume could be used to detect hypovolemia
in an early phase. Measurement of reciprocal hemoglobin values
serves this purpose well. However a procedure of lysis of erythrocytes and oxygenation of hemoglobin has to be followed with the
current technique. The purpose of this study was to evaluate the
value of conductivity measurements of blood for the detection of
hematocrit. The hematocrit values obtained with this method were
correlated with those measured with normal laboratory methods.
Furthermore the course of red cell volume, hematocrit, plasma - and
blood volume during hemodialysis was detected.

PATIENTS AND METHODS

23 patients on maintenance hemodialysis (two times five hours a
week) were studied. At the start of dialysis, after three hours and
at the end of treatment the following parameters were studied:
* conductivity of blood (Y_{bl}) and of plasma (Y_{pl})
* erythrocyte count (ery), hematocrit with normal laboratory (Ht_m)
The conductivity measurements were done in a conductivity cell
with four circular electrodes. The outer two were used to apply an
alternating current of 1 mA r.m.s. at 40 kHz; the inner two to mea-

sure the conductivity. The fluid measured was kept at a constant temperature of 37 degrees Celsius.

The hematocrit was calculated (Ht_c) out of Y_{bl} and Y_{pl} according to an equation based on experimental work of Hanai (1) and modified for this purpose:

$$Ht_c = 1 - \left(\frac{Y_{bl}}{Y_{pl}} \right)^{0.67}$$

Ht_m and Ht_c were correlated. Mean cellular volume of the red cell was calculated according to: $MCV = Ht / ery$. Blood volume (BV) changes were calculated both with reciprocal hematocrit (Ht_c) values (BV_h) and with reciprocal erythrocyte counts (BV_e). The amount of ultrafiltration was recorded.

RESULTS

Ht_m and Ht_c correlated significantly ($Ht_m = 0.98\ Ht_c - 0.48$; $r = 0.97$; $p < 0.001$), the slope of the regression line being close to 1.0. The changes of Ht_c, MCV_c, BV and PV are shown in table 1.

Table 1. The course of some calculated variables during dialysis.

variable	t = 3 hours	t = 5 hours
Ht_c	109.5 ± 6.5	112.1 ± 5.7
MCV_c	98.8 ± 8.3	97.2 ± 2.5
BV_h	91.2 ± 5.4	88.0 ± 3.4
BV_e	90.7 ± 5.2	86.7 ± 2.1
PV	87.6 ± 5.9	82.4 ± 2.4

All values are espressed as percentage of the starting value

The decrease of MCV_c was not significant. The same accounted for the difference between BV_h and BV_e. This means that reciprocal hematocrit values are just as good for blood volume calculation as reciprocal erythrocyte counts.

The fall of BV (dBV) and of PV (dPV) showed a significant correlation with the amount of fluid that was withdrawn from the patient by means of ultrafiltration (UF): $dBV = 4.9\ UF - 1.6$; $0.025 < p < 0.05$ and $dPV = 6.8\ UF - 1.3$; $0.01 < p < 0.025$. (UF is in liters).

A high percentual fall of BV and PV was more often seen in patients suffering from frequent episodes of hypotension than in normotensive patients.

DISCUSSION

This study shows that conductivity measurements make an accurate determination of hematocrit possible. As reciprocal hematocrit values are a measure for blood volume changes, these conductivity determinations offer us the possibility to monitor blood volume during hemodialysis. This study must be seen as a pilot study for further investigations. The described method can not be used in this form for continuous monitoring because plasma has to be measured separately. In order to overcome this handicap ultrafiltrate can be measured instead of plasma. Combined conductivity measurements of blood at low and high frequencies may also enable us to overcome this problem. This multi-frequent technique is in development and might make it possible to calculate hematocrit out of blood conductivity alone.

CONCLUSIONS
1. conductivity measurements of blood and plasma make accurate calculation of hematocrit possible.
2. as MCV remains fairly constant during hemodialysis, reciprocal hematocrit values are a measure for blood volume changes.
3. changes of blood- and plasma volume depend on ultrafiltration and were found to be 13 and 18 per cent respectively.
4. continuous blood volume monitoring during hemodialysis might be possible with the described conductivity method in the future.

REFERENCES
1. Hanai, T. In: Sherman (ed): Emulsion science. London, Acad. Press, 1968.

A NEW HEMODIALYSIS SINGLE PATIENT UNIT IN THE SHORT DIALYSIS
TREATMENTS

B.AGAZIA,F.ANGOLETTA,L.GUARDA,C.LOMBINI,S.LORENZI,P.MARCHINI,M.NORDIO
and E.SAPORITI
Department of Nephrology,Santi Giovanni e Paolo Hospital,VENICE,Italy

INTRODUCTION

In the last years new highly permeables membranes have been
introduced in dialysis practice, in order to improve the treatment
effectiveness(1,2);moreover,the dialysis schedule has been often
shortened(3,4).Both the innovations require a strict control of
ultrafiltration (UF) during regular dialysis treatment(RTD),thus
various automatic-UF-control monitors have been set up in order to
ease new dialysis systems(5,6).The present study aims to test a new
hemodialysis single patient unit (Monitral-S$^{®}$,Hospal) in a little
group of subjects who underwent short dialysis treatment.

MATERIALS AND METHODS

Four RTD outpatients(3 males,1 female;mean age 57.5 yrs,range
49-72;mean dialytic age 37.7 mo,range 13-59)entered the study,after
informed consent.All were well-estabilished on 4 hrs,three times a
week RTD and previously considered as candidate for fast dialysis.
Two of them underwent high-flux-bicarbonate short dialysis (Q_B 350
ml/min,Q_D 500 ml/min,time 180 min) and two underwent soft-hemodia-
filtration,or biofiltration(Q_B 300 ml/min,Q_D 500 ml/min,Q_R 6 1).The
Monitral-S unit was evaluated during 7 mo (Nov.86-May 87); 364 treatments were performed and the results recorded in opportune sheets.

The following parameters were considered: 1) the mean weight
loss by direct balance-bed measurements; 2) the achievements of

scheduled dry weight,as previously; 3)the scheduled total weight loss
both at the beginning and at the end of each treatment,as reported in
Monitral-S display; 4)the total weight loss reported on display vs
the total true weight loss as measured on balance-bed; 5)the sodium
dialysate concentration $[Na]_d$ as reported on display(mS/cm)vs direct
Na determination(mEq/l); 6)the pH dialysate value on display vs
direct pH measurements(pH-meter,pbi Milano); 7)the bicarbonate dialysate theoric concentration $[HCO_3]_d$ vs the measured one ($[HCO_3]_d =$
$TCO_2 - pCO_2 \cdot 0.031$; TCO_2 Corning 965 Analyzer); 8)the fluid replacement rate(Q_R) on display vs the direct measurement of the fluid
restitution; 9)eventual technical problems.

RESULTS

The mean weight loss was $2,928 \pm 569$ ml/HD($4 \pm 0.8\%$ of the dry bwt).
The scheduled dry weight was achieved in 31.1% of all treatments,
while in 47.3% there was a discrepancy of 50-150 ml and in 21.6% of
200-300 ml.The total weight loss scheduled at the start of each HD
was equal to the value depicted on display at the end in 60% of case,
while there was a little negative difference(-106 ± 83 ml) in 40%.Table
1 shows the differences among the values on display of considered
parameters and the measured ones.

Table 1. Parameters evaluated

	display	measured	t	p	
Weight loss	$2,856 \pm 540$ ml	$2,859 \pm 583$ ml	0.16	ns	
$[Na]_d$	14.0 ± 0.1 mS/cm	140.7 ± 1.8 mEq/l	-	-	(*)
$[HCO_3]_d$	35 mmol/l	36.4 ± 0.5 mmol/l	4.93	<0.05	
	33 mmol/l	35.5 ± 0.4 mmol/l	1.47	ns	
pH	7.28 ± 0.08	7.09 ± 0.24	2.11	<0.05	

The real Q_R was evaluated during the biofiltration:$1,990 \pm 56$ml(1st hr)
$2,020 \pm 14$ml(2nd hr),$1,960 \pm 14$(3rd hr).Technical problems:there were 2
temperature alarms and the unit was 4/182 days out of order.

(*)Statistical analysis was impossible for different measurement U.

DISCUSSION

Uptodate three systems are used in dialysis monitors to achieve an exact UF control:i)volumetric, ii)gravimetric and iii)fluximetric dialysate balancing.Each method offers advantages and disadvantages and none can be considered ideal,even if some Authors(7)state that volumetric dialysate balancing is the best one.

Monitral-S used a further improvement of the well-know closed volumetric system:the amount of UF,that is checked through two valves, is strongly reduced(two 20 ml cavities)versus the previous model(1 1 cavity),thus permitting UF control at the beginning of dialysis session.Our"in vivo"data confirm the goodness of UF system in various clinical situations,due to the different degrees of weight gain.The tolerance of the system(real wt loss-wt loss on display/real wt loss·100) was always less than 5%. Another characteristic of the equipment is an online conductivity control of dialysate; the measured values were stable all over the treatment, close resembling the programmed ones, except for pH control. Pyrogenic reactions were not observed in our patients, in spite of a theoric possibility of back-filtration, that anyway must be considered in the closed volumetric systems.

REFERENCES
1. Granger A., Vlecheck D. Proc. First American AN 69 Membrane Scientific Exchange, Atlantic City, pp 5-13, 1982.
2. Gohl H., Kostantin P. In: Hemofiltration (Eds. Henderson L.H., Quellhorst E.A., Baldamus C.A., and Lysaght M.J.) Springer-Verlag Berlin 1986, pp 41-82.
3. Zucchelli P., Santoro A., Degli Esposti E., Sturani A. Abstracts 2nd Workshop of the Int Soc Hemofiltration,Milano, p 21, 1984.
4. Albertini B. von, Miller J.H., Gardner P.V., Shinaberger J.H. Trans. Am. Soc. Artif. Intern. Organs 30: 227-231, 1984.
5. Berden J.H.M., Wokke J.M.P., Koene R.A.P. Abstracts XXIInd E.D.T.A. Congress, Brussels, p 99, 1985.
6. Ronco C., Albertini B. von, Frigato G., La Greca G. Abstracts ASAIO 16: 36, 1987.
7. Roy T., Ahrenholz D., Falkenhagen D., Klinkmann H. Int. J. Artif. Organs 5: 131-135, 1982.

PAIRED FILTRATION DIALYSIS (PFD):BETTER PURIFICATION THAN CONVENTI-
ONAL HEMODIALYSIS (HD)

D.Koutsikos,B.Agroyannis,B.Bleta,C.Iatrou,M.Frangos,H.Tzanatos,P.Zi-
royannis,A.Diamantopoulos

Nephrological Dept. of Athens General Hospital, Hellas

INTRODUCTION

Shortening of dialysis time and better removal of small and middle
molecular weight (MW) uremic toxins are main targets of dialytic
methods. PFD,introduced by Ghezzi et al(1983)(1),has been used for
9 hours per week (3x3) with excellent results, in respect to small
and middle MW solutes removal (2,3).

PATIENTS AND METHODS

Twenty-two chronic renal failure patients, aged 18-71 years,under
HD for 3-84 months, 13.5 hours per week (3x4.5), transfered to PFD
for 9 hours per week (3x3).
We used a device containing in separate compartments, a polysulfone
hemofilter of 0.4 or 0.5 m^2 surface area (SA) and a Hemophan dialyser of 1.1 m^2 SA (Fig. I). The ultrafiltration rate was kept
constant at 43±2.8 ml/min. The substitution fluid (NaCl 0.9%) was
administered at a rate of 22.00±3.70 ml/min. The dialysate used
was bicarbonate at a flow of 500 ml/min.

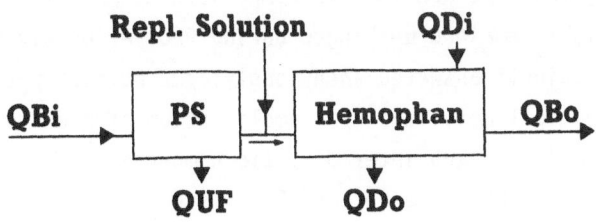

Figure I. Schematic representation of PFD.

Midweek and after HD and PFD values of blood urea,creatinine,uric
acid,phosphates,Ca and Mg (total,free,protein bound), pH and bicarbonates, were determined with standard methods. Six months after
initiation of PFD treatment, patients answered anonymously in respect
to physical rehabilitation.
The estimation of results was done with the student's t-test.

RESULTS

The midweek and after treatment values of creatinine, uric acid and
phosphates were lower in PFD in comparison to HD (Table 1).

Treatment	urea mmol/1	creatinine µmol/1	uric acid µmol/1	phosphates mmol/1
HD/270 min PRE	33.7±5.5	1009±181	392±81	1.87±0.48
		b	b	b
PFD/180 min	34.7±6.1	857±184	321±58	1.52±0.35
HD/270 min POST	16.3±3.8	438±145	136±33	1.00±0.33
	c	c	a	c
PFD/180 min	15.6±4.1	339±152	83±21	0.77±0.34

Table 1. Values before (PRE) and after (POST) a single HD and PFD
session (a:$P<0.001$, b:$P<0.01$, c:$P<0.05$)

In contrast, the values of blood urea,total,free and protein bound
Ca and Mg,pH and HCO_3 were similar with both treatment modalities.
The plasma phosphates remained low in 8 patients, even after a 50%
reduction of phosphate binders administration. The hypotensive
episodes during PFD were 35% less in comparison to HD. Blood pressure and body weight remained unchanged during PFD. After six months
of PFD the 22 patients answered anonymously:7/22 better appetite,
10/22 better physical activity, 8/22 amelioration of pruritus,
10/22 decrease of intra-and inter dialytic number and severity of
muscle cramps and 20/22 preference of PFD instead of HD.

DISCUSSION

PFD is an alternative to Hemodiafiltration (HDF), proved to be

equally effective with HD in removing small MW solutes and superior
for removing middle MW uremic toxins (1,2,3).:
The expediture of convection and diffusion simultaneously but in
different compartments offers some advantages in comparison to classical HDF,such as:no diffusion obstacle to convection or vice versa;
the smal volume and simple composition of reinfusion fluid carries
reduced contamination risks and low cost; the passage of bicarbonates
from dialysate to plasma is not hindered by the convective flux
across the membrane in the opposite direction; PFD can be performed
with "normal" blood flow without hemodynamic problems; the size of
the protein cake in Hemophan compartment is smaller, due to practically absence of ultrafiltration; the constant ultrafiltration rate
permits accurate evaluation of body weight loss. The better clearance obtained in this study in comparison with the first clinical
trials of PFD (2,3), perhaps is due to the larger SA of polysulfone
membrane and to the use of Hemophan instead of Cuprophan. Indeed
our results show that 9 hours per week (3x3) with PFD offer better
detoxification in comparison to 13.5 hours (3x4.5) with HD, in
respect to Creatinine,Uric Acid and Phosphates, and better rehabilitation of patients.

REFERENCES

1.   Ghezzi P.M., Frigato G., Fantini G.F., Dutto A., Meinero S.,
     Gento G., Marazzi F., D'Andrie V., Grivet V. Life Support
     Systems 1:suppl. 1:S271-S274, 1983.

2.   Ghezzi P.M., Zucchelli P., Botella J., Koutsikos D.,Marazzi F.,
     Canepari G., Nigrelli S., Spongano M., Ziroyannis P., Santoro
     A. (Abstract),Blood Purification 2:196, 1985.

3.   Koutsikos D., Hadjigeorgiou G., Agroyannis B., Ziroyannis P.,
     Perakis K., Ghezzi P.M. (Abstract), Kidney Int., 31:578,1987.

MODIFICATION OF BIOHUMORAL AND ELECTROMYOGRAFIC FEATURES
PATIENTS ON PFD: 12 MONTHS FOLLOW-UP RESULTS

F. DELLA GROTTA, L. FRANCESCHELLI, L. POLIMENO, F. AMBROSINI
Servizio Emodialisi Ospedale Provinciale Anzio, Italy

INTRODUCTION

In the last few years, technology has put different dialytic membranes at our disposal some of them have shown us
to have depurative performances, much better than traditional cuprophan membranes (1). Similarly, the continually improving performances of the equipment have made the achievement of high-efficiency dialytic treatments possible shorter. PFD is one of these treatments. In this system convection and diffusion through the membranes occurs simultaneously, thanks to a depurative system consisting of an
haemophilter and a dialyser.

MATERIALS AND METHODS

Out of six patients treated with PFD, only one has had
peripherical neuropathy with strong intradialytic hypotension. Because of that no advantages have been gained by
changing from an acetate to a bicarbonate dialysis. The
other 5 patients are young people, aged from 22 to 42, and
all waiting for transplantation. This treatment has been
tried with them with the intent, above all, of improving
their clinical situation and not of shortening their treatment period. For that the following features have been considered: - At the beginning and at the end of each month:
azote, creatinine, uric acid, protein, albumin, calcium,
phosphorus, alkaline phosphatase, cholesterin, triglycerides, haemoglobin, B2 microglobulin in the blood,electrocar-

diogram, a cardiology examination and cardiac-thoracic index. - Once a year: electromyography in order to study the conduction speed of median and external popliteus nerve. Besides, the following have been considered: intradialytic arrhythmia, pre, intra and post dialysis pressure values, the interdialytic increases as well as eventual technical complications. Adding to that, psychological subjective remarks on the patient have been noted. A bath of dialysis with acetate and some reinfusion liquid with bicarbonate ($Na+$ 140 mEq/l - HCO_3^- 40 mEq/l) has been utilized. So: Q_D has been 500 ml/m; Q_B has been 300 ml/m; medium Q_F has been about $41^{\pm}$ 2 ml/m.

The following technical characteristics refer to a haemodiafiltration devige used in our Centre:

unit for haemofiltration	unit for haemodialysis
active surface 0,4 m^2	1,06 m^2
hollow fibre polysulphone	haemophan
thickness of the wall 40 μmol	8 μmol
number of fibres 6750	6900

RESULTS

The arterial pressure values in PFD system, compared with the traditional extracorporeal one, have increased in 66% of the cases. In the remaining 33%, they have remained quite unchanged. The incidence of intradialytic symptomatic hypotension has amounted to 2,4% against 29,2% in haemodialysis. As for the haemato-chemical analysis, it must be pointed out that many values (in particular azote, creatinine, and phosphorus) have remained reasonably unchanged, except for one case. On the contrary, there has been a strong decrease on B_2 microglobulinaemia which, not being influenced by alimentary habits, demonstrates a better depuration of the membrane. In particular the average rate of. varations of B_2 microglobulinaemia has amounted to 10,2%. The EC graphic remarks have remained unchanged and, as expected, there have been no variations in cardio-thora-

cic index with those patients treated with PFD system,
when compared with the traditional dialysis. On the contrary, there has been also a decrease in intradialytic arrhythmia which is mostly due to the patients young age. As
for the electromyographic diagram, the signs of neuroge-
nous suffering of SPE and median nerve, represented in the
dialysis with cuprophan filter, have now become sub-inter-
ferential ones, with relevant improvement on max conduction
speed (42 m/second in every cases, with starting overage
values amounting to 40,9 m/sec). From the subjective point
of view, every patients tested, have improved their cenae-
sthesia that is: increasing appetite, decreasing sense of
thirst, regularization of the rythm waking-sleep, decreasing of adynamia and asthenia. Such an inprovement has
been testified by a recovery of muscolar trophism as well
as a ponderal intradialytic increase. Besides, it has been
assured by every patients an increase in libido. To be precise, in one case there has been an increase in the sper-
miogram such as to allow a conception, longed a lot.

Furthermore out of 850 cases of dialysis in a year there has never been any accident which may be ascribed to
the dialyser.

CONCLUSIONS

A long term selection of young patients who are waiting
for nephric transplantation has derived advantages out of
the PFD treatment from the objective and subjective point
of view. If those elements have all contributed to give
PFD a positive sense, high costs still hinder its usage.

REFERENCES
1. Gotch F.A.,Sargent J.A.: A mechanistic analysis of the
    national cooperative dialysis study. Kidney Intern.,
    28, 526-534, 1985

RESTORATION OF THE STRENGTH OF ESRF PATIENTS BY PFD

DIAMADOPOULOS A., GOGOS H., HINARY E., THEOTHOROPOULOS P., LAFI N.,
APOSTOLOPOULOS A., TRIANTAPHYLLOU G., AND ZOUBOS H.,

Renal unit, Patras State Hospital " St. ANDREWS " and Patras University Department of Haematology

INDRODUCTION

Chronic renal failure (C.R.F) causes a significant depression of cell mediated immunity (C.M.I.) (1), not largely improved by haemodialysis (2). This study investigates the influence of paired haemodiafiltration (P.F.D) on the CMI of end stage renal failure (E.S.R.F) patients.

MATERIAL AND METHODS

Twenty seven patients (11 F and 16 M, mean age 54,4 ± years) and twelve healthy volunteers (7 F and 5 M, mean age 56,7 ± years)were included in the study. The patients had been on H.D. from 11 to 82 months (M 35,9 months). At the beginning of the study, the patients were still on H.D. with a cuprophan dialyser 14 hours, a week. The strenght of their CMI was then tested by a) the contact sensitivity skin test using Dinitrochlorobenzene as antigen (3) b) the number of T4 + and T8 + -T lymphocyte subpopulations c) The number of the NK cells and their activity. The patients were then transferred to P.F.D. treatment for 9 hours a week with the model Spiraflo SG2- 1108 Supplied by Sorin. The DNCB test was repeated four months later, while the T-lymphocyte Subpopulations and the NK cells and their activity were estimated 20,40, and 120 days later. when we also estimated the T-lymphocyte transformation from healthy volumenteers. These were incubated with PHA and radioactive thymidine and drainage fluid after a) H.D. with a cuprophan dialyser of ten patient on chronic HD b)PFD with a polysulphon filter of nine patients on four months PFD c)PFD of five patients on chronic HD who were treated only the day of the experiment with PFD.

RESULTS

The results of the DNCB test are shown in Fig 1. The results of the
T-lymphocytes sulpopulation are shown in Table 1, the NK activity
in Table 2, and the lymphocyte transformation in Table 3.

Table 1

	Before PFD	120 Days on PFD
Total T-cells	61,85 ± 3,56	67,2 ± 3 (P<0.01)
Helper- cells	37,13 ± 2,18	46,4 ± 21(P<0.005)
Suppressor-cells	26,12 ± 1,94	24,9 ± 1,6 (N.S.)
Ratio H/S	1,42 ± 0,13	1,86 ± 0,2 (P<0.005)
NK - cells	14,25 ± 1,7	14,68 ± 2.00 (N.S.)

Table 2

	NK%	Interferon Stimulation
HD	9,40 ± 2,28	23,20 ± 4,42
PFD	11,75 ± 2,86	21,25 ± 4,90
Controls	60 ± 3,10	70 ± 2,85

HD / PFD = N.S.

Table 3

Percentage of Suppresion of lymphocyte transformation with drainage
fluid of:

	No PATIENTS		
a) HD	10	58,72%	1/2 P < 0.005%
b) PFD	9	18,13%	2/3 P < 0.001%
c) HD - PFD	5	87,8 %	1/3 P < 0.05 %

Fig. 1

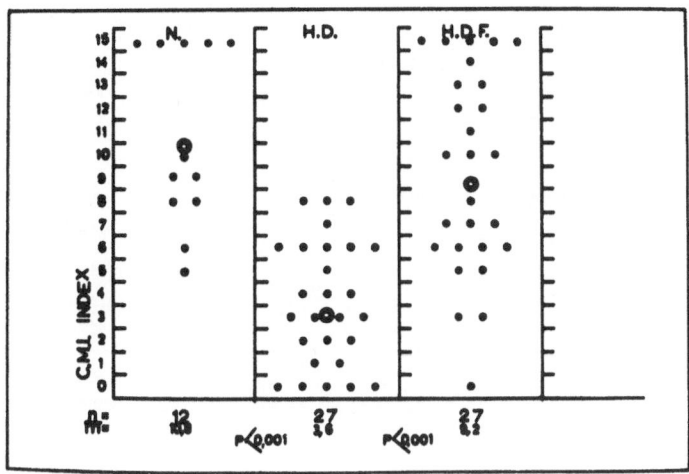

DISCUSSION

It is obvious from our results that PDF restores CMI by improving
mainly the T4/T8 Ratio, through a better blood purification than
usual H.D. Thus drainage fluid from chronic PFD patients causes less
suppression than the same fluid from chronic HD patients presumably
because the first group has been " Purified " during the four months
reriod. When HD patients rich in immunodepressing agents, were treated once with P.F.D. their drainage fluid had an extreme immunodepressing potency. The profound increase of the strength of immune
skin reaction to DNCB from patients sensitized while on HD and
then transferred to PFD indicates that in uraemia only the efferent
Branch of CMI is damaged. We conclude that PFD restores back to
normal CMI in uraemic patients.

BIBLIOGRAPHY

1.Boulton-Jones J.M., Vick R., Cameron J.S., and Black P.J. (1973)
  Clinical Nephrology, 1,351-360

2.Watson M., Diamandopoulos A., Briggs D., Hamilton D. and Dick H.(1979)
  Lancet, 2,1323-1326

3.Diamandopoulos A., Hamilton D., and Briggs D. (1978).
  Proc. Eur. Dialysis Transp. Association 15: 283-88

Beta-2-Microglobulin

RELATION BETWEEN RED BLOOD CELL FUNCTION AND B2-MICROGLOBULIN CONCENTRATION IN HEMODIALYSIS.

R. L. LINS, P. ZACHEE*, R. DAELEMANS, E. VANDEN BROECKE, M. BOGAERTS*, M. E. DE BROE

Department of Nephrology-Hypertension, A.Z. Stuivenberg and University of Antwerpen, Antwerpen. *Department of Hematology, U.Z. Gasthuisberg, Leuven, Belgium.

INTRODUCTION

It has recently been recognized with increasing frequency that patients maintained on regular hemodialysis develop amyloid arthropathy after several years (1,2,3). It was reported that a major constituent of this amyloid is a new form of amyloid fibril protein homologous to β_2-microglobuline (β_2M) (4).

Whether lack of removal or release of β_2M as the consequence of acute-phase activation by regenerated cellulose membranes are important pathogenetic mechanisms is yet unknown (2).

Local production in endothelial cells of the lung and other tissues as a consequence of acute phase activation with endothelial injury due to the contact of blood with bioincompatible membranes have possibly to be considered as an additional pathogenetic factor in this syndrome. Granulocytes producing toxic radicals have been implicated in the generation of this endothelial injury in different conditions (5). Red blood cells have shown to inhibit the damage induced by free oxygen radicals in lung injury models (6).

Therefore we studied the possibility that red blood cells may serve as endogenous free radical scavengers during hemodialysis in situations where granulocytes are immunologically triggered, preventing to some extent endothelial damage and release of endothelial enzymes and proteins.

MATERIALS AND METHODS
Patients.

41 hemodialysis patients, mean age 59,7 years, ± 12,6 years, (range 4-76 years),17 men and 24 women on chronic hemodialysis (mean duration 37,5 ± 18 months) were studied. Patients were treated with single-needle dialysis, bicarbonate or acetate dialysate, and cuprophane membranes.

Methods.

The experiments were done during a regular dialysis procedure with ultrafiltration as needed. Each experiment was done twice in each patient. Blood samples were obtained from the arterial line during complete stop of both pumps. Because of previous results of a kinetic study (7) sampling was restricted to time 0, 15 and 180 min. The change in $\beta_2 M$ ($\Delta \beta_2 M$ %) between the start (T0') and 180 min (T180'), corrected for plasmavolume was compared with the reduced glutathion content (Δ GSH %) at T0' and T15'.

Laboratory methods

White blood cells (WBC) and Red blood cells (RBC) were counted with a coulter S+4. β_2- microglobuline ($\beta_2 M$) was measured using a radioimmunoassay (β_2-micro RIA 100,Pharmacia, Uppsala), and corrected for plasma volume using the procentual change in hematocrit. Reduced glutathion (GSH), the principal reducing agent in RBC was measured by an earlier published method (8).

Statistics.

The results are presented as mean ± s.e.m. or ± confidence intervals (C.I.) Statistical analysis was performed using the Spearman Rank Correlation Test. The level of significance was set at .05.

RESULTS

In the 41 patients the mean drop in WBC after 15' of cuprophane dialysis was 67,8 ± 15,2, the mean elevation of $\beta_2 M$ after 180 ', corrected for hematocrit, was 11,3 ± 14,71 % and the drop in GSH after 15' was - 0,8 ± 13,6 %. We found no correlation between $\beta_2 M$ and GSH for the whole group (R = -.12, n.s.). If we take into account the variability between the two experiments in the same patient of 13,0 ± 4,5 % and set the level of significant elevation of $\beta_2 M$ at 15 % (n = 12) (see Fig. 1), a correlation of R = -.61, P < .05 becomes evident. The correlation becomes more striking if we set the level of elevation of $\beta_2 M$ at 20 % : R = -.90, P < .05(n = 5).

DISCUSSION

Contact of blood with a cuprophane membrane results in activation of complement and granulocytes, which adhere to and degranulate in the first capillary bed they encounter after the dialyzer, i.e. the microcirculation of the lung, releasing oxygen-free radicals, enzymes, and inflammatory mediators (5).

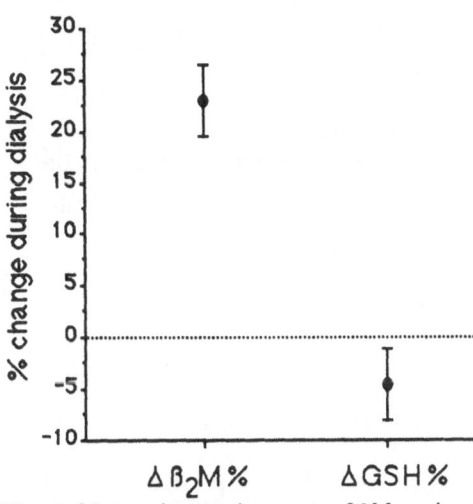

Fig. 1. Mean change in serum ß2M and GSH during dialysis. (n = 12, increase ß2M ≥ 15 %, mean ± 95 % C.I.

This causes local inflammation, edema formation, increase in alveolar arterial oxygen tension difference and hypoxaemia (5,9). As a consequence of the inflammation proteins like human placental alkaline phosphatase and ß2M localised at the plasma membrane of pneumocyte I and the endothelial cell of the capillary bed can be released in the circulation (10). These two cell types are well documented to be highly susceptible to oxygen-free radicals produced in the process of acute inflammation. At least to some extent, complement activation can be involved in the pathogenesis of amyloidosis.

In different situations like in hyperoxic lung models, where granulocytes are activated with production of oxygen free radicals, enzymes and inflammatory mediators, it has been shown that erythrocytes can inhibit oxygen-free radical induced damage to endothelial cells (6). In a previous study the role of the erythrocytes in hemodialysis was demonstrated by measuring the oxydative sensitivity and the amount of reduced glutathion before and during dialysis (11). This is an important reducing agent that can prevent the oxidation of hemoglobin to methemoglobin and the lipid peroxidation of erythrocyte membranes.

If we suppose that endothelial damage is a response not only depending on the type of membrane but also on individual variations - for which there is experimental evidence (7) -, then it can be expected that the RBC scavenger function becomes only important in those patients with a significant release of B_2M. This is suggested by the lack of correlation between WBC drop and changes in B_2M and GSH in the whole group and correlations of .61 and of .91 between B_2M and GSH respectively in those patients with a net increase of B_2M of more than 15 % and 20 %. These levels were chosen because experiments in the same patient show a variation of 13 %. This suggests generation of B_2M in some patients during dialysis and a protective role of RBC during this procedure.

The exact role of the RBC- and other scavengers in dialysis has to be further evaluated by defining there relation to membrane biocompatibility and to different endproducts of complement activation.

REFERENCES
1. Bardin, T., Zingraff, J., Shirahama,T., et al. Am. J . Med.83:419-424,1987.
2. Flöge., J., Granolleras., C., Bingel, M., et al. Nephrol. Dial. Transplant. 1: 223-228, 1987.
3. Chanard, J., Lavaud, S., Toupance, O., et al. Lancet i: 1212, 1986. 4. Gejyo, F. Biochem. and Biophys. Research Comm. 129:701-706,1985.
5. Craddock, P.R., Fehr, S., Brigham, K.L., et al. N. J.Med.296:769-773,1977.
6. Van Asbech, B.S., Hoidal, J., Vercelotti, G.M., et al. Science 227:756-759, 1985.
7. De Roeck, M., Lins, R.L., Hautekeete, M., et al. Abstracts 5th Annual Meeting of the International Society of Blood Purification, pp 40, Stockholm 1987.
8. Beutler, E., Duron, O., Kelly, B. J. Lab. Clin. Med. 61:882, 1963.
9. De Backer, W.A., Verpooten, G.A., Borgonjon, D.J., et al. Kidney Int 23: 738-743, 1983.
10. De Broe, M.E., Nouwen, J., Van Waeleghem, J.P. Nephrol. Dial. Transplant. 2: 124-125, 1987.
11. Zachée, P., Emonds, M.., Goossens W., et al. Clinical Hemorheology 7: 413, 1987.

BETA-2-MICROGLOBULIN (B2m) ADSORPTION ON ACTIVATED CHARCOAL (AC)

A. Anelli, M. Gallieni, P. Padovese, G. Colantonio, S. Barbesti,
D. Brancaccio

Renal Units, Ospedale S. Paolo, Milano, Ospedale S. Anna, Como, Italy

Hemoperfusion (HP) has proven to be an useful instrument in treating several clinical problems related mainly to acute poisoning, liver failure an uremia (1). It has been suggested that sorbents could induce a high clearance for molecules in the middle molecular weight range (2), thus it has been thought that activated charcoal (AC) could have a role in removing B2m. However prior attempts have been reported to be unsuccessful (3, 4).

The aim of our study was to evaluate the possible removal of B2m by combined hemodialysis-hemoperfusion (HD-HP) in an in vivo study. Further which B2m removal by AC was studied in an ex vivo experiment using ^{125}I labelled B2m.

MATERIAL AND METHODS

Ten uremic patients were submitted to a four hour treatment with HD-HP using two different coated carbons:
1) 100 g of peat-based extruded carbon covered with methacrylic hydrogel coupled with 1.2 sqm cellulose acetate dialyzer
2) 100 g of a petroleum based spherical charcoal coated with cellulose nitrate coupled with 1.2 sqm cuprophane dialyzer.

As control a further group of patients was treated with conventional hemodialysis using the same dialyzers. Blood samples were taken at times 0, 15, 30, 60, 120, 240 min and plasma B2m was measured by RIA method (Phadebas, Pharmacia). In the ex vivo experiment 2500 ml of dialysate were matched with 500 ml of normal human blood enriched with cold B2m an ^{125}I labelled B2m so as to obtain a concentration of 10-12 mg/L. The HD-HP device was made of 100 g of collodion coated AC and a 1.2 sqm cuprophane dialyzer. Dialysate and blood samples were taken at times 0, 15, 30, 60, 90, 120 min and counted with a solid scintillation counter (NaI(Tl)). At the end of the experiment the HD-HP device was counted in a body counter as well. The results were corrected for ECV reduction (5).

RESULTS

Fig. 1 shows the results observed in the in vivo study. The two AC behave in a quite similar way inducing a decrease of 17% (methacrylic coated AC) and 16% (collodion coated AC) of the initial plasma B2m concentration. It is noteworthy that a step decrease is observed during the first thirty minutes, afterward no significant changes occur. When HD alone was performed using the same dialyzers only a slight variation in B2m plasma levels was observed.

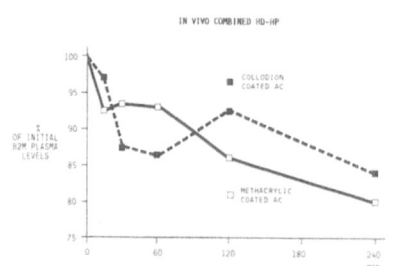

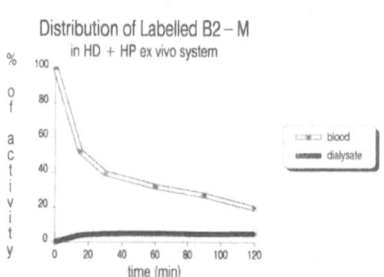

Fig. 1: see text   Fig. 2: see text

Fig. 2 shows the results obtained in the ex vivo experiment. After 120 min of treatment 20% of the initial radioactivity was present in the blood, while only 5% was detected in the dialysate, thus suggesting that no clearance of B2m occured. The counting of the residual radioactivity on the HD-HP device showed that 63% of labelled material was bound to AC.

CONCLUSION

B2m has been identified as being concerned in dialysis related amyloidosis; therefore it is presumable that its removal could be of benefit in dialysis patients.

High flux membranes can remove consistent amount of this protein expecially when used with convective mechanisms. However the removal during each dialysis is far less than the protein generation rate (8). Our ex vivo results demonstrate that AC has a high affinity toward B2m, since all the labelled material which disappeared from blood at the end of the experiment was detected on AC. However the in vivo studies show that the amount of B2m removed by AC is smaller than the one by high flux membranes, because of a quick saturation of AC by B2m and other plasma molecules. In conclusion, although hemoperfusion "per se" is not as efficient as high flux membranes its use could be considered as an additional therapeutic measure in lowering B2m plasma levels in uremic patients.

REFERENCES

1. Klinkmann H., Falkenhagen D. and Courtney J.M. Int. J. Artif. Organs. 2: 1-13, 1979.
2. Castro L.A., Hampel G., Gebharat R., Fateh A. and Gurland H. In: Artificial kidney, artificial liver and artificial cells (Ed T.M.S. Chang), Plenum Press, New York 1978, p 193
3. Ackrill P., Robinson E.L., Hill K. and McClure J. Abstracts XXIII Congress EDTA-ERA, Budapest 1986, p 106.
4. Kinugasa E., Akizawa T., Kitaoka T. and Koshikawa S. Artif. Organs. 12:11-15, 1988.
5. Bergström J. and Wehle B. Lancet. i: 628-629, 1987
6. Gejyo F., Odani S., Yamada T., Honma N., Saito H., Suzuki Y., Nakagawa Y., Kokayashi H., Maruyama Y., Hirasawa Y., Suzuki M., Harakawa M. Kidney Int. 30: 385-391, 1987.
7. Anelli A., Brancaccio D., Barbesti S., Padovese P., Gallieni M., Sabbioni E., Pietra R., Ubertalli L. and Berlin A. Nephrol. Dial. Transplant. 2:446, 1987.
8. Revillard J.P. and Vincent C. Abstracts X International Congress of Nephrology, London 1987, p 168.

CLINICAL CHARACTERISTICS OF BETA 2 MICROGLOBULIN ASSOCIATED
AMYLOIDOSIS IN CHRONIC HAEMODIALYSIS PATIENTS

S.Kaplan-Pavlovčič[1], J.Drinovec[1], M.Koselj[1], V.Jevtič[2], A.Vizjak[3],
M.Malovrh[1]
[1]Department of Nephrology, University Medical Center, Ljubljana
[2]University institute of radiology, Ljubljana
[3]Institute of Pathology, Medical faculty, Ljubljana, Yugoslavia

INTRODUCTION

The range of osteoarticular diseases in patients with chronic
renal failure treated with long term haemodialysis (HD) has recently
been broadened by description of a new clinical entity: beta 2
microglobulin associated dialysis amyloidosis. It is mainly reflected by clinical syndromes such as   the carpal tunnel syndrome
(CTS) and dialysis arthropathy (DA) (1).

PATIENTS AND METHODS

81 patients, who had received HD for six or more years at our
dialysis center were reviewed to establish the incidence, clinical
picture and radiological features of dialysis amyloidosis. A
detailed clinical hystory of all musculosceletal complaints was
taken. Physical examination included inspection of all joints,
measurements of motion and determination of synovitis. Regular
radiographic bone surveys were available of all patients and consisted of radiography of hands,wrists,long bones, scull and pelvis.
Tissue removed at the time of operative carpal tunnel release and by
synovial biopsies was analysed by light microscopy (two special
amyloid stains: Congo red and Thioflavin T) and, imunohistoche-
mically by anti-human beta 2 microglobulin.

RESULTS

14 patients had CTS, both clinically and electromyographically
(all were operated on); three of them also had DA. Clinical

characteristics and histological findings of patients with CTS are
shown in Table 1.

Table 1. Clinical characteristics of patients with CTS and
histologic findings.

Patient	Age	Sex	HD (yr)	Pain onset after HF (yr)	Site of CTS	Amyloid	Beta 2 microglobulin
1*	55	m	12	9	bilateral	+	+
2	55	f	8	7	right side	−	−
3*	64	f	10	9	right side	+	+
4	60	m	13	12	right side	+	+
5	60	f	9	7	left side	not done	not done
6	52	f	8	6	right side	not done	not done
7*	65	f	12	10	right side	+	+
8	60	f	10	9	right side	+	+
9	61	f	10	8	bilateral	+	+
10	53	f	10	8	bilateral	−	+
11	51	f	8	8	bilateral	+	−
12	57	f	8	6	right side	not done	not done
13	45	m	12	11	right side	−	−
14	57	f	10	8	right side	+	+

*dialysis arthropathy also

7 patients had clinical and or radiologic signs of DA. Clinical
characteristics are presented in Table 2.

Table 2. Clinical characteristics of 7 patients with DA.

Patient	Age (yr)	Sex	HD (yr)	First Symptoms after HD (yr)	Early Symptoms	Affected areas
1	55	m	12	9	pain	hips
2	65	f	14	12	swelling	shoulders
3	55	m	8	7	pain	lumbal spine
4	64	f	10	9	pain	hips
5	66	m	10	9	pain	shoulder
6	57	f	10	8	swelling	knee
7	55	m	6	6	pain	lumbal spine

Radiological changes included erosions, radiolucent defects, destructive arthropathy and erosive spondylarthropathy. On serial rentgeno-
grams, x-ray lesions of shoulders and femoral head preceded clinical
symptoms by 2-3 years. Small radiolucent defects in the hand and
wrist bones were always asymptomatic. Except in one case,

(destructive arthropathy of the shoulder) there was no true relationship between clinical symptoms and radiological changes. Amyloid and
beta 2 microglobulin positive deposits were shown in three synovial
biopsy samples (two from shoulders, one from hip), one synovial
fluid (from knee) and in two radiolucent defects (pseudocysts).

DISCUSSION

The epidemiology of dialysis amyloidosis is stil poorly defined
because there are no clear relationships among clinical picture,
rentgenographic changes and deposition of beta 2 microglobulin
associated amyloid.
Females predominanted in our group of patients with CTS; of 27 women
treated with HD 8 years or more, 11 had CTS, while of 32 men treated
with HD 8 years or more, only 3 developed CTS. Other authors did not
find a predominance of women in the dialysis group with CTS (2).
There was no sex predomination in our group of patients with DA. The
most common radiographical changes included erosions and radiolucent
defects of various size, as it has been reported (3). Radiologic
changes were suspicious, but not specific to DA and did not correlate
with clinical symptoms, of which pain was the most common.
Biopsy of suspicious rentgenographic changes is stil the only
definite method for diagnosing DA, but it is difficult to propose it
to patient, since the diagnosis of DA has no specific therapeutic
implication as yet.

REFERENCES

1. Charra,R., Calemard,E., Uzan,M., Terrat,J.C., Vanel,T., Laurent,
   G. Proc Eur Dial Transplant Assoc Eur Ren Assoc.21: 291-295, 1985.
2. Walts, A.E., Goodman,M.D., and Matorin, P.A. Am J Nephrol 5:
   225-226, 1985.
3. Munoz-Gomez, J., Gomez-Perez, R., Llopart-Buisan, E. and Sole-
   Arques, M. Ann Rheum Dis 46: 573-579, 1987.

PLASMA B$_2$-MICROGLOBULLIN (B$_2$M) CHANGES INDUCED BY DIFFERENT DIALYSIS MEMBRANES.

G. SAKELLARIOU, E. KOKOLINA, P. MARGARI, B. PASTOURMATZI, M. PAPADIMITRIOU.

Departement of Nephrology Hippokratio General Hospital, Aristotelian University of Thessaloniki-Greece.

INTRODUCTION

An increased incidence of carpal tunnel syndrome in patients on long term heamodialysis treatment has been recently reported.[1,2] Amyloid deposition has been observed in the perineural tissue of the mediam nerve in the majority of these patients at time of surgery.[2,3] Recent evidence indicate that β_2-microglobulin (β_2M) is the major precursor protein in this new form of amyloid. The pathogenesis has been related to the persistenly raised plasma β_2M concentrations, observed in CRF patients and its possibly low clearance during hemodialysis.[2-5]

The purpose of the present study was to compare the efficiency of removal of serum B$_2$M by various dialysis membranes and the kinetics of β_2M removal during haemodialysis (HD) haemofiltration (HF) and haemodiafiltration (HDF).

PATIENTS AND METHODS

Criteria for patient selection were the absence of acute or chronic infection, autoimmune disease and cancer.

The study was divided in two sections;

I. Influence of HD membranes on serum β_2M.

The study comprised 6 consecutive dialysis treatments in 7 patients with a mean age 47.7 yrs/range 22-59 yrs, and mean time on HD of 49,7 mos (range 12-127 mos).The artificial membranes used consisted of a 1,2m^2 cuprophan capillary (GF 120 Gambro), a polysulphone capillary (F40 Fresenius), a 1,2m^2 modified cuprophan capillary Hemofan (Biodec, HISPANDIAL), an acetate cellulose capillary (FB 110 Nipro), a polyacrilonitrile capillary (PAN 150 ASAHI), a polyamide capillary (HF 77 GAMBRO) and a double capillary filter (Hemofan + polysulphone, SPIRAFLO SG2 SORIN).

Dialysis was performed for 4 hrs using standard technics. Serum samples for β_2M were taken from the arterial line before and after the sesssion of HD. For the kinetic of serum β_2M during HD serum samples were odtained from the arterial line each at times 0,15', 60', 120' and 240 minutes of each HD session.

II.Comparison of changes of β_2M on HD, on HDF and HF.

HD was performed in 8 pts (6 male, 2 female; mean age 51.1 yrs, (Range: 25-68 yrs); mean time on HD was 48.3 ± 23.7 months utilizing a 1.2 m^2 capillary (GF 120 Gambro). HDF was performed in 8 pts (7 males, 4 females), mean age 60.3 yrs, (Range: 50-76), mean time on HD 63.7 ± 32.6 months utilizing a polysulphone capillary (F40 Fresenius) and polyacrilonitrile (PAN 200 ASAHI) Hemofiltration was perfomed in 5 pts (4 male, 4 females, mean age 46.8 yrs, (Range: 25-64); mean time on HD 50 ± 24.4 months (± SD) with a polyamide capillary. HDF and HF were performed for 4 and 5 hrs respectively using the postdilution mode, (mean exchange volume 12L and 18L respectively). β_2M levels were determined in serum samples before and after treatment. and were measured by Phadezym β2-microtest enzyme immunoassay (provided by Pharmacia) corrected for haemoconcentration during treatment. The results are expressed as mean ± SD. Significance was assessed by means of the student's test for paired or unpaired data.

Results

Study I. A 20% and a 5,3% increase of serum β_2M was observed after HD with cuprophane and cellusose acetate membranes respectively. In contrast a 26% reduction of serum β_2M was observed after HD with polyamide, 11,7% with Hemofan, 15% with polyacrilonitrile, 25% with Polysulfone and 7% with polysulfone + Hemofan.

Study II.   The increase of serum β_2M was not statistically significant in hemodialysis with cuprophane membrane. The mean value of serum β_2M concentrations at the beginning of the HDF treatment was 34.3 ± 6.99 versus 21.5 ± 6.3 at the end of the session (p<0.001).

The reduction of serum β_2M concentrations during polyacrilonitrile HDF was not statistically significant . A significant decrease in β_2M levels was observed from 45,5 ± 7,8 to 25,9 ± 3,99 (p<0.001) in HF with polyamide membrane.

DISCUSSION

In the present study it is clearly shown that β_2M levels remain high during HD with a cuprophane or a regenerated cellulose membrane. In contrast, significant removal of β_2M is observed during HD with more porous and higher permeable membranes such as polyamide, polysulfone and polyacrilonitrile. These findings suggest that removal of serum β_2M depend on the membrane permeability characteristics of the dialyzer.[5,6,7] Our data also demonstrate that HF is more efficient in lowering serum β_2M levels than HD due to its efficiency of convective transport removal of large molecular weight substances. The daily elimination of β_2M by a healthy individual is estimated at 150mg per day and it appears that a similar effectiveness in its removal can be achieved during HD with higlly permeable membranes or HF. The biocompatibility of the membrane is also important. β_2M levels rise during cuprophane HD due to its small pore size which restricts passage of proteins, and also its poor membrane biocompatibility with activation of complement and mononuclear cells. The latter phenomenon is due to the release of β_2M from its cellular localization induced by any nonbiocompatible membrane. This release could merely be the concequence of the stress to which the circulating blood cells are submitted to in the extracorporeal circuit or it could be part of the general biocompatibility reaction triggered by cellullosic membranes.[8] Thus effective plasma elimination of β_2M is obtained using a high permeable and biocompatible membrane. Some authors suggest that partial absorption of β_2M[4,6,7] onto the membrane is the third mechanism which in combination with removal and generation during HD determine the intradialytic evolution of β_2M plasma levels. The theurapeutic implications of these observations for the prevention of dialysis associated amyloidosis are of great importance.

In conclusion we suggest that the best treatment for dialysis athropathy which is one of the most disabling complications of long-term HD, is its prevention. The use of highly permeable and biocompatible membranes or HF treatment are effective in preventing dialysis amyloidosis in end stage renal disease. For patients with established arthropathy transplantation may lead to improvement in joint symptoms.

REFERENCES
1.Brawn, E.A. Cower, P.E. Clin Nephrol, 18:247-250.
2.Brawn, E.A. Arnold, I.R. Cower, P. E. Br Med J 292:163-166, 1986.
3.Bardin, T. Kuntz, O. et al. Arth Rheum 28:1052-1058, 1985.
4.Nakazawa, R. Hamaguchi, K. et al. Nephron, 44:379-380, 1987.
5.Vincent, C. Rewillard, J.P. et al. Nephron 21:260-268, 1978.
6.Zingraff, J. Beyne, P. et al Abst Am Soc Nephrol 91A, 1986.
7.Floge, M.A. Granolleras, C.et al. Nephrol Dial, Transplant, 1:223-227, 1987.
8.Hakim, R,M. Fearon, D.T. Lazarus, J.M. Kidney Int, 26:194-200,1984.

INTRADIALYTIC BEHAVIOUR OF β-2-MICROGLOBULIN DURING ACETATE DIALYSIS (HDac), BIOFILTRATION (BF) AND PAIRED FILTRATION DIALYSIS (PFD)

V. SAVICA, G.BELLINGHIERI[1], A.MALLAMACE[2], B.RICCIARDI[2], F.TORRE[2], A.SAPORITA[2], C.GIARDINA[2], M.L.RESTA[2], M.EGITTO[2], G.CAVALLARO[3]

Cattedre di Nefrologia Sperimentale, Nefrologia[1], Clinica Medica 1[2]- Clinica Chirurgica[3] - Università di Messina .

INTRODUCTION

Literature data report   the presence of a like-amyloid substance in the tendons, synovias and in the bones of the patients undergoing long term dialytic treatment(1,2,3,4). The β-2-microglobulin, produced by lynphoid cells and by the mastocytes when the blood comes into contact with the dialytic membranes, was identified as the most impor tant component of the like-amyloid substance. Many autors(1,2,3,4) re fer that the above substance plays a negative role on the bones alte gation progression of the dialyzed patients and it may be considered as an index of the adequate dialysis. The above considerations and the introduction of the PFD among the new dialytic strategies, sugge- sted us to carry a study on the intradialytic behaviour of β-2-micro globulin during standard haemodialytic treatment using cuprophan mem branes during BF and during PFD using respectively AN 69 S and Cupro phan associated to Polisulphone membranes.

MATERIALS AND METHODS

Fifteen patients, 9 males and 6 females, undergoing periodic haemo- dialytic treatment three time per week for 180 minutes since at least 12 months(range 12-168), aging 33 to 65 years(mean 48,2) without nutri tional impairement were studied. None of them, previously dialyzed with cuprophan membranes, had residual diuresis. The patients were divided in 3 groups of five subjects according to the various dialytic treat ment and various dialytic membranes used: - one group was dialyzed with cuprophan membranes of 1,2 mq.surface for 180 minutes; -the se- cond group was dialyzed for 180 minutes utilizing the BF technique with AN69S membranes and infusion of a 3 liters of 40 mEq/lt bicarbo nate solution; -The last group was dialyzed by PFD for 180 minutes with a cuprophan membrane of 1,06 mq.surface associated with a poli- sulphone of 0,4 mq surface membranes and a dialisate solution costi- tued by bicarbonate. During dialysis, to all patients were administe-

red 5.000 U.I. of eparine continuously.Blood samples were obtained at
times 0,15,30,60,120,180 minutes during the middle week treatment,from
all fasting patients(pts),to dose by RIA technique,the serum β-2-mi-
croglobulin levels using Eiken Chemical Co.Kits. The results were sta
tistically evalued by t of student.

RESULTS

During the standard dialytic treatment using cuprophan membranes the
β-2-microglobulin serum levels significantly increased at the various
times (Fig. 1).Using the biofiltration technique,with AN69S membrane
was noted a significant decrease of the β-2-microglobulin at the end
of the dialytic treatment(Fig.1) while from 0 to 15 minutes an increase was registered. Using paired filtration dialysis technique with
cuprophan and polisulphone associated membranes,a β-2-microglobulin
serum levels decrease was registered at the end of the dialysis while
an increase was reported from 0 to 30 minutes starting dialysis(Fig.1)

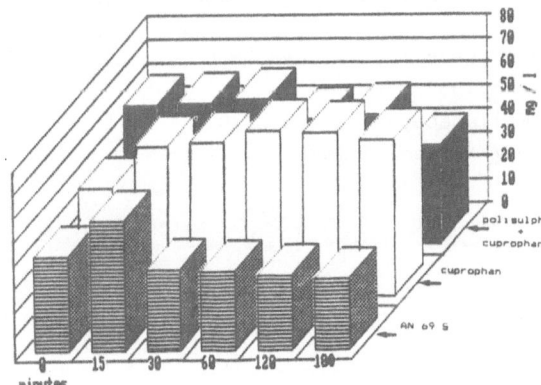

Fig.1 : β-2microglobulin
serum levels during HD
with polisulphone + cupro
phan,cuprophan,AN69S mem-
branes.

Conclusions

   Our results show that:
- The behaviour of the β-2-microglobulin during BF and PFD is better
than standard dialysis to remove β-2-microglobulin from the serum of
the dialyzed patients;
- The decrease is due to the dialytic membranes used and not to the
dialytic treatment technique,because the AN69S and polisulphone membranes have a good clearance for the β-2-microglobulin.
- The cuprophan membranes increase the β-2-microglobulin serum levels
during dialysis,for activation of leucocytes interleukin 1 and complement mediated.In fact we and other autors report a significant activation of the complement during dialysis(5).
- Today is reported thet the β-2- microglobulin may be considered as

an index of adequate and biocompatible dialysis,therephore it is possible to affirm that the AN69S and polisulphone membranes are two membranes more biocompatible than others.The polisulphone membrane,however,suffers the negative effect of the cuprophan association in PFD. It is important to consider that a new membranes association for PFD technique,in order to a better answer to biocompatibility criteria is necessary.A solution could be or the realization of a new association between polisulphone and a more biocompatible membrane or the variation of the surface ratio between the associated membranes advantaging the polisulphone and avoiding,however,back-filtration phenomena.

References

1.Gejo,F.,Yamada,T.,Odani,S.,Nokagana,Y.,:Bioch.Biophys Res Comm,129: 701÷706,1985
2.Vanderbrouke,J.M.,Jadoul,M.,Maldagne,B.,Huaux,J.P.,Noel,H.,van Yper sele de Striou,C.,:The Lancet i:1210-1211,1986
3.Haglustaine,D.,Waer,M.,Michielse,P.,Goebbels.J.,Vandeputte,M.,: The Lancet i,1211,1986
4.Bommer,J.,Seelig,P.,Seelig R.,Geerlings,W.,Bommer,G.,and Ritz,E.,: Nephrol Dial Transplant 2:22-25,1987
5.Savica,V.,Bellinghieri,G.,Mallamace,A.,Ricciardi,B.,: Arch. Att. Med. Chir. Me,Anno XXX,fasc.II,1986

IN VITRO INFLUENCE OF SIX DIALYSIS MEMBRANES ON BETA-2-MICROGLOBULIN BEHAVIOUR.

D. Bonucchi, L. Lucchi, G. Cappelli, A. Stefani, A. Baraldi, E. Lusvarghi.
Nephrology and Dialysis Department, University Hospital, 41100 Modena, Italy.

INTRODUCTION

In 1987 Beta-2-Microglobulin (ß2M) was reported to increase during dialysis and was suggested as an index of membrane biocompatibility (1). The issue is still controversial and different mechanisms have been proposed: according to De Broe, ß2M generation might occur in lung vascular bed (2), while others suggest ß2M production by white blood cells stimulated by cuprophan (CU) and contaminants (3).
We therefore studied ß2M behaviour in a simplified dialysis system containing the membrane under investigation and the blood components necessary in bioincompatibility reactions. In this experimental model we previously demonstrated complement activation and leukocyte oxidative metabolism stimulation (4): in addition, we chose to use fresh normal blood so as to enable even very small variations in ß2M concentration to be detected.

MATERIALS AND METHODS

Six different commercially available hollow fiber membranes were used in the study. We tested 6 dialyzers for each membrane that included: CU (BL 612M, 1.2 sqm, Bellco, Mirandola, Italy), cellulose acetate (CA) (CDAK 4000, 1.4 sqm, Cordis-Dow Corp., Miami, Fl, U.S.A.), hemophan (HE) (BL 613HB, 1.3 sqm, Bellco), polyacrylonitrile (PAN) (Filtral AN-69HF, 1.15 sqm, Hospal, Basel), polymethylmetha-crylate (B2-150, 1.26 sqm, Toray Industries, Tokio, Japan), polysulphone (PS) (BL 627, 1.3 sqm, Bellco). The closed loop dialysis system consisted of PVC lines and the dialyzer under investigation immersed in a water bath at 37°C, and of a peristaltic blood pump allowing blood flow of 150 ml/min. The circuit was filled with 180 ml of fresh heparinized (1 I.U./ml) blood from healthy donors; dialysate compartment contained 200 ml of a sterile and pyrogen free solution similar to plasma water (Ca^{++} 1.3 mM/l) and was closed to avoid ultrafiltration.

ß2M was measured with Enzyme Immunoassay (Enzygnost ß2-Microglobulin. Behringwerke AG, Marburg, W. Germany), with a lower limit of detection of 0.003 mg/l. Blood samples were drawn at 0, 60 and 120 min.; dialysate was tested for ß2M at the end of any experiment.

Student's t test was used for statistical handling of data.

RESULTS

Mean basal values of ß2M were 1.65 ± 0.10 mg/l. As shown in Table 1, cellulosic membranes and PMMA caused ß2M to fall at 60 and 120 min., but, as expected, no ß2M was found in dialysate.

Using PAN and PS, ß2M disappeared from blood at 60 as at 120 min., and was absent in dialysate.

Table 1. In vitro ß2M levels (mg/l).

Time(min)	Plasma			Dialysate
	0	60	120	120
CU	1.65 ± 0.16	1.26 ± 0.24*	1.21 ± 0.23**	<0.01
CA	1.69 ± 0.12	0.72 ± 0.08**	0.66 ± 0.08**	<0.01
HE	1.54 ± 0.15	0.83 ± 0.06**	0.88 ± 0.17**	<0.01
PMMA	1.77 ± 0.19	1.00 ± 0.15**	0.67 ± 0.16**	<0.01
PAN	1.73 ± 0.21	<0.01	<0.01	<0.01
PS	1.52 ± 0.19	<0.01	<0.01	<0.01

* = $p < 0.02$; ** = $p < 0.01$ vs. basal value.

DISCUSSION

Previous studies by some of us demonstrated increased levels of C3a and polymorphonuclear resting chemiluminescence in our system (4); nevertheless, ß2M does not increase in this experiment.

The significant fall in ß2M concentration observed in this study also with cellulosic membranes might be explained by the high membrane surface/blood volume ratio, causing a small adsorption, as demonstrated by Sakai (5). On the other hand, membranes able to adsorb proteins effectively, like PAN and PS, clear ß2M completely at 60 minutes. The conclusion can be drawn that a system effective in anaphyla-toxin production and oxidative metabolism stimulation (4), fails to generate ß2M.

Wherease uremic retention of ß2M is firmly established and

inversely related to GFR, the influence of dialysis procedure on ß2M metabolism is still under investigation. Effective removal, even if lower than daily generation, is achieved by using highly permeable membranes (6).

Data about plasma ß2M behaviour during dialysis using different membranes are controversial, but some groups have claimed a rise in ß2M with CU dialysis. ß2M generation might result from the so-called "release phenomena": our data seem to exclude a direct influence of dialysis membranes on ß2M generation by circulating leukocytes, in spite of C3a increase. The possibility that extradialytic target-cells, like type I pneumocytes, could be activated by anaphylatoxins and oxygen-free radicals is indirectly confirmed by our findings.

If in vivo ß2M generation occurs during dialysis, this would take place outside the dialyzer, possibly caused by cells other than leukocytes.

REFERENCES

1. Deuber, H.J., Mühlbaur, H.G., Schulz, W. and Frank, R. BLood Purification 5: 278, 1987.
2. De Broe, M.E., Nouwen, J. and Waeleghem, J.P. Nephrol. Dial. Transplant. 2: 124-125, 1987.
3. Yamagami, S., Mori, K., Sugimura, T., Nishimoto, K., Kishimoto, T., Maekawa, M. and Naito, H. Nephrol. Dial. Transplant. 2: 442, 1987.
4. Lucchi, L., Cappelli, G., Acerbi, M.A., Spattini A. and Lusvarghi, E. Blood Purification 5: 276, 1987.
5. Sakai, K., Nagase, M. and Tsuda, S. Nephrol. Dial. Transplant. 2: 449, 1987.
6. Kaiser, J.P., Hagemann, J., von Herrath, D. and Schaefer, K. Nephron 48: 132-135, 1987.

BEHAVIOUR OF BETA2MICROGLOBULIN IN CRF PATIENTS STARTING BLOOD PURI-
FICATION.
CHIMIENTI S., MELE G., PERRONE F., DISTRATIS C., MUSCOGIURI P. &
CRISTOFANO C.
Nephrology Department, Manduria (TA) - ITALY

INTRODUCTION

Beta2microglobulin (B2m) has been shown play a causal role in
amyloidosis of long term hemodialyzed patients. Many authors demonstrated that increased levels of B2m and amyloid deposition are dire
ctly correlated with the use of cuprophane dialysis membranes (1).
This findings led several authors to study the capacity of different
membranes to generate or to remove this protein (2). Less is known
about the behaviour of B2m in CRF patients beginning hemodialysis
treatment. The purpose of this study is to compare B2m in patients
dropped out conservative therapy with artificial diet supplemented
with ketoanalogues and essential aminoacids (AD) (3), beginning different types of blood depuration, monthly until six months.

MATERIALS AND METHODS

9 male subjects with chronic glomerulonephritis and CRF, drop-
ping out AD, were introduced to this study. 3 pts underwent chronic
conventional hemodialysis (HD) with hollow fiber cuprophane membrane
(1.3 mq. SA). 3 pts on chronic hemofiltration (HF) with polyamide
membrane (2 mq. SA). 3 pts on once a week hemofiltration (OWHF) with
polyamide membrane (2 mq.SA) and AD.Serum and urinary B2m levels were
measured when patients started the first treatment and monthly until
six months(B2m radioimmunoassay kit -Eiken chemical Co.,LTD).Curves
and statistical analysis performed by IBM computer.

RESULTS

Serum B2m levels in HD are:

15mcg/ml before the first treatment

25mcg/ml at two months,30mcg/ml at

four months,33mcg/ml at six months

$(Y=20e^{7.2x};r=0.99;P=0.001)$.In HF

are:13mcg/ml before the first treat-

ment,22mcg/ml at two months,24mcg/ml

at four months,23mcg/ml at six mon-

ths $(Y=17e^{4.4x};r=0.94;P=0.01)$.In

OWHF are:15mcg/ml before the first

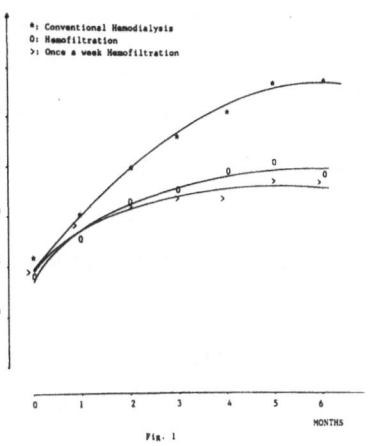

Fig. 1

treatment,22mcg/ml at two months,22mcg/ml at four months,23mcg/ml at

six months $(Y=17.9e^{3.2x};r=0.94;P=0.01)$.(Fig.1).Urinary B2m reaches

zero in HD or HF subjects after few days of treatment,for the contra-

ction of diuresis. In OWHF B2m urinary elimination is 228mg/day.

DISCUSSION

Results show that B2m increases in subjects on HD treated with

cuprophane membrane in earlier phases of treatment reaching in an

exponential way at six months twice the initial values, far from HF

values;moreover the calculated values of B2m at ten years for the

curve of conventional hemodialysis are similar to values obtained by

patients on conventional cuprophane HD for ten years (55mcg/ml Vs.

60mcg/ml respectively,PNS).

In HF patients B2m levels reach the steady state and is similar

to patients on OWHF that have residual diuresis.

We conclude that the early use of membranes that can remove B2m

and HF technology can play an important role to resolve amyloidosis,

now an unresolved problem.

REFERENCES

1) Gejyo F., Homma N., Suzuki Y., Azakawa M.; Serum levels of Beta2-
microglobulin as a new form of amyloid protein in patients undergoing
long-term hemodialysis.New. Eng. J. Med. 314,9,585-586(1986).

2) Hanglstaine D., Waer M., Michielsen P.,Goebels J., Vandeputte M.:
Hemodialysis membranes, serum Beta2microglobulin dialysis amyloidosis. Lancet 1,8491,1211(1986).

3) Barsotti G., Guiducci A., Ciardella F.,Giovannetti S.: Effects
on renal function of a low nitrogen diet supplemented with essential
aminoacids and ketoanalogues and of hemodialysis and free protein
supply in patients with chronic renal failure. Nephron 27:113-117
(1981).

Nutrition

STANDARDS FOR NUTRITIONAL ASSESSMENT IN DIALYSIS

JOEL D. KOPPLE

Division of Nephrology and Hypertension, Harbor-UCLA Medical Center and UCLA Schools of Medicine and Public Health, Torrance, California 90509

This paper will discuss the strengths and limitations of methods for assessing the nutritional status of maintenance dialysis patients. Virtually every survey of the nutritional status of patients undergoing maintenance hemodialysis, intermittent peritoneal dialysis, or continuous ambulatory peritoneal dialysis (CAPD) indicates that they frequently suffer from wasting or protein-calorie malnutrition (1-5). The evidence includes decreased relative body weight (the patient's body weight divided by the weight of normal people of the same age, height, sex and frame size), skinfold thickness (an estimate of body fat), arm muscle diameter or surface area (a reflection of total muscle protein mass), total body nitrogen, decreased serum concentrations of many proteins (including albumin, prealbumin, transferrin and certain complement proteins), low muscle alkali soluble protein, and low growth rates in children. The plasma amino acid pattern, which is unique to chronic renal failure, shows many similarities to the amino acid pattern in protein calorie malnutrition. Total body potassium tends to be low in patients with chronic renal failure and normal in individuals undergoing maintenance hemodialysis (data are reviewed in references 1-6).

In most individuals, the wasting would be classified as mild or moderate. However, in the author's experience, approximately 10 to 15 percent of maintenance hemodialysis patients suffer from more severe wasting. It should be emphasized that many patients undergoing maintenance hemodialysis are not wasted, and that it is only when comparing groups of chronic renal failure patients to age and sex matched controls that the evidence for wasting is clearly apparent. Indeed, many individual parameters of malnutrition are often within normal limits; however, the values are often at the lower range of normal.

Although the nutritional disorder most commonly associated with maintenance dialysis patients is protein-calorie malnutrition, other nutritional deficiencies may also occur if the patient does not receive supplemental nutrients. For example, in unsupplemented maintenance dialysis patients, deficiencies are not uncommon for 1,25-dihydroxy-cholecalciferol, vitamin B_6, folic acid, iron and possibly carnitine and zinc (7-13).

There are many causes for wasting and malnutrition; these have been reviewed elsewhere (6,14). In brief, the causes include inadequate nutrient intake, the presence of underlying illnesses (e.g., heart, lung, or liver failure, lupus erythematosus), the frequent occurrence of superimposed illnesses (e.g., sepsis) and the catabolic effects of the dialysis procedure itself. Other possible but less well documented causes of wasting include increased levels of catabolic hormones, uremic toxins and altered cellular function due to the uremic environment or, in the diseased kidney, to loss of renal parenchyma. Thus, wasting is caused not only by inadequate nutrient intake but also by other metabolic and clinical disorders. It also follows from this observation that the parameters for assessing nutritional status usually do not distinguish between the effects of inadequate nutrient intake and the effects of catabolic stresses caused by underlying or superimposed illnesses or the other above mentioned factors.

It is not clear to what extent poor nutritional status of uremic patients causes adverse or undesirable effects. Most clinicians would agree that it is probably undesirable for chronically uremic patients to have even mild malnutrition. However, the evidence that mild or moderate malnutrition impairs the health, quality of life or longevity of uremic patients is very sparse. Indeed, there are few studies concerning the relationship between nutritional status and clinical outcome in patients with renal failure.

Shapiro and associates reported that maintenance hemodialysis patients who had an average serum urea nitrogen (SUN) level below 60 mg/dl had greater mortality rates than patients who had average SUN levels greater than 80 mg/dl (15). The mean of 10 SUN values were taken to define the different groups. For a given hemodialysis regimen, low SUN levels are often reflective of a decreased protein intake. Hence, the results of this study have been interpreted to indicate that low protein intakes are associated with increased mortality in maintenance hemodialysis patients. Acchiardo and coworkers examined this question by assessing the relationship between net protein degradation, an indicator of protein intake, in a group of maintenance hemodialysis patients who were monitored for 12 months (16). Net protein degradation was determined by dialysis urea kinetic techniques. Their results in 98 nondiabetic patients indicated that those individuals with the lowest protein intake, as indicated by the lowest net rate of urea generation, had the higher incidence of hospitalization and mortality.

Anderson and Wochos reported that of 47 patients admitted to a nephrology service, those individuals with a low serum albumin (less than 3.4g/dl) had a significantly longer duration of hospitalization than those with higher serum albumin levels (17). We evaluated the relationship between nutritional status and the number of days that patients spent in the hospital in a group of patients undergoing self-care maintenance hemodialysis or intermittent peritoneal dialysis (reference 2, unpublished observations). The nutritional parameters were assessed at the time that patients were beginning maintenance dialysis therapy. The results indicated that there was an inverse relationship between the number of days that patients spent in the hospital and each of the following parameters: protein intake, energy intake (each determined from dietary interviews), relative body weight and mid-arm muscle diameter. Unexpectedly, serum transferrin levels correlated directly with the number of days of hospitalization.

A number of investigators have examined whether giving nutritional supplements to maintenance hemodialysis or CAPD patients will improve the nutritional status of these patients (18-22). Patients either received amino acid infusions intravenously or into dialysate during the course of dialysis treatments or were given oral supplements to ingest daily. Outcome usually was assessed in terms of nutritional parameters rather than overall clinical status. In these studies, there was, in general, no attempt to distinguish the response of the malnourished patients separately from the more well nourished individuals. Individual studies usually evaluated only small numbers of patients. Moreover, there was no evidence presented as to how much of the oral nutritional supplement, in the patients prescribed oral rather than intravenous nutrition, and how much of the patient's usual food intake was actually ingested by the patients during the study. These limitations in the experimental design of the studies may explain why the results do not clearly indicate improvement in the nutritional status or clinical course of maintenance dialysis patients given nutritional supplements.

We monitored the nutritional status of adult patients undergoing self-care maintenance hemodialysis or intermittent peritoneal dialysis and children undergoing CAPD (2,23, also unpublished observations). The results of these studies indicated: 1. That patients frequently exhibited wasting and malnutrition and (in children) growth retardation at the commencement of maintenance dialysis therapy. 2. The patients' nutritional status at the onset of dialysis treatment was a good predictor of their nutritional status one to three years later. On the other hand, we also evaluated nondialyzed adult patients with advanced chronic renal failure who were treated with dietary therapy. These individuals maintained good nutritional status even though their average estimated glomerular filtration rate (GFR) (i.e., mean of creatinine and urea clearances) at the end of the study was only 5.2 ml/min.

These observations suggest that patients may be at greatest risk for developing wasting and malnutrition immediately before and during the time that they commence maintenance dialysis (i.e., when the GFR is less than 5.0 ml/min and immediately afterwards). Since most patients who are wasted at the onset of dialysis remain so for at least one to three years afterwards, the most effective way to avoid wasting in dialysis patients may be to prevent it during the small "window" between the time when patients have clinically stable chronic renal failure and when they are in need of maintenance dialysis.

Methods that potentially could reduce the incidence or ameliorate the severity of wasting or malnutrition during the period when patients commence dialysis therapy include the following:

1. Maintain good nutritional intake during this

period.

2. Earlier commencement of dialysis therapy. This usually requires careful planning to arrange for the smooth transition from the conservative management of renal failure to maintenance dialysis treatment. The patient will need to have vascular access prostheses placed earlier, when the GFR is sufficiently great so that patients are in no imminent need for dialysis treatment.

3. Rigorous attempts to avoid superimposed catabolic illnesses.

4. Vigorous treatment of superimposed illnesses including nutritional support.

It is our impression that during and immediately before the time when most patients begin dialysis treatment, their food intake is decreased (2). A large proportion of our patients who are beginning maintenance dialysis treatment describe the loss of nonedematous weight during the preceding weeks or months. The following factors contribute to the reduced food intake and weight loss: anorexia caused by uremic toxicity, frequent employment of diagnostic or therapeutic procedures that require the patient to fast (e.g., radiographic studies, vascular access placement), and superimposed illnesses. Not uncommonly, in a clinically stable patient with advanced renal failure who has not been prepared for maintenance dialysis, a superimposed illness precipitates a sudden decrement in renal function, engenders the development of uremic toxicity, and causes a sudden need for dialysis therapy. Careful preparation of patients who have stable advanced renal failure (e.g., GFR of about 6 to 10 ml/min/1.73m^2) for maintenance dialysis and attention to the nutritional intake of these patients should enable the physician to inaugurate dialysis when it is needed and to maintain better nutritional status.

It should be emphasized that these recommendations for avoiding wasting are based upon hypotheses that must be confirmed by careful prospective clinical trials. It is possible, for example, that the polyendocrinopathy that occurs in advanced renal failure may also cause wasting at the time when patients begin dialysis therapy. Such a cause of wasting might not be preventable with better nutritional intake and earlier onset of maintenance dialysis.

The standards that can be used to assess and monitor the nutritional status of patients may be classified into two groups: Those that can be used under clinical conditions and those which may have particular value for research purposes. Tables 1 and 2 contain proposed lists of methods for nutritional assessment that could be used for clinical or research activities. The measures indicated in Table 1 may be used for research studies as well as the clinical management of patients, whereas the techniques shown in Table 2 are generally only used for research investigations. It should be emphasized that this list is rather arbitrary. In any individual laboratory, the combination of familiarity, expertise, and ready availability of a given method for assessing nutritional status could convert a technique which is usually utilized as a research tool into a one that could be used for the clinical management of patients.

Unfortunately, the precision, reproducibility, and sensitivity of most methods of nutritional assessment are not good. These techniques usually are able to discriminate cases of advanced malnutrition from normal individuals. However, the methods are least reliable in identifying mild or impending malnutrition, and it is these latter, subtle cases of malnutrition where identification is most difficult and specialized testing is most needed. This problem exists for the assessment of vitamin and mineral malnutrition and the evaluation of lipid disorders and altered lipoprotein metabolism as well as for the examination of protein-calorie malnutrition. The effects of uremia per se on some of the methods of nutritional assessment have not been well defined. Renal failure could alter the measurements independently of the presence of wasting or malnutrition. For example, it is not known whether altered body electrolyte content in uremic patients will influence electrical impedance determinations.

Table 1. Use of nutritional parameters for clinical monitoring of maintenance dialysis patients[a]

I. Nutrient intake
1. Urea nitrogen appearance - urea kinetic analyses
2. Dietary diaries, interviews

II. Serum concentrations
1. Proteins (albumin, transferrin)
2. Minerals - electrolytes - especially P, K, Na, HCO_3^-
3. Lipids - cholesterol, triglycerides, HDL-cholesterol

III. Body composition
1. Subjective global nutritional assessment
2. Body weight (edema free)
3. Desirable body weight
4. Relative body weight
5. Percent of preillness weight
6. Interdialytic weight gain, edema status
7. Skinfold thickness (triceps, biceps, subscapular) and estimated body fat
8. Mid-arm muscle area
9. Height, weight and height and weight gain (children)

---

[a]References 2, 23-26 discuss the techniques for using many of these parameters and their strengths and limitations.

Table 2.   Use of nutritional parameters for research
           activities[a,b]

   I.   Serum or tissue concentrations
        1.   Other serum proteins (e.g., prealbumin,
             cholinesterase, pseudocholinesterase)
        2.   Plasma amino acids
        3.   Muscle alkali soluble protein, RNA:DNA
             ratio, free amino acids, electrolytes
        4.   Serum lipoproteins
        5.   Vitamin assays
        6.   Trace element analyses
  II.   Body composition or pools
        1.   Total body nitrogen, potassium
        2.   Isotope dilution studies - D_2O, Br or Cl
             spaces
        3. Na_e/K_e ratio
        4.   Electrical impedance
        5.   Radiographic measurement of compartments
             (e.g., size of muscle mass in arm or leg)
        6.   Magnetic resonance imaging
        7.   Nitrogen and mineral balances
 III.   Functional parameters
        1.   Energy expenditure
        2.   Protein or amino acid turnover
        3.   Immune function (e.g., skin tests,
             lymphocyte count, polymorphonuclear
             leukocyte mobility, phagocytosis and
             killing)
        4.   Muscle contractility

---

[a]These are in addition to the parameters listed in
Table 1 which can also be used for scientific
investigation involving nutritional status.
[b]References 2 and 25 discuss the techniques for use
and the strengths and limitations of many of these
parameters.

It also should be emphasized that many of the factors that cause wasting and malnutrition in patients with renal failure are not nutritional (see above); superimposed catabolic stress or underlying debilitating illnesses (e.g., chronic heart, liver or lung failure) may contribute to these disorders. It therefore follows that the parameters listed in Tables 1 and 2 provide information concerning both the nutritional status and the overall clinical condition of the patient with renal failure. The extent to which these parameters can be used exclusively to 1. assess nutritional status, 2. determine whether the nutritional intake is optimal or 3. evaluate whether changing the nutrient intake may improve the patient's nutritional status is often limited and will vary from patient to patient. As in virtually all matters related to the medical care of patients, the physician ultimately will have to use judgement in interpreting the results of nutritional assessment.

The degree to which parameters of nutritional status will identify malnutrition, predict morbidity or mortality, or identify patients who may improve with better nutritional intake may be enhanced by multivariate analyses of these outcome measures. These techniques have been used in sick patients who do not, as a rule, have renal disease. Mullens and coworkers have developed a linear predictive equation of outcome of hospitalized patients, referred to as the prognostic nutritional index (27). Their equation is as follows: Percent risk of complications = 158 - 16.6 (serum albumin) - 0.78 (triceps skinfold thickness) - 0.20 (serum transferrin) - 5.8 (delayed cutaneous hypersensitivity). Dempsey and Mullen have recently reviewed the literature concerning nutritional indices, and they have analyzed the advantages and limitations of these methods (28). The development of prognostic nutritional indices for nondialyzed patients with chronic renal failure, patients undergoing maintenance hemodialysis or peritoneal dialysis, and individuals who have received a renal transplant would seem to be a fruitful area for further investigation.

In summary, this paper has briefly reviewed published data that indicates that maintenance dialysis patients frequently are wasted and malnourished. There are many causes for the wasting; some of these causes are not strictly nutritional. Most parameters for assessing nutritional status are not very sensitive, specific or reproducible. Evidence is accumulating that the presence of parameters of wasting or malnutrition indicate an increased risk for morbidity and mortality in maintenance dialysis patients. However, this relationship may reflect the fact that illnesses which cause morbidity and mortality also reduce nutritional intake and promote wasting. It is not established that providing more calories or protein to such individuals will improve their prognosis. Further research is necessary to 1. establish more sensitive and reliable indicators of nutritional status, 2. to examine the relationships between parameters of nutritional status and clinical outcome, and 3. to assess under what conditions improving nutritional intake may improve the nutritional and clinical status of patients with renal failure.

Supported by the UCLA Clinical Nutrition Research Unit Grant # 5 PO1 CA 42710.

REFERENCES:

1. Attman, P.O., Ewald, J. and Isaksson B.   Am. J. Clin. Nutr. 33:801-810, 1980.

2. Blumenkrantz, M.J., Kopple, J.D., Gutman, R.A., Chan, Y.K., Barbour, G.L., Roberts, C., Shen, F.H., Gandhi, V.C., Tucker, C.T., Curtis F.K. and Coburn J.W. Am. J. Clin. Nutr. 33:1567-1585, 1980.

3. Young, G.A., Swanepoel, C.R., Croft, M.R. and Hobson S.M. Kidney Int. 21:492-499, 1982.

4. Schoenfeld, P.Y., Henry, R.R., Laird, N.M. and Roxe D.M. Kidney Int. 23:S80-88, 1983.

5. Wolfson, M, Strong, C.J., Minturn, D., Gray, D.K. and Kopple J.D. Am. J. Clin. Nutr. 37:547-555, 1984.

6. Kopple, J.D. In: Nephrology Volume II. (Ed R.R. Robinson), Springer-Verlag, New York, 1984, pp. 1498-1515.

7. Gray, R.W., Weber, H.P., Dominguez, J.H. and Lemann J. Clin. Endocrinol. Metab. 39:1045, 1974.

8. Kopple, J.D., Mercurio, K, Blumenkrantz, M.J., Jones, M.R., Tallos, J., Roberts, C., Card, B., Saltzman, R., Casciato, D.A. and Swendseid M.E. Kidney Int. 19:694-704, 1981.

9. Whitehead, V.M., Comty, C.H., Posen, G.A. and Kaye, M. N. Engl. J. Med. 279:970-974, 1968.

10. Kopple, J.D. and Swendseid, M.E. Kidney Int. 7:S79-S84, 1975.

11. Lawson, D.H., Boddy, K., King, P.C., Linton, A.L. and Will G. Clin. Science 41:345-351, 1971.

12. Mahajan, S.K., Prasad, A.S., Lambujon, J., Abbasi, A.A., Briggs, W.A. and McDonald F.D. Am. J. Clin. Nutr. 33:1517-1521, 1980.

13. Guarnieri, G., Toigo, G., Crapesi, L., Situlin, R., Del Bianco, M.A., Corsi, M., LoGreco, P., Paviotti, G., Mioni, G. and Campanacci L. Kidney Int. 32:S116-S127, 1987.

14. Kopple, J.D. Kidney Int. 14:340-348, 1978.

15. Shapiro, J.I., Argy, W.P., Rakowski, T.A., Chester, A., Siemsen, A.S. and Schreiner G.E. Trans. Am. Soc. Artif. Intern. Organs 29:129-134, 1983.

16. Acchiardo, S.R., Moore, L.W. and Latour P.A. Kidney Int. 24:S199-S203, 1983.

17. Anderson, C.F. and Wochos, D.N. Mayo Clin. Proc. 57:181-184, 1982.

18. Heidland, A and Kult, J. Clin. Nephrol. 3:234-239, 1975.

19. Hecking, E., Port, F.K., Brehm, H., Zobel, R., Brandl, M., Prellwitz, W. and Opferkuch, W. Kidney Int. 12:482, 1977.

20. Ulm, A., Neuhauser, M. and Leber H.-W. Am. J. Clin. Nutr. 31:1827-1830, 1978.

21. Williams, F.P., Marliss, E.B., Anderson, G.H., et al. Perit. Dial. Bull. 2:124-130, 1982.

22. Feinstein, E.I., Collins, J.F., Blumenkrantz, M.J., Roberts, M., Kopple, J.D. and Massry S.G. Progress. Artif. Organs. 1:421-426, 1984.

23. Salusky, I.B., Fine, R.N., Nelson, P, Blumenkrantz, M.J. and Kopple J.D. Am. J. Clin. Nutr. 38:599-611, 1983.

24. Sargent, J., Gotch, F., Borah, M., Piercy, L., Spinozzi, N., Schoenfeld, P. and Humphreys, M. Am. J. Clin. Nutr. 31:1696-1702, 1978.

25. Guarnieri, G., Kopple, J.D. and Furst, P. (Eds.) J. Parent. Enter. Nutrit. 11:33S-137S, 1987.

26. Detsky, A.S., McLaughlin, J.R., Baker, J.P., Johnston, N., Whittaker, S., Mendelson, R.A. and Jeejeebhoy, K.N. J. Parent. Enterl. Nutr. 11:8-13, 1987.

27. Mullen, J.L., Buzby, G.P., Waldman, M.T., Gertner, M.H., Hobbs, C.L. and Rosato E.F. Surg. Forum 30:80-82, 1979.

28. Dempsey, D.T. and Mullen, J.L. J. Parent. Enteral. Nutr. 11:109S-114S, 1987.

IS MALNUTRITION A CLINICALLY EVIDENT CONDITION IN PATIENTS UNDERGOING HEMODIALYSIS?

B.Cianciaruso, A.Capuano, F.Marcuccio, L.A.Reed°,
F.Contaldo°, A.Nastasi°°, V.E.Andreucci

Division of Nephrology,Div.of Internal Medicine°,Dietetic
Service°°,II Faculty of Medicine,Univ.of Naples,Naples.

Several studies have indicated that patients undergoing hemodialysis (HD) may develop protein-energy malnutrition (1,2). However,few attempts have been made to assess if wasting may occur in HD patients even when they
appear healthy by a simple clinical examination. The purpose of this study was to evaluate the occurrence of malnutrition in a selected group of healthy patients considered in good nutritional status by clinical judgement.

METHODS

Fortysix HD patients were examined (33 males and 13
females, age 36±13 years) and 233 normal subjects (132 males,101 females,age 39±7years) of the same geographic area
Patients were selected on the basis of good dialysis tolerance and good nutritional status,as judged by the staff
of the dialysis unit. Were excluded diabetics,patients
with chronic respiratory and gastrointestinal diseases and
patients who had recent surgery or acute illnesses in the
last 6 months. Nutrient intake was estimated with dietetic
diaries and interviews. Anthropometric measurements included body weight,height,tricipital,bicipital,subscapular
and suprailiac skinfolds (Lange Caliper,Cambridge,Maril.)
and middlearm circumference. All measurements were carried

out after dialysis, blood specimens were collected before dialysis. Data are reported as mean and standard deviation.

RESULTS

Nutrient intake showed a rather high calories (total calories:41 ± 11,Kcal/kg/day) and proteins (1.7 ± 0.7gr/kg/day) intake. Body Weight (BW),Body Mass Index (BMI=BW/H^2) and Body Fat are reported in Table 1.

	BW (kg)		BMI		BF (%)	
	M	F	M	F	M	F
U	61 ± 10**	56 ± 8*	23 ± 2**	24 ± 5*	23 ± 6	32 ± 8*
C	75 ± 12	65 ± 10	27 ± 4	27 ± 5	24 ± 6	36 ± 7

Uremic vs Control:$p<0.05$(*), $p<0.001$ (**)

Tricipital(TSF),bicipital(BSF),suprailiac(SISF), subscapular(SSSF) skinfolds are reported in Table 2.

	TSF		BSF		SISF		SSSF	
	M	F	M	F	M	F	M	F
U	11 ± 5	21 ± 7	6 ± 3*	11 ± 6	17 ± 9	18 ± 10*	15 ± 6*	16 ± 10**
C	11 ± 4	22 ± 8	8 ± 4	13 ± 6	18 ± 8	25 ± 10	18 ± 7	26 ± 10

Uremic vs Control:$p<0.05$ (*),$p<0.005$ (**). SF units are cm.

Serum albumin(g/dl),prealbumin(mg/dl),retinol binding protein (R.B.P.,mg/dl),arm musce circonference (A.M.C.,cm),transferrin (g/L), lynphocyte count (n/mm^3) are reported in Table 3.

	ALB.	PREALB.	R.B.P.	A.M.C.	TRANSF.	LYNF.COUNT
M	3.9 ± 0.5	40.9 ± 11.3	25.7 ± 6.3	25 ± 2.5	2.4 ± 0.5	1932 ± 951
<NR	15%	0%	0%	36%	18%	38%
>NR	0%	33%	100%	0%	0%	0%
F	3.7 ± 0.5	36.7 ± 9.7	24.5 ± 6.5	23 ± 3.6	2.4 ± 0.9	1659 ± 499
NR	38%	0%	0%	8%	31%	45%
NR	0%	8%	100%	0%	8%	0%

M=males;F=females. NR=normal range.

DISCUSSION

Several studies have shown that wasting and malnutrition are common in HD patients (1-3). In these patients, however, malnutrition may be masked by extracellular volume expansion. Often the true degree of malnutrition may not be obvious until extracellular volume expansion has been reduced by ultrafiltration during dialysis therapy. The patients selected for this study are representative of the healthy dialysis population, nevertheless our data indicate that they also are at risk of wasting. Body mass index,infact, was significantly decreased in HD patients as compared to normal subjects. Both men and women HD patients tended to have less fat stores than controls;body fat was significantly decreased in HD females and two skinfolds were lower in both males and females patients. Biochemical indices tended to be in the lower normal range,except for prealbumins and R.B.P. which are metabolized by the kidney.

In conclusion malnutrition is a subtle condition in chronic renal failure and may be present even in apparently healthy HD patients.

REFERENCES

1. Attman, P.O., Ewald, J. and Isaksson B. Am. J. Clin. Nutr. 33: 801-810, 1980.
2. Blumenkrantz, M.J., Kopple, J.D., Gutman, R.A., Chan,Y.K., Barbour, G.L., Roberts, C., Shen, F.H., Gandhi, V.C., Tucker, C.T., Curtis, F.K. and Coburn J.W. Am. J. Clin. Nutr. 33:1567-1585, 1980.
3. Wolfson, M., Blumenkrantz M.J., Coburn,J.W., Kopple, J.D. Abstract Book 11th Mtg West Dial Trans Soc. 1980;7.

SERUM BRANCH-CHAIN AMINO AND KETO ACIDS IN THE NUTRITIONAL AND IMMUNOLOGICAL ASSESSMENT OF UREMICS ON CONSERVATIVE AND DIALYSIS TREATMENT.

P. Cappelli, *K. Langer, M. Evangelista, P.F. Palmieri, S. Marzan, G. Del Rosso, B. Di Paolo and A. Albertazzi.

Institute of Nephrology, University of Chieti, Italy; *Institute for Experimental Nutrition, Erlangen, FRG.

INTRODUCTION

Defective cell-mediated immunity (CMI) is well documented in patients with chronic renal failure (CRF) due to many factors (1). The aim of our study was to examine the effects of CRF on serum branch-chain amino and keto acids (BCAA-BCKA), visceral proteins and CMI.

MATERIALS AND METHODS

We examined 4 groups of male patients affected with CRF of different degree, due to various renal diseases. We excluded patients with nephrotic syndrome, diabetes or other systemic diseases. Group 1 (G1) consisted of 20 patients, 25-72 years of age, with creatinine clearance (Cr.C.) of 41.6 ± 13.1 ml/min on free diet. They followed a standard conservative pharmacological treatment. Group 2 (G2) consisted of 20 patients, 32-68 years, Cr.C. 10.6 ± 3.3 ml/min. For 9-20 months all had been on a conventional low-nitrogen diet (CLND: 0.6 g/kg/day of proteins, 700-800 mg/day of phosphorus, 35 kcal/kg/day). Group 3 (G3) consisted of 12 patients, 32-61 years, Cr.C. 8.2 ± 2.4 ml/min. For 8-23 months they had all been on a very low-nitrogen diet (0.3 g/kg/day) supplemented (2) with a mixture of essential amino acids and ketoanalogues (Alfa-Kappa[R], Farma-Biagini), with 35 kcal/kg/day and 300-400 mg/day of phosphorus (SD). Group 4 (G4) consisted of 34 patients, 18-78 years, on standard acetate RDT from 54.5 ± 46.0 months. All were on a completely free diet.

We carried out the following examinations on all patients: skin tests using several recall antigens (Multitest[R] CMI-Institut Mérieux); serum

BCAA (cation exchange chromatography on an analyzer LC 5001) and BCKA (HPLC-method); albumin, transferrin, BUN, PTH. Multitest CMI enables the calculation of a score (MS n.v.: > 10 mm.) (3).

RESULTS

The MS was always normal in G1 (15.7$\pm$3.9) and in G3 (12.1$\pm$1.7) while it was significantly lower ($p < .001$) in G2 (7.7$\pm$2.0) and G4 (3.8$\pm$2.6). The serum values of BCAA and BCKA are reported in Table 1. The BCAA/BCKA ratio gradually increased in all 4 groups and the highest values were observed in RDT patients. In addition, this ratio was negatively correlated to Cr.C. in G2 and G3 ($p < .01$ and $p < .05$ respectively) but Leu/K-Leu in G3. Notice that only in G3 are Leu and K-Leu in inverse correlation ($p < .05$). In G2 the MS was in direct correlation to the Leu/K-Leu ratio ($p < .01$).

As regards the nutritional parameters (Table 2), some significant differences were observed only for transferrin, where the lowest values occurred in G4. Differences in BUN and PTH (Table 2) were significant.

DISCUSSION

CRF has an inhibitory effect on cell-mediated immunity as assessed by cutaneous tests. RDT enhances the problem while SD corrects it. Decreasing serum level of BCAA-BCKA may reflect a specific action of uremia, enhanced by a wasting effect of RDT which is exerted also on visceral proteins. SD, although it does allow an adequate nutritional status, does not correct the alterations of BCAA-BCKA, at least in the formula and quantities we used. A low Leu/K-Leu ratio is strictly correlated with defective CMI in CLND patients; SD improves this defect supplying K-Leu which, inducing an anabolic state (4), at intracellular level, could affect the T-lymphocyte function. Moreover SD reduces BUN and PTH markers of uremic metabolic derangements.

Table 1. Serum values of BCAA (umol/l) and BCKA (nmol/ml).

	N.V.	G1	G2	G3	G4
Val.	248.0+38.4	221.7+38.6[a]	204.3+42.6[c]	177.7+27.1[ce]	184.5+50.5[ce]
K-Val.	13.8+5.1	10.9+3.2[a]	9.2+2.5[c]	9.5+3.0[b]	7.9+3.4[cd]
Leu.	142.5+22.5	129.4+26.2[a]	126.7+19.2[b]	117.3+18.3[c]	116.5+35.3[c]
K-Leu.	36.0+10.7	26.3+7.7	22.6+7.4[c]	18.3+3.3[ce]	12.7+5.4[cfhi]
Ile.	72.3+17.0	66.1+16.4	65.9+9.2	63.0+16.8	67.4+22.6
K-Ile.	20.4+6.8	17.7+4.6	14.6+3.8[cd]	15.8+3.3[a]	8.9+3.1[cfhi]

Table 2. Serum values of albumin, transferrin, BUN and PTH.

	G1	G2	G3	G4
Albumin (g%)	4.2+0.4	4.1+0.2	4.1+0.4	4.0+0.3
Transferrin (mg%)	289.5+54.0	252.7+29.6[d]	281.8+39.6[g]	238.3+81.9[e]
BUN (mg%)	41.1+11.9	73.7+27.8[f]	42.6+10.5[h]	84.4+15.6[fi]
PTH (ng/ml)	0.7+0.2	2.1+0.9[f]	1.5+0.7[fg]	6.9+5.1[fhi]

ap < .05 vs n.v.   dp < .05 vs G1   gp < .05 vs G2

bp < .01 vs n.v.   ep < .01 vs G1   ip < .01 vs G3

cp < .001 vs n.v.   fp < .001 vs G1   hp < .001 vs G2   ip < .001 vs G3

REFERENCES

1) Mattern, W.D., Hak, L.J., Lamanna, R.W., Teasley, K.M., Laffell, M.S. Am. J. Kidney Dis. 1: 206-218, 1982.

2) Giovannetti, S. Nephron 40: 1-12, 1985.

3) Kniker, W.T., Anderson, C.T., Roumantzeff, M. An. Allergy 43: 73-79, 1979.

4) Mitch, W.E., Walser, M.K. and Sapir, D.G. J. Clin. Invest. 67: 553-562, 1981.

NUTRITIONAL ABNORMALITIES AS A GUIDE TO PROGNOSIS IN HEMODIALIZED (HD) PATIENTS (PTS)

M.G.CHIAPPINI,G.SELVAGGI,M.MOSCATELLI,S.DEL SIGNORE,R.BARTOLI

Dialysis Unit, Fatebenefratelli Hospital, Isola Tiberina, Roma, Italy

Malnutrition occurs commonly in HD pts. Inadequate dietary intake, loss of nutrients in the dialysate, hormonal abnormalities and delay in the beginning of HD therapy are indicated as the main factors of malnutrition (1,2). It has been suggested that poor nutritional status may affect the clinical course of these pts, promoting an increased morbidity and mortality (1,3). The aim of the present study is to evaluate the clinical consequences of malnutrition in HD pts and to identify the most sensitive markers of the nutritional status of these pts that could be used as prognostic indicators.

PATIENTS AND METHODS

41 pts (male 24, female 17, mean age 50 ± 15 yr) with chronic renal failure undergoing maintenance HD (4 hr,3 time per wk) from at least 6 mo,were studied. Pts with diabetes mellitus, neoplastic diseases, acute intercurrent illnesses were excluded. Nutritional status was assessed by anthropometric parameters:Ideal Body Weight(IBW), Body Mass Index(BMI), Triceps Skinfold Thickness (TST), Mid Arm Muscle Circumference (MAMC),%Body Fat(BF); biochemical determinations: serum Albumin(Alb), Prealbumin (Pre),Transferrin(Trf), C_3; Immunological assay:Total Lymphocyte Count (TLC),intradermal skin test with Multitest(MT) CMI-Merieux; dietary intake by 3-day dietary diaries to calculate %Basal Energy Expenditure(BEE) and %of recommended protein intake (PI). Blood samples for biochemical determinations were obtained before HD. Anthropometric measurements were performed at the end of dialysis. Values of serum proteins,TLC and MT were expressed as % of the mean normal value,

anthropometric parameters as % of standard value (4). From the measured parameters a short number of synthetic indices was obtained: Antropometric Index(AI)=(TST+MAMC)/2; Visceral Protein Compartment Index(VPCI)=(Alb+Pre+Trf+C_3)/4; Immunological Index(II)=(TLC+MT)/2; Nutritional Index(NI)=(AI+VPCI+II)/3; Dietary Index(DI)=(%BEE+%PI)/2. All pts were followed up for 36 months.

RESULTS

Among the anthopometric parameters, the more striking abnormalities were observed in TST and BF,decreased in 66% of cases. A very high correlation was found between TST and BF(r=.94,p ‹.001). IBW and BMI were normal in the majority of pts. In regard to biochemical parameters a marked reduction was observed in Pre,Trf and C_3.TLC and MT were abnormal respectively in 78% and 44% of cases. As far as synthetic indices are concerned, AI was reduced in 54% of pts,VPCI in 56%,II in 73% and DI in 32%. AI correlated inversely with duration of HD therapy(r=-.40,p ‹.05)and with duration of pre-HD low protein diet(r=-.55,p ‹.01).No correlation was found between nutritional parameters and dietary intake. According to their nutritional status pts were arbitrarily subdivided in Normal(N=21,NI 85)and Malnourished(M=20, NI 85). During the follow up period 16 pts died:3(14%)N and 13(65%)M(p .001). Survival rate was significantly lower in M as compared to N pts (mean value respectively 24.6+10.2 and 33.2+7.3, p ‹.001)(Fig.1).M pts had also the highest incidence of complications(Tab.1).

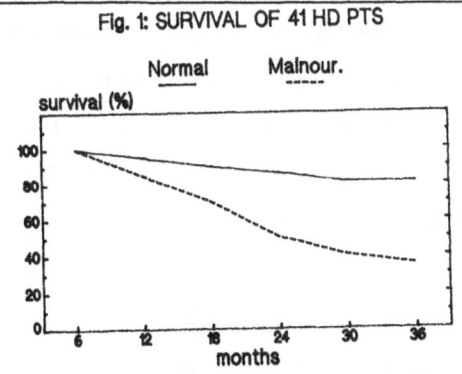

Fig. 1: SURVIVAL OF 41 HD PTS

Normal   Malnour.

survival (%)

months

Low values of MAMC,Pre,Trf,TLC were significantly related to the highest incidence of complications. Survival correlated with TLC(r=.39,p‹.01),Pre (r=

Tab. 1	%M	%N
Hospitalizations	90	33**
Infectious illnesses	70	24*
Non-infec.illnesses	90	48*
Peripheral Neurop	70	14**
Hyperparathyroidism	65	4°

*p ‹.05; **p ‹.005; °p‹.001

.54,p<.001),BEE(r=.40,p<.01),P1(r=.37,p<.05).

DISCUSSION

The results of the present study, according to literature data,confirm that malnutrition is frequently observed in HD pts (1,2,3,5).The more striking abnormalities are in biochemical and immunological parameters.The importance of nutritional status in influencing the outcome of these pts has been recently pointed out(1,6).Our findings indicate that malnutrition negatively affect the cli- nical course of HD pts.During the follow-up M pts had the greatest incidence o complications and the highest mortality rate.Conversely,it is true that superim- posed illnesses per se may promote malnutrition and affect the outcome of these pts.The majority of M₂pts showed severe clinical and laboratory signs of hyper parathyroidism,per se one of the main causes of malnutrition in these cases. We were unable to demonstrate a correlation between nutritional status and die- tary intake.However,inadequate protein and caloric intake negatively influence< the prognosis of our pts.Because of the relationsheep between malnutrition and the outcome of HD pts, it may be necessary to identify,among nutritional parame ters,the most specific markers for these pts that could be used as prognostic ir dicators.In the present study low values of MAMC,Pre,Trf,TLC were significa tly related to the highest incidence of complications; TLC and Pre correlated with survival rate. Therefore we conclude that: malnutrition is associated with increased morbidity and mortality in HD pts; synthetic indices may be useful to early and simply identify malnourished pts at risk; MAMC,Pre,Trf and TLC see to be the most sensitive nutritional markers;low values of TLC and Pre may be considered significant predictors of mortality in these pts.

REFERENCES

1)E.I.Feinstein,J.D.Kopple,Am.J.Nephrol. 5:398-405, 1985
2)B.J.Thunberg et al.,Am.J.Clin.Nutrition 34:2005-2012, 1981
3)M.Wolfson et al.,AM.J.Clin.Nutrition 37:547-555, 1984
4)D.B.Jeliffe, WHO Monograph Series N°53,Geneva:World Health Organization 1966
5)M.J.Blumenkrantz et al.,Am.J.Clin.Nutrition 33:1567-1585, 1980
6)N.Cano et al.,Kidney Int 32(S22):178-180, 1987

RELATIONSHIP BETWEEN PHYSICAL ACTIVITY AND NUTRITIONAL STATUS IN PATIENTS ON MAINTENANCE HEMODIALYSIS.

B.CIANCIARUSO,F.MARCUCCIO,A.CAPUANO,V.BELLIZZI,N.FERRARA, G.GIGLIOTTI,E.D'AMARO,V.E.ANDREUCCI.
Division of Nephrology, II Faculty of Medicine, University of Naples,Naples,Italy.

Gutman and coworkers have recently reported that only 60% of non-diabetic patients on maintenance hemodialysis are capable of physical activity beyond caring for themselves and even fewer are able to work outside home(1). Other common characteristics of dialysis patients which may directly affect rehabilitation are malnutrition and psychic depression.

The purpose of this study was to evaluate the level of physical activity and the presence of depression in well nourished hemodialysis patients.

METHODS

Therty patients were studied (22 males,8 females) with mean age of 46 for males and 35 for females and serum urea nitrogen of 76 ± 30 mg/dl. Patients were selected on the basis of good nutrient intake (total calories:41 ± 11 Kcal/Kg/day;proteins:1.6 ± 0.4 gr/Kg/day) as indicated by dietetic diaries and interviews; serum total proteins (7.1 ± 0.6 gr/dl), serum albumin (3.5 ± 0.4gr/dl),transferrin (2.7 ± 0.8 gr/L), and anthropometric measurements.

Physical activity was estimated with a questionnaire developed by the Psycology Istitute of the University of Naples. A final scoring was obtained, taking into account different kinds of physical activity such as: work outside home, housework, free time activity.

Depression was evaluated with the IPAT Depression Scale (2).

RESULTS

On the basis of physical activity scoring, four groups of patients were obtained as shown in Table 1.

Physical Activity	Score	N°Patients	%
Only Selfcare	0-5	8	27
Low Rare Activity	6-10	4	13
Low Continous Act.	11-19	15	50
Good Continous Act.	≥20	3	1o

The depression score for each group of physical activity is shown in Table 2.

Phys.Act.Group	Depr.Score<8(N°)	Depr.Score>8(N°)
I	1	7
II	3	1
III	12	3
IV	2	1

The presence of serious depression, as indicated by a score higher than 8, was more often observed in the group of patients with lowest physical activity.

DISCUSSION

The clinical outcome of maintenance hemodialysis has mainly focused on morbidity and patient survival. Only recently Gutman et al have studied physical rehabilitation and employment status in a large multicenter survey (1). The results of this study suggested that a large proportion of dialysis patients are severely debilitated.

283

There are many reasons why a patient undergoing hemodialysis may have a poor physical and social rehabilitation. In this study we focused on malnutrition and psychic depression as possible factors directly affecting physical activity. A various degree of wasting and protein-energy malnutrition has been shown in hemodialysis patients (3). The severity of depression in many dialysis patients is comparable to that of patients seeking psychiatric treatment for depression (4). These preliminary data were collected only in well-nourished dialysis patients in order to rule out malnutrition as a possible cause of poor physical activity. Our data in well nourished dialysis patients indicate that only 60% of these patients had a good degree of physical rehabilitation; 27% of these patients,however carried out only activities involving selfcare. Psychic depression was more often observed in patients with the lowest levels of physical activity.

In conclusion nutritional status does not seem to be the major determinant of physical activity in well nourished dialysis patients.

REFERENCES

1. Gutman, R.A., Stead, W.W., Robinson, R.R. New England J Med 304: 309-313, 1981.
2. Krug, S.E., Laughlin, J.E.,Insttitute for Prsonality Testing , Champaign, Illinois,1976.
3. Blumenkrantz,M.J., Kopple J.D., Gutman,R.A., Chan,Y.K., Barbour, G.L., Roberts, C., Shen,F.H., Gandhi,V.C., Tucker,C.T., Curtis, F.K. and Coburn J.W. Am.J Clin. Nutr.33:1567-1585,1980
4. Finkelstein,F. Steele,T. Dial.Trasplant.7:877,1978.

RISK FACTORS OF MALNUTRITION IN RDT PATIENTS

M.Gonella, G.Calabrese, A.Mazzotta, G.Vagelli, G.Pratesi.
Servizio di Nefrologia e Dialisi, Casale Monf.to, Italia.

INTRODUCTION

The patients on chronic hemodialysis (RDT) are known to be prone
to wasting (1). Thus, in the attempt to find the causative factors
of this condition, parameters and clinical status were evaluated in
a group of patients on apparent steady state and on the same dialytic
schedule maintenance.

PATIENTS and METHODS

A group of 33 patients (F 9, M 24, mean age 61 ± 11 yrs) on RDT for
a 51 ± 29 months period was considered in this study. 19 of them were
on HD with cuprophane membrane (CU) and acetate (4-4.30 h 3 times a
week); 11 on HDF with PAN or PMMA membrane and acetate (3.15-4 h with
more than 20 l of substitution fluid in postdilution mode, 3 times a
week); 3 on HF with polyamide membrane and acetate (30 l in postdilution mode, 3 times a week). More or less wide vascular calcifications
(VC) were present at x-ray in 19 of the studied patients. At the beginning of the observation period, all the patients had a dialytic
age of more than 8 months and were then followed for a 28 ± 10 months
period. In the middle of this, each patient completed a dietetic dia-
ry for 3 days including the dialytic midweek day, maintaining his die
tary habits, in order to evaluate the caloric and protein intake and
the protein catabolic rate (PCR) according to the Sargent's formula.

The dry body weight (BW) was estabilished according to the following parameters: normal cardiac volume, complaint of transient postdialytic mild cramps, normal blood pressure (BP) with a few episodes
of severe postdialytic hypotension whenever the programmed weight
loss was slightly exceeded. The mean value of BW and BP was compared
between the first and the last month of the observation period.

BUN, sCr, RBCs and lymphocytes count, serum albumin and proteins,
PTH, IgG, C_3 and C_4 were determined every month and the means of 3
consecutive measurements at the beginning and at the end of the obser
vation period were compared, as well as other hormonal parameters (T_3
T_4, TSH, Insulin, Cortisol), measured as a mean of 2 determinations
(by radioimmunoassay or immunoenzimatic method).

RESULTS

Urea generation (mean value 8.1 ± 1.8 g/day) was closely correlated
($r=0.69$, $p < 0.001$) with the declared protein intake, whose mean value
was 1.03 ± 0.25 g/Kg. The mean PCR was 63 ± 12 g/day and the caloric inta
ke 31 ± 7 kcal/Kg B.W./day.

BW decreased from 66 ± 9 to 63 ± 8 Kg ($p < 0.001$) in 12 patients (Group
I) and was stable or increased (64 ± 16 and 67 ± 16 Kg) in 21 patients
(Group II).

During the observation period, BUN decreased significantly in both
groups (from 78 ± 15 to 67 ± 18 mg/dl, $p < 0.001$, and from 74 ± 12 to 68 ± 13
mg/dl, $p < 0.01$, respectively) and sCr in the Group I (from 11.4 ± 1.8
to 10.3 ± 2 mg/dl, $p < 0.01$), because of the progressive increase of the
dialyzers surface and/or substitution fluids amount; the failure of a
significant sCr decrease in the Group II (11.3 ± 3 and 10.9 ± 2.1 mg/dl)
could be attributed, at least partially, to the concomitant increase
of the muscle mass. However the significant increase, detected at the
end of the observation period, of RBCs count and of Hb (from 10.4 ± 2.4
to 11.7 ± 2.4 g/dl, $p < 0.01$, in the Group I, and from 9.8 ± 2.3 to $10.9 \pm$
2.2 g/dl, $p < 0.01$, in the Group II) supported a better removal of

uremic toxins in both groups. Anagraphic and dialytic age, weight index, BP,   nutritional and hormonal parameters (which were in the normal range, except PTH which ranged between 2.8 ± 0.9 - 3.2 ± 1.2 ng/ml in the Group I, and 2.5 ± 1.1 - 2.7 ± 1.2 ng/ml in the Group II) were not significantly different between the 2 groups; moreover, the parameters, evaluated at the beginning and the end of the observation period, did not change significantly within each group.

A difference was found in the prevalence of CU use (11/12 vs 8/21) and VC presence (11/12 vs 8/21) in the wasting group with respect to the no wasting group. Moreover, the use of CU and the VC existence were contemporarily found in 10/12 in the Group I and in 1/21 in the Group II.

Furthermore, among the 19 patients on CU, VC were present in 10/11 wasting patients and 1/8 no wasting patients. In addition, among the 19 patients with VC, the CU was used in 11/12 wasting patients and not used in no wasting patients. In both cases no significant difference of the other examined parameters was found between the 2 groups

DISCUSSION

These results point out that CU dialysis seems to favour wasting in RDT patients, expecially with concomitant severe vascular disease. The possible role of CU in resulting in this condition is supported by previous studies (2) which explained it by the catabolic effect due to the lower biocompatibility of the membrane (1,2). However the present finding of PCR adequate to the protein intake questions this hypothesis, thus requiring further studies. Similarly the role of artherosclerosis should be further investigated to find out whether it may be responsible for wasting by itself.

REFERENCES
1. Kopple J.D.,Feinstein E.I.:Severe wasting and malnutrition in a patient undergoing maintenance dialysis.Am.J.Nephrol.5:398-405(1985).
2. Colton C.K.:Analysis of membrane processes for blood purification. Blood Purification 5:202-251(1987).

DIETETIC SUPPLEMENTS IN MALNOURISHED PATIENTS UNDERGOING CHRONIC
HEMODIALYSIS.

Peláez E., Orofino L., Marcén R., Matesanz R., Quereda C., Herrero
JA., Zamarrón I., Ortuño J.

Department of Nephrology. Hospital Ramón y Cajal. Madrid. Spain.

INTRODUCTION

Malnutrition is common in patients with chronic renal failure.
Despite dialysis therapy, many patients continue with a suboptimal
nutritional status. A mixed, protein-caloric malnutrition, due to a
decreased caloric intake and other factors, is often observed (1-3).
This situation lead to a higher morbidity and mortality (4). We have
evaluated the effect of caloric dietary supplements on the nutritional status in malnourished patients on hemodialysis (HD).

MATERIAL AND METHODS

We studied 10 patients, 6 male and 4 female, treated with periodic HD (3 X 4 hr weekly). Mean age was 51,9 yr (21-64) and mean time
on HD 81,5 mo (5-116). All the patients had a previous chronic malnutrition and a loss of wt during the last 3 mo before the begining
of the study, without any other intercurrent processes. The following parameters were evaluated: (1) Anthropometrics: wt, height, tri
cipital skinfold thickness (TST) and midarm muscle circunference
(MMC), measured according to the standard methods.(2) Biochemics:
hemoglobin (Hb), albumin (A), transferrin (T), prealbumin (PA), re-
tinol binding protein (RBP), total lymphocyte count (TLC), urea (U),
and protein catabolic rate (PCR).All these parameters were evaluated
at the begining of the study and 3 and 6 mo thereafter.

Patients were administered a free base diet, poor in phosphorus
and potassium, and 1000 ml/d of a hydrolyzed maltose with an energe
tic value of 1 Kcal/ml and containing: 4% proteins with 16% essential aminoacids, 4% lipids with 36% essential fat acids, 12% carbo-
hydrates and other vitamins and oligoelements.

RESULTS

After six months of treatment (Fig. 1) the mean recuperated wt
was greater than that lost during the previous 3 mo (1.87 ± 0.45 vs
1.85 ± 0.70 kg). TST improved mildly and MMC did not change significantly during the study. Table 1 shows the biochemical parameters
expressed as $\bar{x}$ ± SD. The PCR increased from 1.2 ± 0.18 to 1.41 ± 0.15
gr/Kg/d (p < 0.01), likewise U was not modified significantly (Fig.2).

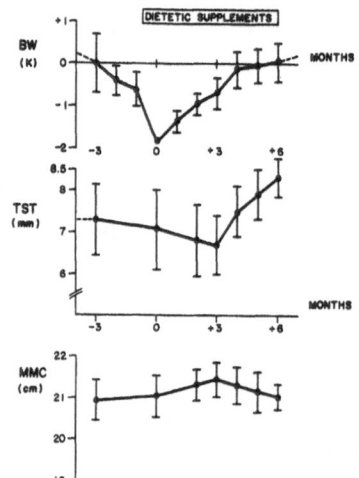

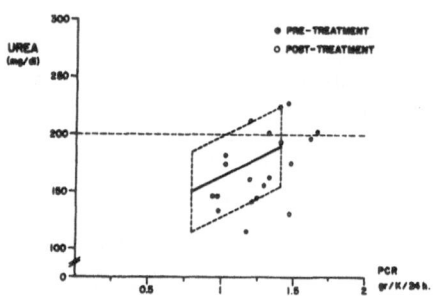

FIGURE 2.- Evolution of urea and PCR
values.

FIGURE 1.- Anthropometric parameters

TABLE 1.- Comparison of biochemical parameters along the study.

PARAMETERS	BEGINING	6 MONTHS	NORMAL VALUE
A	3.18 ± 0.4	3.55 ± 0.32	3.4 – 4.8 gr%
T	269 ± 71	256 ± 83	204 – 360 gr%
PA	29.80 ± 8.5	26.52 ± 4.8	10 – 40 gr%
RBP	21.50 ± 7.0	19.28 ± 6.5	3 – 6 gr%
Hb	9.02 ± 2.5	10.22 ± 2.3	12 – 16 gr%
TLC	1689 ± 70	1692 ± 663	1500 – 4000/mm^3

DISCUSSION

Precise assessment of the nutritional status in HD patients is
sometimes difficult and could be interferred by other intercurrent

processes (3, 5-8). Anorexia, asthenia and a progressive loss of wt can often indicate the presence of a severe malnutrition.

Usually, the treatment consists of the administration, orally or intravenously, of dietary supplements, with a variable caloric value (5, 9, 10). We have used an essentially caloric supplement which have been effective in controlling the loss of wt in our patients. The TST and the MMC did not improve in the same way, perhaps due to the short follow-up period. Visceral protein mass was much less altered than anthropometric parameters. Decreased serum protein concentration is a relative late manifestation of malnutrition, and is frequently altered by recent changes in dietary intake (1, 3).

The tolerance at treatment was excellent and the subjective feeling of well-being increased notably. In conclusion, we think that this type of supplement is an alternative to consider in order to control problem of malnutrition in HD patients.

REFERENCES

1.- Schoenfeld, P. In: Introduction to Dialysis (eds. Cogan and Garovoy), Churchill Livingstone 1985, pp 223-231.
2.- Thumberg, B.J., Swamy, A.P., Cestero, R.V.M. Am J Clin Nutr 34: 2005-2012, 1981.
3.- Schoenfeld, P., Henry, R.P., Laird, N.M., Roxe, D.M. Kidney Int. 23 Suppl. 13: S-80-87, 1983.
4.- Wolfson, M., Strong, C.J., Minturn, D., Gray, D.K., Kopple, J. D. Am J Clin Nutr 37: 547-555, 1984.
5.- Guarnieri, G., Faccini, L., Lipartiti, T., Ranieri, F., Spangaro, F., Giuntini, D., Toigo, G., Dardi, F., Berquier-Vidali, F., Raimondi, A. Am J Clin Nutr 33: 1598-1607, 1980.
6.- Kopple, J.D., Swenseid, M.E., Holliday, M.A., Alfrey, A.C., Gulyassy, P.F. Kidney Int. 7: S-249-252, 1975.
7.- Young, G.A., Swanepoel, C.R., Croft, M.R., Hobson, S.M., Parsons, F.M. Kidney Int 21: 492-498, 1982.
8.- Kopple, J.D.,Swenseid, M.E., Kidney Int. 7, Suppl 2: 64-72, 1975.
9.- Hecking, E., Kohler, H., Zobel, R., Lemmel, E.M., Mader, H., Oplerkuch, W., Prellwitz, W., Keim, H.J., Muller, D. Am J Clin Nutr 31: 1821-1826, 1978.
10.- Phillips, M.E., Havard, J., Howard, J.P. Clin Nephrol 9: 241-248, 1978.

Biocompatibility

CLINICAL ASPECTS OF HEMODIALYSIS BIOCOMPATIBILITY

ALFRED K. CHEUNG

Renal Section, Veterans Administration Medical Center, Salt Lake City, and the Department of Medicine, University of Utah School of Medicine, Salt Lake City, Utah, U.S.A.

General principles

Bio*in*compatibility of the hemodialysis extracorporeal circuit occurs primarily through one of several mechanisms: (a) cell adhesion, aggregation and activation; (b) transformation and adsorption of noncellular elements such as proteins; (c) mechanical shear; and (d) leaching and spallation of substances (1). Many substances are produced in the hemodialysis circuit which have theoretical biological effects. Whether these substances In fact lead to the theoretical effects, however, depend on a number of other factors: the timing and location of the production of the substances as well as the thresholds for the potential consequential events.

Coagulation and platelet activation

Adsorption of plasma proteins to the dialysis membrane occurs immediately upon blood contact. Activation of the intrinsic coagulation pathway follows, which may lead to the obvious problem of thrombosis inside the dialyzer. Activation of the fibrinolytic system also occurs, which participates in counteracting the effects of the clotting proteins.

Platelets are also major contributors to dialyzer thrombosis, as illustrated by the effectiveness of antiplatelet agents used as the sole administered anticoagulant (2). Adhesion of platelets to the dialyzer membrane is promoted by surface-bound fibrinogen and is followed by activation of the cells. In addition, platelets can be activated by mechanical disruption, or by other mediators released into the plasma, such as thrombin, thromboxane and platelet-activating factor. The clinical importance of platelet activation can be illustrated by the occurrence of hemodialysis-induced thrombocytopenia and hemorrhage. Different types of dialysis membranes activate platelets to different extents. Recent studies further suggest that such differences may affect the long term clinical outcome of the dialysis patients (3).

Complement activation

Complement is activated during hemodialysis with cellulosic membranes primarily via the alternative pathway. As a result, anaphylatoxins C3a and C5a are released into the plasma (4). These complement fragments may produce various effects on the patients, such as dialysis-induced peripheral granulocytopenia, pulmonary hypertension, hypoxemia, first use syndrome, structural and functional alterations in neutrophils, stimulation of monocytes to produce interleukin-1 as well as release of histamine and thromboxanes which have potent biological effects on their own. Activation of complement may have other consequences unrelated to anaphylatoxins. For example, some other C3 and C5 fragments are biologically active; their effects on hemodialysis patients are not well understood.

Three potential effects of anaphylatoxins on the hemodialysis patients have been intensely debated in the past few years. One relates to the pathogenesis of the first use syndrome. It appears that what has been called the first use syndrome is a constellation of syndromes with different etiologic agents rather than a single entity (5). Some of the events occurring within the first 1-2 minutes of hemodialysis are likely to be attributed to the direct noxious or allergic effects of leachable products from the dialyzer, one of which is ethylene oxide. Other events occurring later in the first hour may be related to complement activation, the severity of which partially depends on the rapidity of inactivation of the anaphylatoxins by serum carboxypeptidases. The acute cardiopulmonary effects of the anaphylatoxins are probably due to their direct spasmogenic properties on smooth muscles and may be unrelated to their effects on the neutrophils. Both the anaphylatoxins and the IgE released by the ethylene oxide-antibody complex can stimulate mast cells to release histamine and cause hypersensitivity reactions.

The second controversy centers around the pathogenesis of hemodialysis-induced hypoxemia. Acetate dialysate undoubtedly plays a major role in this phenomenon. There is nonetheless ample evidence to support the effects of the dialysis membranes. It is important to point out that membrane effects do not necessarily imply leukocytes or complement effects, although the latter is likely to contribute to dialysis-induced hypoxemia directly or indirectly through other mediators such as arachidonic acid metabolites. Polyacrylonitrile membranes, which are associated with lower plasma C3a antigen concentrations during hemodialysis, are also associated with less hypoxemia than cuprophan, regardless of the types of dialysate used (6).

The third controversy relates to the pathogenesis of dialysis-induced peripheral leukopenia. Although C5a(desArg) has been considered as the primary agent mediating such phenomenon, the role of other mediators such as platelet-activating factor and leukotrienes cannot be discounted (7). This is especially true in view of the fact that close and complex interactions exist among the many systems in the blood and other parts of the body.

Attenuation of complement activation during hemodialysis can be accomplished in several manners. Utilization of noncellulosic membranes, surface modifications or reuse of cellulosic membranes (8) have resulted in decreased complement activation. Cooling of dialysate and infusion of citrate attain similar effects.

Leukocyte alterations

Besides the prominant pulmonary sequestration, neutrophils are altered in several other ways during hemodialysis. Degranulation occurs which may be partially unrelated to complement activation. Release of intragranular proteases have been proposed to cause intradialytic catabolism. In addition, it may be responsible for the decrease in density of neutrophils harvested from patients observed during the first of hemodialysis. Other functional defects of neutrophils have also been described. They include defects in chemotactic response, aggregation and in oxidative metabolism.

Other leukocytes such as natural killer cells are also altered during hemodialysis (9). Such defects of leukocytes have been proposed to contribute to the impaired immunity of dialysis patients, who have higher incidence of infection and malignancy than the nonuremic population. From the limited information available in the literature, it appears that some of these effects are dependent on the types of dialysis membranes used.

Interleukin-1 (IL-1).

IL-1 has been recognized as a potent mediator of acute inflammatory response. Several substances have been found to be stimulants to IL-1 production by monocytes in the hemodialysis setting. These include not only endotoxins and other bacterial cell wall fragments such as muramyl peptides, but also include complement C5a, acetate buffer in the dialysate and the cellulosic dialysis membranes themselves (10). Serum level of IL-1 has in fact been shown to increase during hemodialysis. Although definitive evidence is lacking at present, IL-1 conceivably plays a role in many diseases and abnormalities found in dialysis patients. Cited for example are dialysis-related fever, sleep disturbance, hypozincemia, muscle wasting, osteopenia and periarticular disease.

$\beta_2$microglobulin (β_2MG) as a facet of membrane bioincompatibility

β_2MG has been incriminated as the major component of the AH amyloid found in hemodialysis patients (11). This type of amyloid is primarily localized in carpel tunnels, bones and periarticular tissues, although generalized systemic involvement has also been described. The exact pathogenetic mechanism of AH amyloid is unknown. The persistently high serum concentration of β_2MG may indeed play a role. In turn, retention of the molecules as a result of renal failure is undoubtedly a major factor in the hyper-$\beta_2$microglobulinemia. Of significant interest, however, is the increase in serum β_2MG concentration during hemodialysis with cuprophan membranes. Despite some controversy, studies have demonstrated such an increase even after correction for hemoconcentration. The tissue origin and the stimuli to the β_2MG release during hemodialysis are unknown.

Leaching and spallation

Leaching refers to the release of soluble substances into the fluid phase. The elution of the sterilant ethylene oxide (ETO) from the hemodialyzer is an example of this phenomenon. ETO and its derivatives have been incriminated in the pathogenesis of the first use syndrome, especially those with hypersensitivity-like manifestations. Cellulose derivatives are another class of materials elutable from certain hemodialyzers. These substances are of potential significance from several standpoints. They react positively in the *limulus* amebocyte lysate (LAL) assay; as such, they produce a state of pseudoendotoxemia in the patients. Secondly, they may elicit IgG/IgM production and form immune complexes which can potentially activate the classical pathway of complement. Finally, they may serve as carriers for the ETO hapten to stimulate IgE production.

Spallation usually refers to the release of particulate matters, of which silicone is a well-recognized example in the hemodialysis setting (12). Silicone particles released from the roller pump segment of blood tubings have been found in various visceral organs of dialysis patients. Their accumulation causes granuloma formation and can manifest clinically as hepatitis and hypersplenism. The plasticizer phthalate is yet another substance released from blood tubings which can cause liver damage.

Conclusions

Multiple phenomena occur inside the body and in the extracorporeal circuit during hemodialysis. Many of them are interrelated in complex manners such that they have to be considered together in the pathogenesis of some of the observed events. Careful studies of these phenomena and their interactions should lead to the design of more biocompatible circuits and to better understanding of the functions of the body.

297

References

1. Leonard EF: Dialysis membranes. Proc Eur Dial Transplant Assoc 21:99-109, 1984.
2. Zusman RM, Rubin RH, Cato AE, Cocchetto DM, Crow JW, Tolkoff-Rubin N. Hemodialysis using prostacyclin instead of heparin as the sole antithrombotic agent. N Engl J Med 304:934-939, 1981.
3. Simon P, Ang KS, Cam G: Enhanced platelet aggregation and membrane biocompatibility: possible influence on thrombosis and embolism in hemodialysis patients. Nephron 45:172-173, 1987.
4. Chenoweth DE, Cheung AK, Henderson LW: Anaphylatoxin formation during hemodialysis: Effects of different dialyzer membranes. Kidney Int 24:764-769, 1983.
5. Cheung AK, Henderson LW: Effects of complement activation by hemodialysis membranes. Am. J. Nephrol. 6:81-91, 1986.
6. DeBacker WA, Verpooten GA, Borgonjon DJ, Vermeire PA, Lins RR, DeBroe ME: Hypoxemia during hemodialysis: effects of different membranes and dialysate compositions. Kidney Int 23:738-743, 1983.
7. Camussi G, Pacitti A, Tetta C, Bellone G, Mangiarotti G, Canavese C, Segoloni G, Vercellone A: Mechanisms of neutropenia in hemodialysis (HD). Trans Am Soc Artif Intern Organs 30:364-368, 1984.
8. Chenoweth DE, Cheung AK, Ward DM, Henderson LW: Anaphylatoxin in formation during hemodialysis: Comparison of new and re-used dialyzers. Kidney Int 24:770-774, 1983.
9. Kay NE, Raij LR: Immune abnormalities in renal failure in hemodialysis. Blood Purification 4:120-129, 1986.
10. Luger A, Kovarik J, Stummvoll H-K, Urbanska A, Luger TA: Blood-membrane interaction in hemodialysis leads to increased cytokine production. Kidney Int 32:84-88, 1987.
11. Gejyo F, Odani S, Yamada T, et al : ß2-microglobulin: a new form of amyloid proteins associated with chronic hemodialysis. Kidney Int 30:385-390, 1986.
12. Bommer J, Ritz E: Spallation of dialysis materials: problems and perspectives. Nephron 39:285-289, 1985.

CELLULAR ASPECTS OF BIOCOMPATIBILITY

W.H. Hörl

Department of Medicine, Division of Nephrology, University of
Freiburg, D-7800 Freiburg, FRG

In hemodialysis patients, the anaphylatoxins C3a and C5a can be
generated as a result of dialysis membrane-induced activation of the
alternate pathway of the complement system. Complement activation
was temporally correlated with hemodialysis leukopenia using cuprophan dialyzers. By contrast, patients dialyzed with polyacrylonitrile
dialyzers failed to exhibit hemodialysis leukopenia and displayed
only modest increases in their plasma C3a levels (1). C5a mediates
the expression of a granulocyte-adhesion-promoting surface glyco-
protein on granulocytes providing leukoaggregation, sequestration of
granulocytes, and neutropenia during hemodialysis (2). A specific C5a
receptor on human polymorphonuclear leukocytes has been demonstrated
(3). On the other hand, polymorphonuclear neutrophils and monocytes
obtained from chronic dialysis patients have a significant reduction
in their ability to bind C5a (4).

Studies from our laboratory challenged the concept that neutrophil activation during hemodialysis occurs solely via the activation
of the complement pathway (5). For example, only 50 % of the patients
dialyzed with dialyzers made of cuprophan displayed a remarkable
elevation of plasma levels of granulocyte elastase as a result of degranulation of azurophilic granules (6). Very little complement
activation occurs in patients dialyzed with polymethylmethacrylate
dialyzers but markedly elevated plasma levels of elastase and lactoferrin were observed indicating degranulation of azurophilic and
specific granules under these conditions (7). Similarly, plasma
lactoferrin levels are also markedly elevated in patients dialyzed
with dialyzers made of polyacrylonitrile (8). Furthermore, plasma

levels of granulocyte elastase were significantly higher in patients dialyzed with the polycarbonate compared with the cuprophan membrane. Conversely plasma C3a levels were higher in patients dialyzed with the cuprophan dialyzer (9). Finally, plasma levels of main granulocyte components were significantly increased during dialysis with flat sheet dialyzers compared with hollow-fiber dialyzers. With respect to suface area, larger dialyzers tend to cause more release of granulocyte constituents, compared with dialyzers with smaller surface areas, irrespective of the configuration of the dialyzer used. Activation of the complement system, however, did not differ with both types of configurations. The same held true for initial leukopenia (10).

Recently, several authors also presented evidence for cell activation during hemodialysis not correlated with corresponding level of complement activation. For example, in vitro studies of Schultze and coworkers (11) showed that the release of PGE_2 and TXB_2 from blood cells was not pronounced due to exposure to polycarbonate, followed by polyacrylonitrile and cuprammonium cellulosic (CAC) membranes. By contrast, the highest C3a levels were found in the presence of CAC (11). These authors also demonstrated higher release of ß-thromboglobulin using the polycarbonate dialyzer compared to the other tested membranes (12). Mahiout et al. (13) determined significantly higher plasma platelet factor 4 levels in patients dialyzed with dialyzers made of polymethylmethacrylate than in those patients dialyzed with regenerated cellulose membranes. Tetta et al. (14) showed that only cationic, but not anionic or neutral, polymethylmethacrylate membranes activate polymorphonuclear neutrophils.

Foidart and coworker (15) measured production rate of 12-hydroxyeicosatetrarenoic acid (12-HETE) by platelets during hemodialysis with cuprophan or polyacrylonitrile membranes. 12-HETE production rate by platelets from patients dialyzed with dialyzers made of cuprophan was 2 to 3 times higher than that measured with platelets obtained from patients dialyzed with polyacrylonitrile dialyzers. It was suggested that stimulation of 12-HETE synthesis by platelets resulted whether from a complement-neutrophil-platelet interaction or a cell-membrane interaction. These authors (15) measured also 12-HETE synthesis by platelets collected before hemodialysis in the presence of autologous plasma samples harvested during hemodialysis. Plasma samples collected after 15 minutes of hemodialysis with cuprophan dialyzers caused higher 12-HETE production rate than plasma samples obtained after 15 minutes of hemodialysis with polyacrylonitrile membranes. The authors assumed both polyacrylonitrile and cuprophan membranes are capable of generating humoral factors which are unrelated to biologically active complement breakdown (15).

In-vitro experiments on human monocytes, polymorphonuclear neutrophils or platelets incubated with cuprammonium membranes demonstrated non-complement dependent stimulation of these cells. It was suggested that Ca^{++}-dependent pathways are involved (16).

The effect of the calcium channel blockers nifedipine (9 and 18 µg kg^{-1} h^{-1}) and verapamil (19 µg kg^{-1} h^{-1}) continuously infused during hemodialysis on granulocyte and complement activation was investigated (17). Plasma levels of lactoferrin, elastase in complex with α_1-proteinase inhibitor (E-α_1PI) and C3a were measured in patients dialyzed with dialyzers made of cuprophan, polymethylmethacrylate and polyacrlyonitrile. Calcium channel blockers caused no change of blood pressure during hemodialysis in all patients. There was no effect of nifedipine, diltiazem or verapamil on plasma lactoferrin, E-α_1PI or C3a levels in patients dialyzed with cuprophan. However, plasma lactoferrin and E-α_1PI values were significantly reduced by all calcium channel blockers in patients dialyzed with polymethylmethacrylate, and also by nifedipine and verapamil in patients dialyzed with polyacrylonitrile. Our data indicate that calcium channel blockers inhibit granulocyte activation occuring in dialyzers with very little anaphylatoxin formation. These drugs, however, are ineffective in patients dialyzed with cuprophan where complement activation takes place. Therefore, granulocyte activation during hemodialysis in the absence of complement activation seems to be mediated by calcium ions. Continuous infusion of nifedipine (5.91 $\pm$ 0.53 µg kg^{-1} h^{-1}) caused also significantly lower E-α_1PI and lactoferrin but not anaphylatoxin levels (18) during cardiopulmonary bypass.

Studies of Bingel et al. (19) demonstrated that healthy human donor monocytes (MNC) may be induced to release interleukin-1 under the experimental conditions of in vitro closed loop dialysis in the presence of purified endotoxin in the dialysate loop. A plausible explanation was suggested for the mechanism of the febrile response seen in the dialysis patient when the dialysate has been heavily contamined by bacteria. It was recommended that in vitro MNC-Il-1-production provides a more reliable and relevant assay to determine dialysis membrane permeability for pyrogene than the limulus test (20).

Chronic interleukin-1 production in long-term hemodialysis patients may be associated with headache, lassitude, hypotension, muscle wastage or myalgia (for review see (21)). Recent qualitative and quantitative studies of Colton (22) support the interleukin-1 hypothesis. Monocytes are activated by C5a and endotoxins. Therefore, it was concluded that both C5a generation by the membrane and endotoxin in the dialysate must be eliminated for an observable improvement in the acute and chronic complications of hemodialysis to be observed (22). Finally, further studies are necessary to find out the importance of cell activation during hemodialysis not correlated with corresponding level of complement activation.

REFERENCES

1. Chenoweth, D.E., Cheung, A.K. and Henderson, L.W. Kidney Int. 24:764-769, 1983.
2. Arnaout, M.A., Hakim, R.M., Todd, R.F., Dana, N. and Colton, H.R. N. Engl. J. Med. 312:457-462, 1985.
3. Chenoweth, D.E. and Hugli, T.E. Proc. Natl. Acad. Sci. USA 75: 3943-3947, 1978.
4. Lewis, S.L., Van Epps, D.E. and Chenoweth, D.E. Clin. Nephrol. 26:37-44, 1986.
5. Hörl, W.H., Steinhauer, H.B. and Schollmeyer, P. Kidney Int. 28: 791-796, 1985.
6. Hörl, W.H. and Heidland, A. Clin. Nephrol. 21:314-322, 1984.
7. Hörl, W.H., Riegel, W., Schollmeyer, P., Rautenberg, W. and Neumann, S. Clin. Nephrol. 25:304-307, 1986.
8. Riegel, W., Leverenz, K., Schollmeyer, P., Wilms, H. and Hörl, W.H. Nephron 46:161-166, 1987.
9. Hörl, W.H., Riegel, W. and Schollmeyer P. Nephron 45:272-276, 1987.
10. Schaefer, R.M., Heidland, A. and Hörl, W.H. Am. J. Nephrol. 7: 121-126, 1987.
11. Schultze, G., Wagner, K., Neumayer, H.H. and Molzahn, M. Contr. Nephrol. 59:44-50, 1987.
12. Schultze, G., Wagner, K., Fitzner, R., Neumayer, H.H. and Molzahn, M. Kidney Int. 33 (Suppl. 24):S-82-S-83, 1988.
13. Mahiout, A., Lajous-Peter, A.M., Jörres, A., Meinhold, H. and Kessel, M. Kidney Int. 33 (Suppl. 24):S-75-S-79, 1988.
14. Tetta, C., Camussi, G., Segoloni, G. and Vercellone, A. Kidney Int. 29:609, 1986.
15. Foidart, J.B., Davin, J.C., Malaise, M., Saint-Remy, M. and Mahien, P. Kidney Int. 33 (Suppl. 24):S-80-S-81, 1988.
16. Betz, M., Hensch, G.M., Rauterberg, E.W. and Ritz, E. Kidney Int. 31:228, 1987.
17. Haag-Weber, M., Schollmeyer, P. and Hörl, W.H. Eur. J. Clin. Invest. (in press).
18. Riegel, W., Spillner, G., Schlosser, V. and Hörl, W.H. J. Thorac. Cardiovasc. Surg. 95:1014-1019, 1988.
19. Bingel, M., Lonnemann, G., Shaldon, S., Koch, K.M. and Dinarello, C.A. Nephron 43:161-163, 1986
20. Lonnemann, G., Bingel, M., Floege, J., Koch, K.M, Shaldon, S. and Dinarello, C.A. Kidney Int. 33: 29-35, 1988.
21. Dinarello, C.A., Koch, K.M. and Shaldon, S. Kidney Int. 33(Suppl. 24):S-21-S-23, 1988.
22. Colton, C.K. Kidney Int. 33(Suppl. 24):S-27-S-29, 1988.

HEMODIALYSIS-ASSOCIATED NEUTROPHIL ABNORMALITIES AND GENERATION OF LEUKOTRIENE B_4

H. Schiffl, TH. Strasser, J.H. Hohnloser, P.C. Weber+
Medizinische Klinik Innenstadt der Universität München, + Harvard
Medical School Massachusetts, General Hospital, Boston, MA

Clinical hemodialysis has provided a particularly comprehensive model for the study of acute modulations of granulocyte function.

CHANGES OF GRANULOCYTE COUNT AND FUNCTION DURING HEMODIALYSIS

The most striking effect of the hemodialysis procedure on leukocytes is the profound leukopenia (primarily limited to neutrophils and monocytes) that occurs during the early phase of treatment. The duration of the fall in neutrophils (PMNS) is short with the nadir between 10 and 20 minutes after commencement of treatment, and is followed by a gradual return to predialysis levels by the end of the first hour. The main cause of this leukopenic event is the sequestration of leukocytes into the pulmonary vasculature. The return of the white cell count to pretreatment values can be attributed to either the recirculation of neutrophils from lungs and/or to bone marrow release of immature PMNs into the circulation (1, 2).

Neutrophils that remain in the peripheral circulation during the leukopenic period associated with hemodialysis are functionally defective as compared to the same patient's predialysis PMNs. Functional responses that have been shown to be altered in the intradialysis period include chemotaxis, aggregation, adherence and degranulation (3).

These changes in neutrophil count and function are dependent on the type of dialysis membrane, with cuprophane being the strongest offender. Leukopenia occurs minimally with the poly-acrylonitrile membrane, and rarely whenever dialyzers are reused.

COMPLEMENT ACTIVATION IN EXTRACORPOREAL CIRCUIT DURING CLINICAL HEMODIALYSIS

Interaction of the dialyzer membrane with the patient's blood causes activation of the alternate pathway of complement to generate the biologically active compound C_{5a}. Detection of complement products in plasma occurs maximally at 15 minutes. As dialysis proceeds, the rate of complement activation decreases. The number and reactivity of surface groups on the membrane that initiate complement activation may play a critical role in the regulation of membrane activation events, but factors that affect anaphylatoxin distribution would also be expected to modify patient exposure to C_{5a} that is produced within the extracorporeal circuit. Complement activation by the dialyzer membrane might be blocked as a result of surface-bound proteins masking potentially reactive groups and/or binding of inhibitory factors (H and I).

The mechanism of complement activation has been proposed to account for the early hemodialysis-induced alterations in granulocytes (4). However, as reasonable as this hypothesis seems, a number of studies have questioned it (2). Complement activation is not proportional to the neutropenia, since polyacrylonitrile membranes cause marked total complement activation with minimal neutropenia, whereas polycarbonate membranes are associated with the opposite effects. There is also a divergence between complement activation and the adverse symptoms of certain patients. Moreover, the role of the complement compounds may not be direct and may involve the concomitant generation of other biologically active products (5). Unfortunately, no concrete knowledge exists regarding the final mediators of the complement pathway, nor regarding the importance of other chemotactic factors.

GENERATION AND LIBERATION OF BIOLOGICALLY ACTIVE LEUKOTRIENES DURING THE EARLY PHASE OF HEMODIALYSIS

The leukotrienes are constituents of a general biological control system based on arachidonic acid as the precursor. Human polymorphonuclear leukocytes convert arachidonic acid after release of cellular phospholipids to leukotriene B_4 (LTB_4) via the 5-lipoxygenase pathway. LTB_4 ist a potent multifunctional neutrophil stimulus, inducing chemotactic, aggregatory and degranulation responses in neutrophils, and is therefore a prime candidate for the intradialytic neutrophil abnormalities (6).

We have obtained first evidence that LTB_4 participates in the hemodialysis-associated leukopenic event. When plasma LTB_4 levels are quantified by radioimmunoassay after extraction and purification by HPLC (7), mean values for hemodialysis patients are within the normal range. When using cuprophane membranes, patients show a transient generation and resultant liberation of LTB_4. LTB_4 rapidly accumulates during the first 10 minutes of dialysis in blood flowing from the dialyzer to the patient. Maximum liberation occurs at 10 minutes as evidenced by a peak, that's more than 17-fold higher than predialysis levels. During the remainder of the four hour dialysis session, plasma LTB_4 gradually declines and normalizes by the end of the treatment. Regression comparison of the relative venous white blood cell counts with the corresponding venous plasma LTB_4 concentrations at each time interval during dialysis demonstrates a close relationship between these two parameters. In contrast, the use of polysulfone membrane only caused a mild generation of LTB_4.

CONCLUSIONS
Granulocyte functional abnormalities associated with clinical hemodialysis are the measurable end products of a complex series of activated pathways. None of these bioregulators acts independently, but they all interact with each other. Synergistic effects of the products of the complement pathway and of the arachidonic acid metabolism have been shown experimentally, and may also

operate during the situation of clinical hemodialysis. The model that emerges from these considerations is therefore one in which neutrophils first recognize the classical chemotactic factor C_{5a}. This compound induces, probably in a Ca^{2+}- dependent manner, the generation and release of Leukotriene B_4. The fatty acid then interacts with specific binding sites or receptors on (or in) neighbouring cells. By inducing essentially the same events as complement C_{5a}, leukotriene B_4 then increases cellular responsiveness. The essential function of generated LTB_4 would therefore be to amplify or stabilize the chemotactic gradients.

Detailed knowledge of the mechanisms underlying hemodialysis-associated leukopenia will permit rational design of more biocompatible membranes.

REFERENCES

1) Hammerschmidt, D.E., Goldberg, R., Raij, L., Kay, N.E.:
Seminars Nephrol 5, 91-103, 1985

2) Hoenich, N.A., Levett, D., Fawcett, C., Woffindin, C., Kerr, D.N.S.:
J Biomed Eng 8, 3-8, 1986

3) Lewis, S.L., Van Epps, D.E.:
Am J Kidney Dis 9, 381-395, 1987

4) Craddock, P.R., Hammerschmidt, D., White, J.G., Dalmasso, A.P., Jacob, H.S.:
J Clin Invest 60, 260-264, 1977

5) Hakim, R.A.:
Proc EDTA-ERA, 22, 163-170, 1985

6) Bray, M.A.:
Br Med Bull 39, 249-254, 1983

7) Sellmayer, A., Strasser, TH., Spelsberg, F., Weber, P.C.:
J Clin Endocrinol Metab 64, 387-390, 1987

AN IMMUNOHISTOCHEMICAL TECHNIQUE FOR THE STUDY OF PLASMA PROTEINS ADSORBED ON DIALYSIS MEMBRANES.

V. PANICHI, A.M. BIANCHI, L. CASAROSA, M. PARRINI, G. GRAZI, A. BARONTI, C. CIRAMI, E. MONTAGNANI, R. PALLA.

2nd Medical Clinic, University of Pisa, 56100 Pisa, Italy.

INTRODUCTION

A protein layer coats the dialysis membrane on the first contact with blood: the nature of this layer may influence the following biological, immunological and clinical events such as intrinsic coagulation system and complement cascade activation (1). The nature of adsorbed protein on dialysis filters has been studied by the use of SDS-PAGE following various desorption procedures. Unfortunately results seem not easily reproducible among different studies: protein-surface interaction depends upon membrane chemical structure and varies among in vitro experiments and in clinical use. In order to better characterize the nature of the protein layer we have developed a new immunohistochemical method with the fluorescent antibody technique already used for the kidney biopsy. Biocompatibility of four different dialysis membranes was evaluated comparing protein cake deposition, plasma anaphilatoxin generation an platelet degranulation as B-TG release.

MATERIALS AND METHODS

Patients : 24 pts in RDT were studied during a single 4 hours acetate bath dialytic seance with an hollow fiber filter. 6 pts were dialyzed with Cu (Spiraflo, 1sqm) 6 with PAN (ASAHI HDF 30 1.3sqm), 6 with PMMA (TORAY B2-150 1.5sqm) and PS (Bellco BL 624 1sqm). All patients received the same dosage of heparin.

Blood samples and sample assays : Whole blood samples were drawn from the patients' arteriovenous fistula prior to dialysis (T0) and at 20 minutes (T20) from the arterial and the venous line for leukocyte count and complement levels (RIA Kits - Upjohn, Kalamazoo, Michigan). Blood samples for platelet count and B-TG levels (RIA Kits - Radiochemical Center, Amersham, UK) were drawn from the arterial line at T0, T20, T60.

Immunohistochemical method (IMM) : At the end of the dialytic seance the hollow fiber devices, rinsed with saline, were frozen at -70°C and later cut in cryostate. All membranes were tested with isothiocyanate coniugate antibodies for IgG, IgA, IgM, C3c, C1q, Fibrinogen, Plasminogen, Fact VIII, Fact XIIIa, Fact XIIIs, AT III and FDP. Protein deposition was evaluated by direct immunofluorescent technique.

RESULTS

Tab.1: Immunofluorescent pattern.

	IgG	IgA	IgM	C3c	C1q	Fibr	FXIIIa	FXIIIs	FVIII	ATIII	FDP	Plasm
Cu	+	+	+-	++	-	+	++	++	+	+	+	+
PS	+	+-	+	+	+-	+	++	++	++	+	++	+
PMMA	+	+	+	+	+	+	+	-	-	+	+	+
PAN	+	+	+	+-	+-	+	+	+	+	+	+	+

C3a increased from 471.9 ± 135 to 4655 ± 176 ng/ml with Cu (p 0.01); from 406.9 ± 30 to 2426 ± 625 with PMMA (p 0.05); from 729 ± 583 to 1818 ± 1079 with PS and from 580 ± 340 to 1394 ± 456 with PAN. C5a varied from 10.5 ± 3.7 to 74.4 ± 36 ng/ml with Cu (p

0.05); from 8.4$\pm$2.3 to 51.5$\pm$19.7 with PMMA (p 0.05); from
10$\pm$8 to 9.7$\pm$3.7 with PS and from 3.3$\pm$1.5 to 23.2$\pm$33.1 with
PAN. A profound leukopenia (from 5100 to 1633 GB./mmc p 0.05) was
observed only with Cu. No significative variations were found in
platelets count and B-TG release with all membranes.

DISCUSSION

This IMM offers a good tool for the study of protein layer; a
positive correlation between complement factor adsorbed and C3a-C5a
plasma levels was found. On Cu a large amount of C3 deposition
without Clq was detected suggesting a massive alternative patway
complement activation. Cu induced leukopenia is confirmed but this
phenomena seems not entirely related to anaphilatoxins release as
shown by PMMA C-activation without leukopenia (2). B-TG increase
and leukopenia seems not related phenomena, as recently claimed
(3). PMMA revealed a different pattern of IF with protein
permeation of the capillary and a positivity distributed on the
outer surface of the fibers.

REFERENCES

1) CHENOWETH D.E. et al. Kidney Int. 24:764-9, 1983.
2) ALJAMA P. et al. Proc. Eur. Dial. Trasplant. Assoc. 15:144-153, 1978.
3) MARTIN-MALO A. et al. In : Immune and metabolic aspects of therapeutic blood purification systems. (Eds. Karger/Basel) 1986, pp.18-25.

ADSORPTION OF ANAPHYLATOXINS C3a AND C5a ON AN-69 AND POLYSULFONE
MEMBRANES OF DIALYZER - IN VIVO STUDY

A.KANDUS*,R.KVEDER*,M.MALOVRH*,S.KLADNIK*,P.IVANOVICH**,J.DRINOVEC*

*Departments of Nephrology and Nuclear Medicine, University Medical
 Center, Ljubljana, Yugoslavia, **V.A. Lakeside Medical Center,
 Chicago, Illinois, USA

INTRODUCTION

Different complement activation, which results in formation of
anaphylatoxins C3a and C5a, occurred during contact of plasma with
different dialyzer membranes (1,2,3). It is believed that increase
of plasma C3a and C5a concentrations, after blood passed through
dialyzer, indicates degree of complement activation. Recent "in
vitro" studies confirmed significant adsorption of C3a and C5a on
the AN-69 membrane of plate dialyzer (4). Despite of this
observation, it is believed that slight complement activation by
AN-69 membrane, rather than its adsorption capability, determines
low plasma concentrations of C3a and C5a. The purpose of this
prospective clinical study was to investigate adsorption of C3a and
C5a on AN-69 and polysulfone (PS) membranes during regular
hemodialysis (HD).

PATIENTS AND METHODS

7 stable chronic uremics, 3 females and 4 males, with mean age
of 45 ± 17 years participated in the study. Informed consent was
obtained from each of them. Blood passed first through cuprophan
dialyzer (Hemomed C 1.3 m^2, hollow fiber, Inex Hemofarm) and then
through AN-69 (Filtral AN-69 HF, 1.15 m^2, hollow fiber, Hospal) or
PS dialyzer (Hemoflow F 60, 1.25 m^2, hollow fiber, Fresenius AG);the
latter two were not in contact with dialysis fluid. During HD,blood
flow was maintained at 200 ml/min. Blood samples were drawn from the
afferent blood line of cuprophan dialyzer at the onset, 15,60, and
240 min after the onset of HD, and from the afferent and efferent

line of AN-69 and PS dialyzers at 15th, 60th, and the last (240th) min
of HD, respectively. Plasma C3a and C5a concentrations were
determined by radioimmunoassay (Amersham International). Results are
expressed as mean$\pm$standard deviation. Significance was assessed by
student's t-test for paired data. Significant differences were
defined with a p value of less than 0.05.

RESULTS

The most relevant results are presented in Table 1-4.

Table 1. Plasma C3a concentrations in the afferent and efferent
blood lines of AN-69 dialyzer (n=7)

	min HD	afferent	efferent	p value
C3a	15th	10510$\pm$1290	3703$\pm$1404	< 0.001
(ng/ml)	60th	3689$\pm$1141	1433$\pm$ 356	< 0.01
	240th	2227$\pm$ 729	901$\pm$ 498	< 0.01

Table 2. Plasma C5a concentrations in the afferent and efferent
blood lines of AN-69 dialyzer (n=7)

	min HD	afferent	efferent	p value
C5a	15th	62.6$\pm$18.5	21.8$\pm$6.1	< 0.001
(ng/ml)	60th	27.9$\pm$ 6.1	13.6$\pm$5.5	< 0.02
	240th	12.4$\pm$ 4.8	7.7$\pm$2.7	< 0.05

Table 3. Plasma C3a concentrations in the afferent and efferent
blood lines of PS dialyzer (n=7)

	min HD	afferent	efferent	p value
C3a	15th	10877$\pm$5312	8494$\pm$2977	NS
(ng/ml)	60th	4280$\pm$1341	4956$\pm$1545	NS
	240th	2454$\pm$ 673	2146$\pm$ 978	NS

NS= not significant

Table 4. Plasma C5a concentrations in the afferent and efferent
blood lines of PS dialyzer (n=7)

	min HD	afferent	efferent	p value
C5a	15th	58.5$\pm$35.0	61.4$\pm$45.7	NS
(ng/ml)	60th	27.0$\pm$ 4.1	24.0$\pm$ 7.9	NS
	240th	11.7$\pm$ 2.5	12.1$\pm$ 2.5	NS

Since all the patients had hematocrit value of less than 0.50, it could be calculated that much more than 34,000 µg of C3a and much more than 150 µg of C5a were adsorbed on the AN-69 membrane during HD.

DISCUSSION

Calculated amount of C3a adsorbed on AN-69 membrane was substantially more than 75 times greater than the amount adsorbed on membrane of a similar surface area "in vitro" (4). Contrary to "in vitro" observation, there was no saturation of membrane adsorption capacity in our study. So far there is no reliable explanation for these differences in adsorption. 150 µg of C5a is the amount approximately 15 times greater than the total amount of C5a in plasma at the time of its peak concentration during HD with AN-69 membrane dialyzer (3). It is possible that this high degree of adsorption on the AN-69 membrane prevents significant increase of plasma C3a and C5a concentrations in the efferent blood line during HD with AN-69 membrane dialyzers. Although no significant adsorption of C3a and C5a on PS membrane could be demonstrated, it is possible that their adsorption was equal to their formation. Further clinical studies, involving investigation of C3a and C5a adsorption, apart from their formation, are necessary to clarify the significance of membrane adsorption in preventing the increase of plasma C3a and C5a concentrations.

REFERENCES

1. Chenoweth,D.E., Cheung,A.K., and Henderson,L.W. Kidney Int. 24: 764-769, 1983.
2. Smeby,L.C., Widerøe,T.E., Balstad,T., Jørstad,S. Blood Purif. 4: 93-101, 1986.
3. Kandus,A., Drinovec,J., Kladnik,S., Bren,A.F., Ponikvar,R., Kveder,R. Artif.Organs (in press).
4. Cheung,A.K., Chenoweth,D.E., Otsuka,D.,and Henderson,L.W. Kidney Int. 30: 74-80,1986.

BLOOD COOLING PREVENTS DEGRANULATION OF NEUTROPHILS
DURING HEMODIALYSIS.

C. CATALANO, G. ENIA, W.H. HÖRL *, Q. MAGGIORE.

Centro di Fisiologia Clinica del C.N.R. Reggio Calabria,
Italy.
*University Medical Clinic, Freiburg,FRG.

INTRODUCTION
    Leukocyte activation during hemodialysis (HD) is
associated with marked leukopenia and release of granule
content of polymorphonuclear granulocytes (neutral
proteases, lactoferrin etc) (1,2). Cooling of
extracorporeal blood during HD prevents to a large extent
leukopenia and anaphylatoxin generation (3). The purpose
of the present investigation was to study the effect of
temperature (T) manipulation on the release of
granulocyte content during HD.

MATERIALS AND METHODS.
    Nine patients undergoing regular hemodialysis
treatment three times per week for 1-12 years (average
3.5) were studied. Each patient underwent in randomized
order 1 hypothermic and one control HD treatment with
Cuprophan hollow fiber dialyzer of 1.2 m2.
    For the purpose of this study HD treatments were
carried out with a special extracorporeal line containing
2 serpentine tubes. The first -250 cm long- inserted in
the arterial segment, the second -500 cm long- in the
venous segment. During hypothermic HD dialysate fluid
flowed unwarmed through the dialyzer while the arterial
serpentine was immersed in a bath at the constant T of 12
C. Before reentering into the patient blood was rewarmed
through the venous serpentine immersed in a thermostatic
bath set at 47 C. During control HD both the arterial and
venous serpentine tubes were kept at room T while
dialysate fluid flowed at the T of 37 C.
    T was monitored by means of thermocouple needles.
WBC were determined by a Coulter counter. Granulocyte
elastase in complex with α1-proteinase inhibitor (E- 1PI)
and plasma levels of lactoferrin were determined as
previously described (4). Statistical analysis was
performed by paired t-test. Data are presented as mean
+/- SEM.

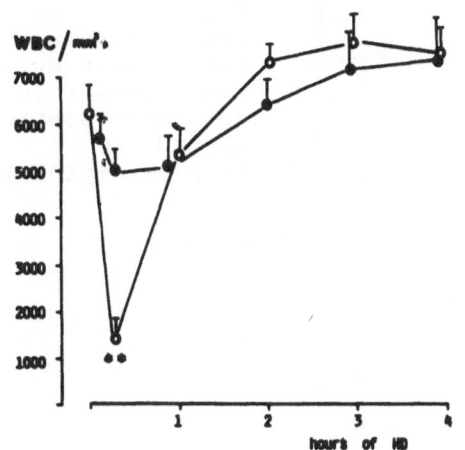

Fig.1:Changes in WBC during hypothermic (●) and control (o) HD. **p<0.001

RESULTS

Blood T within dialyzer (average of pre and post dialyzer blood T) was 22.7 C during hypothermic HD and 33.1 during control HD.

WBC fell by 78 +/- 1.4 % during control HD and this effect was reduced to 19 +/- 3.8 % during hypothermic HD (Figure 1). Control HD caused an increase of plasma E-1PI levels from 128 +/- 7.6 ng/ml to 368 +/- 18. This increase was blunted by hypothermic HD from 112 +/- 7.9 to 200 +/- 15 (Figure 2). The increase of Lactoferrin from 169 +/-27 ng/ml to 629 +/- 105 in control HD was reduced in the hypothermic treatment from 138 +/- 13 to 401 +/- 29 .

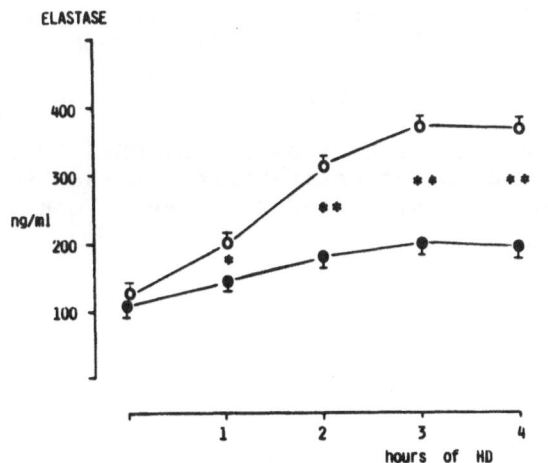

Fig.2:Arterial plasma levels of elastase during hypothermic (●) and control (o) HD
*p<0.01,**p<0.001

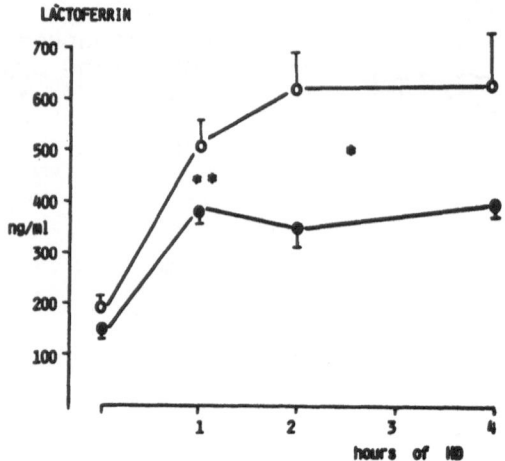

Fig.3:Arterial
plasma levels of
lactoferrin duri-
ng hypothermic
(●) and control
(o) HD.
*p<0.02,**p<0.01

CONCLUSIONS.

Blood cooling reduces elastase and lactoferrin release observed during Cuprophan HD. Blood cooling can be considered as a method of study for evaluating the clinical correlates of biocompatibility, because it offers the unique possibility of employing the same membrane and depurative setting at different levels of biocompatibility.

REFERENCES
1) Craddock PR, Fehr J, Dalmasso AP, Brigham KL, Jacob HS J. Clin. Invest. 59:879,1977.
2) Hörl WH, Riegel W, Steinhauer HB, Wanner C, Thaiss F, Bozkurt F, Haag M, Schollmeyer P, Clin. Nephrol, 26:s-30,1986.
3) Maggiore Q, Enia G, Catalano C, Misefari V, Mundo A Kidney Int. 32:908,1987.
4) Neumann S, Hennrich N, Gunzer G, Lang H In: Hörl WH, Heidland A (eds) Proteases: Potential Role in Health and Disease. Plenum Press, London, New York,p 379,1984.

LONG TERM EFFECTS OF BLOOD-MATERIAL INTERACTIONS.

Stefoni S., Nanni Costa A., Buscaroli A., Bonomini M., Coli
L., Feliciangeli G., Cianciolo G.

Institute of Nephrology, St.Orsola University Hospital,
Bologna

Current knowledge on blood-material interactions is
considerable, mainly with regard to the events which take
place at the interface, to the humoral reactions and to the
acute consequences of contact (1). However, attention
should also be paid to the events occurring at a distance
from the blood-material interface, to the cellular
reactions and to the long-term clinical effects.

In this study the effects of the chronic artificial
dialysis treatment on some structural and functional
characteristics of T-lymphocytes were evaluated: 1) the DNA
"in vivo" synthesis, which is an index of the cell turnover
and reproduction activity (2) and 2) the expression on cell
surface of the specific antigenic determinants (CD3, CD4,
CD8 antigens) which evaluates the antigen recognition and
processing function (3).

Both evaluations were based on the duration of dialysis
treatment. Four groups of patients were considered: the
first group included 20 patients with reduced renal
function (creatinine clearance 25-5 ml/min) not yet on
dialysis; the second 18 patients on regular dialysis
treatment (RDT) for less than 6 months; the third 20
patients on RDT from 3 to 5 years and the fourth 15
patients on RDT from 8 to 12 years. All dialysis patients
were treated with Cuprophan membrane. The tests were
performed by means of a Cytofluorograph (Spectrum III,
Ortho Diagnostic System).

Figure 1 shows the Flow Citometry plot of the DNA "in
vivo" synthesis. In normal subjects only 2.1 ± 0.9% of

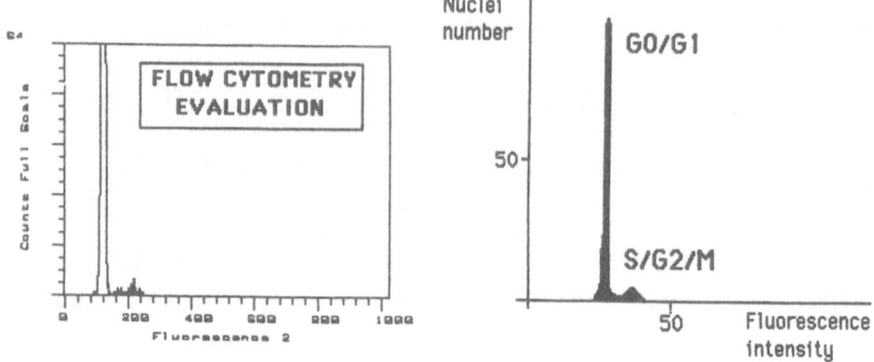

Fig.1:Flow Cytometry plot (on left) of the DNA synthesis "in vivo" and its schematic design (on right).

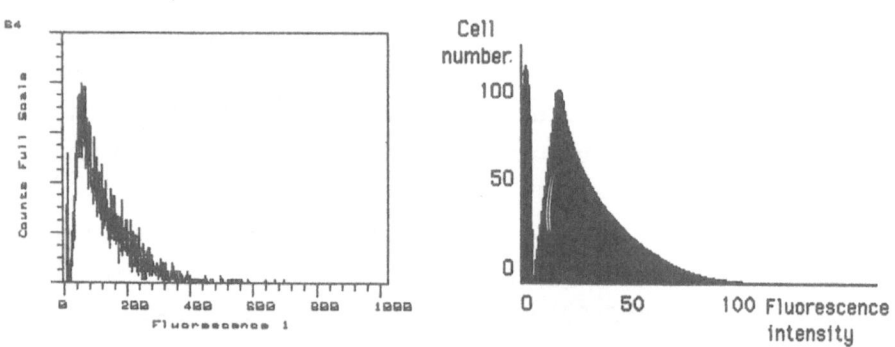

Fig.2:Immunofluorescence analysis of antigens expression on T-cell surface by Cytofluorograph (on left) and its outlining representation (on right).

cells are in the active synthesizing phases (S, G2, M), while the percentage is higher in the uremic patients (6.3 ± 1.7%; p<0.001). The percentage of the DNA synthesizing cells progressively increase from 4.3 ± 1.1% of the patients on conservative treatment to 8.4 ± 1.2% of the patients on RDT from 8 to 12 years (p<0.001).

Figure 2 shows the Cytofluorograph graphic pattern of the surface antigen expression: the fluorescence intensity is related to the density of antigens present on lymphocyte surface. All uremic patients show lower values than normal subjects (CD8: 39.5 ± 26.8 vs.65.1 ± 18.3, p<0.001). The fluorescence intensity increases with the years of dialysis for CD4 antigens and even more for CD8 antigens: 34.5 ± 13.4 for the group on RDT for 6 months vs.48.7 ± 15.2 for the group on RDT from 8 to 12 years (p<0.01).

These data confirm the Uremia related immune-depression (4) and suggest the existence of a chronic activation of the immunocompetent cells in long-term dialysis. This phenomenon could very likely be related to the repeated contacts between blood and artificial dialysis materials.

Supported in part by Grant CNR n°87.01519.04

REFERENCES:

1. Klinkmann, H., Falkenhagen, D., Courtney, J.M. Uremia Therapy; H.J.Gurland (Ed.) 125-140 Springer-Verlag Berlin Heidelberg 1987
2. Stefoni, S., Nanni Costa, A., Scolari, M.P.et al Immune and Metabolic Aspects of Therapeutic Blood Purification Systems (Eds)Smeby, L.C.,Jorstad, S.& Wideroe, T.E. 168-173 Basel Karger 1986.
3. Stefoni, S., Feliciangeli, G., Scolari, M.P., Colì, L., Bonomini, M., Nanni Costa, A., Bonomini, V. Life Support Systems; 5:335-340, 1987.
4. Kurz, P., Köhler, H., Meuer, S., Hütteroth, T., Meyer zum Büschenfelde, K.H. Kidney International 29: 1209-1214, 1986.

BLOOD CONCENTRATION OF PLASTICIZER AT STEADY-STATE IN DIALYSING PATIENTS: A MODEL

P.M. BOSELLI
SISTEMI TERAPEUTICI SIS-TER S.p.A.,
Via Crema, 8
26020 PALAZZO PIGNANO CR - ITALY

The calculation of steady-state plasticizer concentration by blood from a dialysing circuit is based on a few kinetic parameters concerning the distribution, metabolism and elimination. That is very important not only for testing the biocompatibility but to realize both how long for reaching the «plateau level» and the consequent toxicity as well.

INTRODUCTION

The plasticizer extraction by blood from devices is getting more important than before because the best therapeutic conditions must be found. On the other hand plasticizers are still indispensable for making devices. Therefore it needs to look for a method which can help us to know what will be happening if a plasticizer enters the body. Up till now every attempt, just done to compare plasticizers, has not clarified the kinetic processes, about their entry, distribution among the compartiments and way out. We must use that plasticizer which has both lowest toxicity and extraction at all.

AIM OF THE RESEARCH

First purpose is the best fitting of blood plasticizer concentrations. It means us to obtain an equation, the parameters of which can give us some informations about other body's districts, because we are not allowed to know anything into those ones in the experimental way. Second point is about the ability to make a prediction: how long does a patient spend going to the steady-state and what will the blood plasticizer concentration be reached at the plateau?

METHOD

At first an «anatomical model» can be drawn:

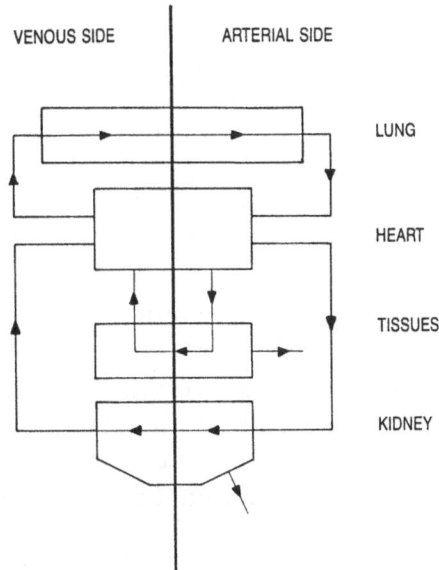

As well as we realise the heart-lung is a system like a tube through of which blood leaves the venous side to flow into arterial side, we can redraw it too:

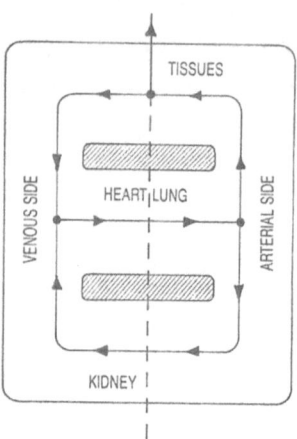

We have two compartments: the venous and the arterial ones.

As blood can run from venous to arterial side straightly through the heart-lung tube, it can run back right passing across another important compartment which includes both organs and peripherical tissues (liver, kidney, ..., fatty tissues, etc.)

At last we can draw:

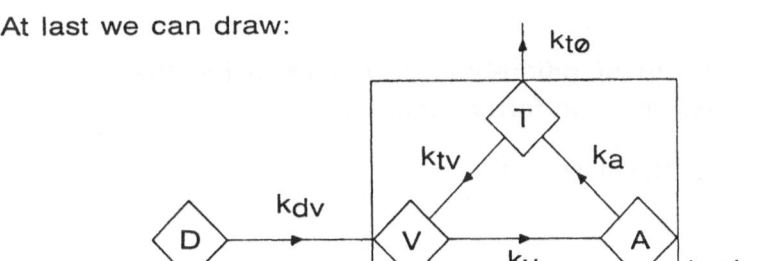

D : disposable compartment
V : venous compartment
A : arterial compartment
T : tissue compartment

k_{dv}, k_v, k_a, k_{tv}, $k_{t\emptyset}$, are transfer constants

At every dialysing treatment an unknown amount of plasticizer enters the venous blood at pre-lung point and
immediately it begins to distribute itself to the tissue
compartment.
Then it goes either back to venous side again or outside the model by excretion and/or metabolism (the model does not exclude the excretion to be possible). Any
way the constant k_{to} represents two exits, kept together.
In order to formal solving of the model we can consider
two analitical adding phases: 1° plasticizer uptake and
2° physiological course

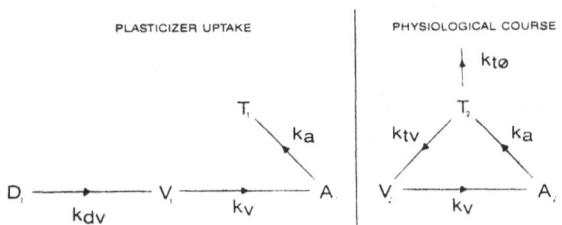

RESULTS

By a system of differential equations using the Laplace transforms the formal solutions are:

1° PLASTICIZER UPTAKE

$$D_1(t) = I\, e^{-k_{dv}t}$$

$$V_1(t) = -\frac{I\,k_{dv}}{(k_{dv} - k_v)}\, e^{-k_{dv}t} + \frac{I\,k_{dv}}{(k_{dv} - k_v)}\, e^{-k_v t}$$

$$A_1(t) = \frac{I\,k_{dv}k_v\, e^{-k_{dv}t}}{(k_{dv} - k_v)(k_{dv} - k_a)} - \frac{I\,k_{dv}k_v\, e^{-k_v t}}{(k_{dv} - k_v)(k_v - k_a)} + \frac{I\,k_{dv}k_v\, e^{-k_a t}}{(k_{dv} - k_a)(k_v - k_a)}$$

$$T_1(t) = I - \frac{I\,k_{dv}k_v k_a\, e^{-k_{dv}t}}{k_{dv}(k_a - k_{dv})(k_v - k_{dv})} - \frac{I\,k_{dv}k_v k_a\, e^{-k_v t}}{k_v(k_v - k_{dv})(k_v - k_a)} + \frac{I\,k_{dv}k_v k_a\, e^{-k_a t}}{k_a(k_a - k_d)(k_v - k_a)}$$

2° PHYSIOLOGICAL COURSE

$$V_2(t) = \frac{T_1(t)\,k_{tv}\,(k_a - \alpha)\, e^{-\alpha t}}{(\alpha - \beta)(\alpha - \gamma)} - \frac{T_1(t)\,k_{tv}\,(k_a - \beta)\, e^{-\beta t}}{(\alpha - \beta)(\beta - \gamma)} + \frac{T_1(t)\,k_{tv}\,(k_a - \gamma)\, e^{-\gamma t}}{(\alpha - \gamma)(\beta - \gamma)}$$

$$A_2(t) = \frac{T_1(t)\,k_{tv}k_v\, e^{-\alpha t}}{(\alpha - \beta)(\alpha - \gamma)} - \frac{T_1(t)\,k_{tv}k_v\, e^{-\beta t}}{(\alpha - \beta)(\beta - \gamma)} + \frac{T_1(t)\,k_{tv}k_v\, e^{-\gamma t}}{(\alpha - \gamma)(\beta - \gamma)}$$

$$T_2(t) = \frac{T_1(t)\,[\alpha^2 - (k_v + k_a)\alpha + k_v k_a]\, e^{-\alpha t}}{(\alpha - \beta)(\alpha - \gamma)} - \frac{T_1(t)\,[\beta^2 - (k_v + k_a)\beta + k_v k_a]\, e^{-\beta t}}{(\alpha - \beta)(\beta - \gamma)} +$$

$$+ \frac{T_1(t)\,[\gamma^2 - (k_v + k_a)\gamma + k_v k_a]\, e^{-\gamma t}}{(\alpha - \gamma)(\beta - \gamma)}$$

Total plasticizer concentrations will be fitted by:

$$
\left[
\begin{array}{l}
D\,(t) = D_1\,(t) \\
V\,(t) = V_1\,(t) + V_2\,(t) \\
A\,(t) = A_1\,(t) + A_2\,(t) \\
T\,(t) = T_1\,(t) + T_2\,(t)
\end{array}
\right.
$$

As we can see, every equation has the general form as following:

$$
C\,(t) = \sum_{i=1}^{m} H_i e^{-k_i t}
$$

During the chronic therapy a patient takes one dose of plasticizer every time and reaches the max level as below:

$$
C_p = \sum_{i=1}^{m} \frac{H_i}{(1 - e^{-k_i t^*})}
$$

Where t^* is the costant time interval of dialysis.

To calcule how long a patient must spend to reach the plateau concentration, we can use:

$$
C_{m,n} = \sum_{i=1}^{h} \frac{H_i\,(1 - e^{k_i n t^*})\,e^{-k_i t^*}}{(1 - e^{-k_i t^*})}
$$

where: n is the number of dialysis.
Therefore the plasticizer concentration levels off ($C_{m,\,n}$) by $n t^*$ time.

IGE ETHYLENE ANTIOXIDE AND EOSINOPHILIA DIALYSIS

J.ARANZABAL, J.GAINZA, R. SARACHO, J.AMENABAR, I.LAMPREABE

Department of Nephrology, Cruces Hospital,Baracaldo, Spain

INTRODUCTION

The appearance of eosinophilia in maintenance hemo-dialysis patients (ED) is a relatively frequent clinical fact. (1) Some of the latest studies carried out point towards a hypersensitivity phenomenon as the cause of ED.(2). Ethylene oxide (ETO) has been mentioned as one of the foreign substances used during hemodialysis which could trigger this hypersensitivity process.

MATERIALS AND METHODS

30 patients (18 men and 12 women)in maintenance hemo dialysis were studied with a follow up for over one year. Ages: 47,3 $\pm$ 14,5 years. Hemodialysis period: 67,4 $\pm$ 33,2 months. Three weekly sessions consisting of four hours each session, using the conventional dialysis tech-nique. Cuprophan capilar dialyzers (non reuseable) and polyvinylchloride tubes sterlized with ETO. Peripheral blood counts were taken with Coulter's counter, and significant eosinophilia was considered when figures were over 450/mm3. Between seven and thirteen extraction were carried out (an average of 9 per patient) during the whole study period. Eosinophilia was considered as per-sistent when it appeared in all the determinations car-ried out and as intermittent when it appeared in more than 30%.

Quantitative determinations of total plasmatic IgE were carried out in all patients by means of direct radioinmunoassay with paper disks as a solid phase (PRIST: Paper Radio Inmunosorbent Test) (Pharmacia). At the same time, specific anti-ETO IgE was also determined by a radioallergosorbent test (RAST) using paper disks with the allergen (ETO) combined with human albumen (Pharmacia).

Statistical method: Variance analysis, Student t in pairs anda calculation of the correlation coefficient.

RESULTS

Three groups emerged from amongst a total of 30 patients. The first of these was made up of seven patients who showed persistent ED (EDP), the second of ten patients with intermittent ED (EDI) and the third by those who had never shown any ED or by a control group (GC).

No important differences were observed between the three groups regarding age, sex or dialysis period.

When using the variance analysis, significant differences were observed in the titers of total plasmatic IgE and anti-ETO IgE between the three groups (EDP, EDI and GC) ($p < 0,001$).

Titers of total IgE and anti-ETO IgE were objectified as significantly greater in the EDP group with respect to the other two ($p < 0,01$, Student t in pairs). Tabla 1.

Table 1. Plasmatic levels of total IgE and anti-ETO IgE in three groups.

	Persistent.E		Intermittent.E		Control.G
Total IgE (U/ml)	365,29	$p < 0,01$	40,60	NS	10,54
Anti-ETO IgE	18,10	$p < 0,01$	1,82	NS	01,16

From a total of 30 patients, we found a correlation coefficient of 0,63 among the number of eosinophile/mm3 and the total IgE plasmatic level (p < 0,001). We also found a correlation coefficient of 0,71 (p < 0,000001) among the number of eosinophile/mm3 and the titer of anti-ETO IgE. Between the total plasmatic IgE level and that of anti-ETO IgE, the correlation coefficient was 0,93 (p < 0,00000001).

We reached the conclusion that an association exists between anti-ETO IgE and ED.

The appearance of a series of reactions during hemodialysis, characterized by bronchospasm, dyspnea, thoracic pain, urticaria, facial edema and/or hipotension, that could even result in cardiac arrest and death, has been described by several aythors. (4) (5). Two main mechanisms have been proposed to explain the etiopathogenesis of these reactions: (1) the activation of the complement and (b) an allergic reaction.

The above makes us think of the possible existence of a relationship between some of the reactions that apear during dialysis, eosinophilia, the total high plasmatic IgE and specific anti-ETO IgE.

As a result, an approach to study those patients showing intrahemodialysis reactions accompanied by eosinophilia would be the realization of total plasmatic IgE and specific anti-ETO IgE.

REFERENCES

1. Hoy,W.E. and Cestero, V.M. J. Dialysis 3:73.87 1.981.
2. Voudiklaris, S.Virvidakis,K.,Kalmantis,T.,Karafoulidou, A. and Mountokalaris, T. Intern Artif Organs 6:195-1981, 1.983.
3. Potthullil, J.Shimizu, A.,Day,R.P. and Wolowich,J.Ann Inter Med 82:58-60, 1.975.
4. Aljama,P.,Brown P.,Turner P., Ward, M.K. and Kerr, D.N.S., Br Med 2:251, 1.978.
5. Hanai,K.,Horiuchi, T.,Hanai, J.,Gotoh, H., Hirasawa, Y.,Gejyo, F., and aizawa, Y.,Nephron 25:247-248, 1.979.

Criteria of Adequacy

CRITERIA FOR ADEQUATE HEMODIALYSIS

FRANK A. GOTCH

Hemodialysis Treatment and Research Center, Davies
Medical Center, Castro & Duboce Streets, San Francisco,
California 94114 USA

CRITERIA FOR ADEQUATE DIALYSIS

The uremic syndrome results in multisystem organ
failure which is only partly responsive to adequate
dialysis. There is variable ongoing morbidity such as
impaired appetite, mild sensory neuropathy, renal osteo-
dystrophy and pruritis in well dialyzed patients and the
mortality rate is strongly dependent on associated illnesses (1). Because of this variable ongoing clinical
morbidity in these patients despite fully "adequate"
dialysis it is very difficult if not impossible to re-
liably optimize the dose of dialysis from empirical
observation of patient symptoms alone.

Calculation of the dose of dialysis is also quite
complicated both conceptually and with respect to practical details. It is useful to consider dialysis dosage
in analogy with pharmacologic therapy. The size of the
maintenance dose of a drug and frequency of administration must be adequate to replace the drug eliminated
from the body and is determined by the fractional rate at
which the drug is cleared from its volume of distribution
through metabolic, hepatic and renal clearance pathways.
In dialysis therapy a clearance pathway is provided to
remove toxic endogenous solutes and, consequently, the
dialysis dose is a dimensionless parameter, the fractional clearance of the volume of distribution of the dialyzed solute. The physical determinants of this definition of dialysis dosage are dialyzer clearance (K),

length of treatment time (t) and solute distribution
volume (V) and the fractional clearance is Kt/V. This
dosage parameter exponentially controls the drop in solute concentration during dialysis and when kinetically
modeled with the frequency of dialysis and the rate of
solute generation can be used to predict solute concentration profiles in body water (2).

The rationale of dialysis therapy of uremia is that
multisystem organ failure in uremia results from the retention of dialyzable solutes which have concentration
dependent toxicity. Rigorous clinical application of
kinetic modeling to optimize the dose of dialysis would
require detailed knowledge of the dependence of clinical
uremic abnormalities on specific toxic solute concentration. Unfortunately knowledge of the molecular toxins in
uremia is far from complete and it is therefore impossible to rigorously model the dialysis prescription for all
toxic solutes.

Since dialyzer solute transport is strongly dependent on solute molecular weight, a marker solute has often
been used for calculation of the dose of dialysis. In
the low molecular weight range urea has been extensively
studied as a marker solute and its utility in this role
verified (3). Development of the urea model for clinical
use (2) results in the mathematically rigorous relationships between midweek predialysis BUN (C02), normalized
protein catabolic rate (NPCR, gm/kg/day) and the dose of
dialysis (Kt/V urea) depicted in Fig. 1. The target
modeling line shown provides a generalized criterion for
the dose of low molecular weight solute transport required for adequate dialysis. Note that the Kt/V requirement is a discontinuous function of NPCR in that
the Kt/V modeled is constant at 1.06 for NPCR $\leq$ 1.1 but
increases in direct proportion with NPCR $>$ 1.1.

It is also important to emphasize that confidence
limits of ± 10% on the prescribed Kt/V and ± 25% on the

actually delivered Kt/V are depicted in Fig. 1. These
confidence limits indicate that the prescribed Kt/V
should be based on kinetic data and that the clinically
administered prescription should be subjected to kinetic
analysis for quality assurance (QA) at regular intervals
(2). Although Kt/V is now widely used as a dialysis dosage parameter for clinical dialysis therapy, kinetic a-
nalysis for prescription calculation and QA of the delivered therapy is far less frequently done in the clinic.
The V is often simply estimated from surface area or
weight rather than determined kinetically and "QA" is
based on monthly measurements of predialysis BUN.

Dialysis is high technology therapy and all components must be well controlled to assure that the prescription is correctly delivered and assessed. Common
clinical problems uncovered by kinetic QA are shown in
Fig. 2. Point 1 depicts an optimal prescribed dose and
point 2 shows it is correctly delivered. Point 3 shows
a high BUN due entirely to high protein intake. Points
4 and 5 clearly show major technical problem(s) with the
delivery of the prescribed dose. The prescribed Kt/V =
1.1 but the delivered doses for points 4 and 5 are only
.6 and .48 indicating one or more major technical problems such as fistula recirculation, excessive dialyzer
clotting or serious blood pump calibration error: note
particularly that the CO_2 values for points 1, 2, 4 and
5 are all very similar and that serious technical problems could not be discerned simply from observation of
the predialysis BUN levels.

Other criteria for adequate dialysis which cannot
be considered here in detail because of space constraint
include: (1) optimal control of Na+ and H2O balance;
(2) optimal control of K+ and H+ balance; and (3) adequate removal of Beta-2 microglobulin to prevent
amyloidogenesis.

References

1. Shapiro F, Umen A. Risk factors in hemodialysis
    patient survival. ASAIO Journal 6:176, 1983.

2. Gotch F. Kinetic Modeling in Hemodialysis, in
    Nissenson A and Gentile D, eds. Clinical Dialysis
    2nd Ed. Appleton & Lange Publishers, in press, 1988.

3. Gotch F, Sargent J. A mechanistic analysis of the
    National Cooperative Dialysis Study (NCDS). Kidney
    Int. 28:526, 1985.

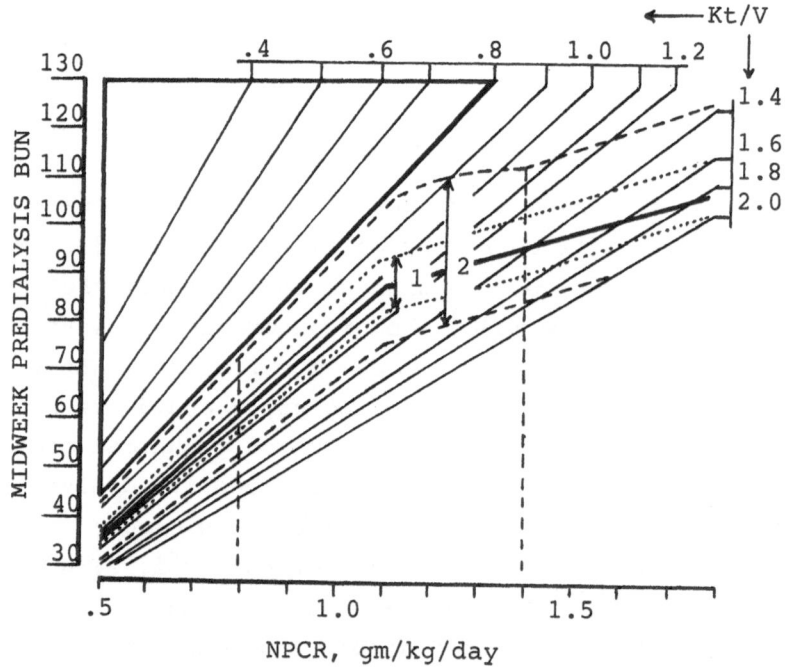

1 = CONFIDENCE LIMITS, ± 10% ON PRESCRIPTION,
    $Kptp/\overline{V}$

2 = CONFIDENCE LIMITS, ± 25% ON EFFECTIVE DOSE,
    $Kete/\overline{V}$

Fig. 1 THRICE WEEKLY DIALYSIS QA MAP.

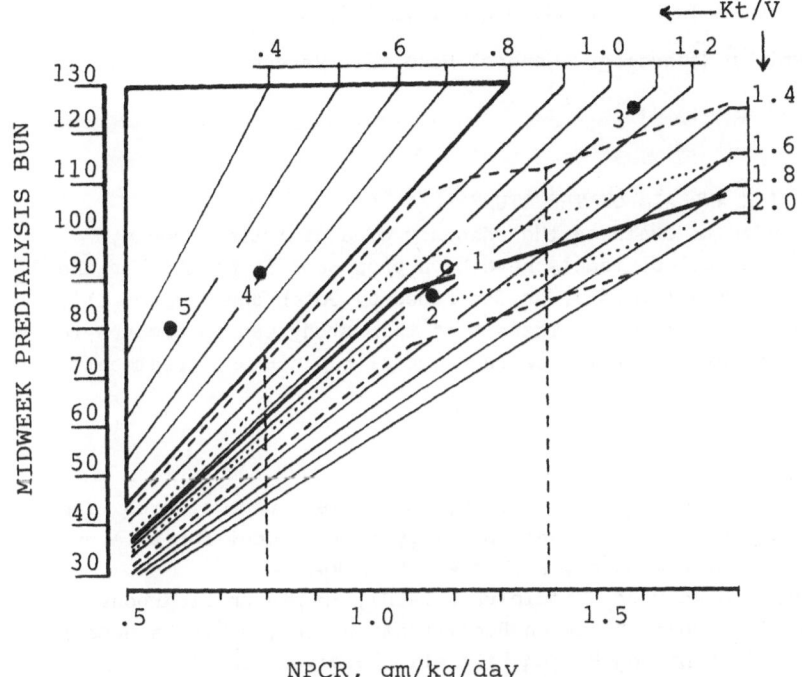

NPCR, gm/kg/day

Fig. 2 DIALYSIS QA: ILLUSTRATIONS OF
(1) OPTIMAL PRESCRIPTION, (2) OPTIMAL
DELIVERY, (3) POOR DIETARY COMPLIANCE,
(4) and (5) TECHNICAL PROBLEMS SEVERELY
COMPROMIZING EFFECTIVE DELIVERY OF
PRESCRIBED DOSE.

DIALYTIC ADEQUACY OF DIFFERENT REPLACEMENT TREATMENTS

P.CERVINI,O.AMATRUDA,F.DOSSI,D.DONATI,L.GASTALDI

Department of Nephrology, General Hospital, Varese

INTRODUCTION AND AIM OF THE STUDY
    In order to evaluate the adequacy of a dialytic program,
various mathematical models have been proposed; in particular the
urea kinetic model (KT/V), as described by Gotch and Sargent (1),
has been widely accepted. The aim of this study was to compare the
dialytic efficiency of the extracorporeal replacement treatments
carried out in our center.

MATERIALS AND METHODS
    101 uremic patients (48 males, 53 females) were studied. Their
mean age was 63.9 yrs and were on dialytic treatment for an average
of 6.7 yrs. Their mean dry weight was 59.3 kg.
42 pts were on Acetate Hemodialysis (AHD); 25 pts on Bicarbonate
Hemodialysis (BHD); 14 pts on Biofiltration (BF); 8 pts on Hemofiltration (HF); 6 pts on Paired Filtration Dialysis (PFD); 6 pts on
Rapid High-efficiency Bicarbonate Hemodialysis (HEHD). Table I
shows some of the major features of an each schedule.

	NoPts	Schedule	Qd	Qb	Membrane	Surface(m^2)
AHD	(42)	4hr30min x 3/wk	500	300	CUPROPHAN	1.0
BHD	(25)	4hr30min x 3/wk	500	300	CUPROPHAN	1.0
BF	(14)	3hr30min x 3/wk	500	300	AN 69 S	1.2
		+ 6 l p.i.(HCO_3^-)				
HF	(8)	30 l x 3/wk		400	PAN	2.1
PFD	(6)	3hr30min x 3/wk	500	300	POLISULFONE	0.4
		+ 9 l p.i.(HCO_3^-)			+ CUPROPHAN	1.0
HEHD	(6)	3hr x 3/wk	700	400	CA	2.1

Table I: Features of the dialytic programs

Each patient was undergoing the reported treatment for at least 12
months (but 7 months for HEHD) and had been previously allocated in
each group for personal, logistic or clinical reasons thus representing an unselected population.
KT/V was employed and computed monthly in the last 6 months on

succession as well as indexes of dialytic tolerance and nutritional status parameters.

RESULTS

The group of patients allocated in each dialytic program were omogeneous as regard to age and dry weight.

Mean values (± SD) of KT/V are shown in Figure 1. In all cases the average value exceeds the limit of 0.80 but it is apparent how the results obtained in HEHD are significantly higher compared to the others. Furthemore in all patients receiving HEHD, KT/V was over 1.10. One-way analysis of variance was performed (Table II).

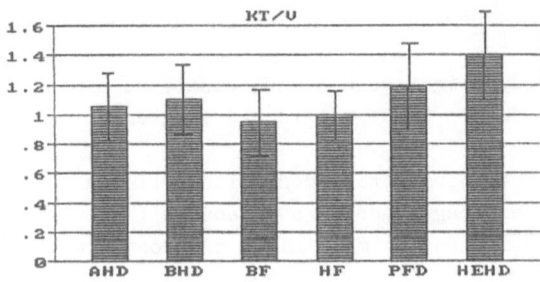

HEHD vs AHD p< 1 e-6
HEHD vs BHD p< 2 e-4
HEHD vs BF p< 1 e-6
HEHD vs HF p< 1 e-5
HEHD vs PFD p< 2 e-2

Table II

Fig. 1: Mean values (± SD) of KT/V

PFD too appears to be more efficient than standard-time dialysises, but the difference is not significant (but vs BF p< 0.05). Midweek urea was 135 (±32) mg/dl in AHD, 139 (±35) mg/dl in BHD, 137 (±28) mg/dl in BF, 134 (±17) mg/dl in HF, 161 (±34) in PFD, 142 (±29) in HEHD.

In Table III data concerning Protein Catabolic Rate (PCR) and other nutritional parameters are reported. The difference among treatments are not significant. Dialytic tolerance was satisfactory and similar in all treatments; it was assessed as number of simptomatic intradia lytic hypotensions, cramps, intradialytic headace bouts, nausea and vomiting per month of treatment.

	Alb	S.T.T.	HCO_3^-	Hct	PCR
AHD	4	309	18.5	29	0.92
BHD	4.1	322	19.8	27	0.94
BF	4.1	388	19.9	29	0.92
HF	4	266	18.6	26	0.96
PFD	4.9	293	19.6	31	1.14
HEHD	4.9	341	21.3	38	1.16
	g/dl	mg/dl	mmol/l	%	g/kg/die

Legend: Alb = Serum Albumine
        S.T.T. = Serum Total Transferrine
Table III: Mean values of nutritional parameters

The mean body weight gain was 4.8 % in AHD, 5.6 % in BHD, 2.8 % in BF, 3.9 % in HF, 2.9 % in PFD, 2.5 % in HEHD.

DISCUSSION

Over the last few years several new dialysis techniques have been applied in order to shorten the lenght and improve the effica- cy. The standard 4-5 hrs x 3/week hemodialysis may probably be no more necessary and often unsuccesful. The new techniques and new membranes available should allow reduction of the single session lenght. It has been suggested that keeping KT/V between 1.0 and 1.3 guarantees the correct dialysis dose provided normal PCR exists (2). In our experience short-time dialysis schedules,namely PFD and HEHD, appear to be adequate in this regard without patient disconfort or metabolic imbalance.

The lesser interdialytic body weight gain cannot easily be explained; it could reflect patients' desire to be maintained on a short dialysis program.

In conclusion although further perspective controlled clinical trials with more patients and longer and more extensive follow-up are required, uremic patients might be maintained on short dialysis schedules.

Among these, HEHD should play a major part in the future trends of renal replacement treatments.

REFERENCES
1. Gotch, F.A. and Sargent, J.A. Kidney Int. 28: 526-534, 1985
2. Gotch, F.A. Dial. Transpl.15: 553-554, 1986

ROUTINE EVALUATION OF Kt/V AND PROTEIN CATABOLIC RATE

F.G. CASINO, V. GAUDIANO, A. SACCO AND T. LOPEZ

Division of Nephrology and Dialysis, MATERA, ITALY

INTRODUCTION

The usual procedure (UP) estimating Kt/V (1) and protein catabolic rate (pcr), requires, as a first step, the measurement of the dialyzer urea clearance (K). It then computes the urea distribution volume (V) and generation rate (G) of the patient, according to the Variable Volume Urea Kinetics Model (UKM)(2).

In order to avoid the measurement of K, we suggest a modified procedure (MP) assuming a theoretical end-dialysis V (VT) and calculating the corresponding value of K and G as a function of VT and BUN values observed (3).

The rationale of MP can be derived from the analysis of a truncated version of UKM, assuming fixed volume, no urea generation during dialysis and a symmetric thrice weekly schedule: with these assumptions, Kt/V and pcr are related to the change in BUN during dialysis by numerical constants (1). This means that when computing K by means of MP, the ratio K/V remains constant with any assumed value of V, the latter being a direct proportional to K.

Aim of this study was to compare Kt/V and pcr obtained from UP with the paired values obtained from MP using the rigourous variable volume UKM in patients with a significant intradialysis volume removal (VR).

PATIENTS AND METHODS

Twenty-nine patients on free diet and thrice weekly hemodialysis (HD) were studied. The mean values ($\pm$ SD) of end-dialysis body wt (BWT) and VR were 58.7 $\pm$ 9.7 Kg, 3.7 $\pm$ 1.0 Kg, and 0.5 $\pm$ 0.9 ml/min, respectively. The session lenght (t) was about 240 min. Blood (Qb) and dialysate flow rate (Qd) were about 300 and 500 ml/min, respectively. The dialyzer surface area ranged between 1.3 and 1.7 m2. Qb, Qd and the ultrafiltration rate (Qf) were kept constant during the session.

Urea Kinetics analysis was performed according to UKM utilizing a specific computer program requiring the following data input: BUN and BW at the beginning, at the end of the session and at the beginning of the next one; time on and off-dialysis; Kr and K.

Kr was measured from the interdialysis urine urea nitrogen output and the averaged interdialysis BUN (2). K was measured two times during the session (at the first and third hour), from Qb, Qf and BUN concentrations at the inlet and outlet of the dialyzer (2): the averaged value of K was used as an input of MP.

For each patient, Kt/V and pcr were computed according to both UP and MP, utilizing the same data input. As regards UP, G and V were computed according to UKM (2). The pcr and Kt/V were calculated as follows:

$$pcr = (9.35G + 0.294VT)/(VT/0.58)$$

$$Kt/V = Kt/(VT + VR/2)$$

where VT + VR/2 is the averaged V during the session. As regards MP, VT was assumed to be 0.58BWT, G was computed according to UKM (2). K was computed by iteration technique using the following formula (3):

$$K = Qf * \left(1 + \frac{\ln \dfrac{CT * (K + Kr - Qf) - G}{CO1 * (K + Kr - Qf) - G}}{\ln (VT/(VT+VR))} \right) - Kr$$

where CO1 and CT are pre and post-dialysis BUN values. Kt/V and pcr were then computed as above.

Data are expressed as means $\pm$ SD. Statistical analysis was done using Student's paired t-test and linear regression analysis.

RESULTS

The results of the statistical analysis are given in table 1 and 2. Units were as follows: VT, 1; VT/BWT, %; K, ml/min; G, mg/min; pcr, g/Kg/day.

Table 1. Student's paired t-test: UP - MP values, N = 29

	UP	MP	Difference	t	P
VT	33.74 $\pm$ 4.33	34.04 $\pm$ 5.60	-0.30 $\pm$ 3.45	-0.23	NS
VT/BWT	58.09 $\pm$ 5.93	58.00 $\pm$ 0.00	0.00 $\pm$ 5.93	0.08	NS
K	220.7 $\pm$ 22.07	222.6 $\pm$ 29.35	-1.93 $\pm$ 19.95	-0.28	NS
G	7.03 $\pm$ 2.32	7.11 $\pm$ 2.39	-0.07 $\pm$ 0.63	-0.12	NS
Kt/V	1.479 $\pm$ 0.202	1.478 $\pm$ 0.201	0.003 $\pm$ 0.020	0.004	NS
pcr	1.324 $\pm$ 0.347	1.323 $\pm$ 0.350	0.001 $\pm$ 0.013	0.019	NS

Table 2. Linear regression analysis:MP vs UP values, N=29

VT   : y = -0.398 + 1.020x   r = 0.787   P < 0.001
K   : y =   7.281 + 0.976x   r = 0.734   P < 0.001
G   : y =   0.129 + 0.992x   r = 0.998   P < 0.001
KT/V : y =   0.007 + 0.995x   r = 0.998   P < 0.001
pcr   : y = -0.009 + 1.007x   r = 0.998   P < 0.001

DISCUSSION

The evaluation of Kt/V and pcr by means of UP is complicated by several technical problems associated with the measurement of K (4). However, the knowledge of the true value of K is required for an accurate estimate of V, but, as shown above, it is not required for an accurate estimate of Kt/V and pcr. In fact, the use of MP, using a theoretical K, gives Kt/V and pcr values nearly identical to the corresponding ones, computed by UP, using the measured value of K: as shown in table 2, the slope and r of the regression line, for both parameters, are close to 1 and the intercept is close to zero. Interestingly, these results were obtained using the rigourous variable volume UKM in a group of 29 HD patients with varying degrees of Kr (0.5 ± 0.9 ml/min) and VR (3.7 ± 1.0 Kg) and in spite of a wide range of distribution of the ratio VT/BWT (46-70%) (table 1).

It should be pointed out that the K value computed by MP is the effective K for an assumed VT/BWT = 0.58, so that it overestimates the true value of K for VT/BWT < 0.58 and underestimates it for VT/BWT > 0.58.

In conclusion, MP is a very accurate procedure which, by avoiding any extra work, allows a routine evaluation of Kt/V and pcr even in busy dialysis units.

REFERENCES
1.Gotch F.A., Sargent J.A. Kidney Int 28:526-534, 1985
2. Sargent J.A., Gotch F.A. In: Replacement of renal function by Dialysis. (Eds. W. Drukker, F. Parsons, J. Maher). 2nd ed., Martinus Nijhoff, Boston, 1983 pp. 53-96
3. Casino F.G. Minerva Urol Nefrol. 36:179-190, 1984.
4. Aebischer P., Schorderet D., Juillerat A., Wauters J.P., and Fellay G. Trans Am Soc Artif Intern Organs 31:338-342, 1985.

ADEQUACY OF BIOFILTRATION: A COMPARATIVE STUDY WITH STANDARD ACETATE HEMODIALYSIS

R.KVEDER, J.DRINOVEC, R.PONIKVAR, A.KANDUS, M.MALOVRH, B.KNAP
University Medical Center, Department of Nephrology, Ljubljana,
Yugoslavia

INTRODUCTION

Biofiltration (BF) represents a new way of renal replacement therapy. The method is simplified hemodiafiltration using highly permeable polyacrylonitrile (PAN) membrane and postdilutional infusion of a bicarbonate containing solution. It possibly favours better control of acid-base status, vascular stability as well as well being of patients (1).

The aim of this study was to estimate the adequacy of BF as an alternative to conventional acetate hemodialysis (AHD) regarding hemodynamic stability, regulation of acid-base balance and purification of small and also larger molecules during 4 months period of either treatment modality.

PATIENTS AND METHODS

Ten patients (5 women, and 5 men; mean age $54^{+}_{-}14$ years) with ERSD due to various renal diseases treated with chronic HD for $90^{+}_{-}30$ months (range 48-137) participate in this study. Four of them had been experienced important cardiovascular instability before they were switched to BF. The patients were on free diet during the whole observation period.

Cuprophane hollow fiber dialysers with standard surface (Hemomed 1.0, Inex Hemofarm) were used during AHD period (3 times per week, session lasting 4-4.5 hours). Blood flow was kept constant 200-300 ml/min, Q_D was about 500 ml/min. High acetate was used in dialysate (42 mmol/L; Na 140 mmol/L).

The same basic condition were maintained during BF period.

Automatic ultrafiltration control system with a reinfusion pump connected with the venous line (Monitral BSM2-Hospal) and PAN membrane (AN-69 S Hospal) were used during BF. The substitution fluid had the following composition (mmol/L): Na^+ 145, Cl^- 45, HCO_3^- 100.

Three liters of infusate were used during each session.

RESULTS

Patients' body weight, amount of fluid intake as well as UFR during whole observation period did not show any significant changes.

Blood pressure values are presented in Table 1.

Table 1. Systolic and diastolic blood pressure during AHD and BF.

	AHD	BF
Systolic: start	147 ± 27	144 ± 26**
(mm Hg) end	148 ± 24*	138 ± 25* **
Diastolic: start	84 ± 1	86 ± 12
(mm Hg) end	85 ± 11	83 ± 13

*$p < 0.01$,   **$p < 0.025$

Systolic blood pressure was significantly lower at the end of BF. We observed also a greater number of symptomatic hypotension during BF (15/176 treatments) when compared to AHD (8/176) but this difference was statistically insignificant.

Significant decrease in the   concentration of small molecules was noticed during BF treatment (Table 2).

Table 2. Some biochemical parameters during AHD and BF treatment.

	AHD	BF	p
Creatinine (μmol/L) (n=25)	1279 ± 263	1077 ± 220	< 0.001
Urea (mmol/L) (n=24)	29.7 ± 6.5	247 ± 4.2	< 0.005
Pi (mmol/L) (n=24)	1.42 ± 0.3	1.52 ± 0.4	NS

Mean total drop of beta-2-microglobulin (BMG) during BF was $30.8^{+}_{-}18$ % (BMG pre BF=$39.8^{+}_{-}5.6$ mg/L, BMG post BF=$27.7^{+}_{-}8.6$).

The influence of BF on acid-base parameters and serum Na is shown in Table 3 (the measurements were done in the second half of BF treatment period).

Table 3. Influence of BF on acid-base parameters and serum sodium.

	pre BF	post BF	p
pH	$7.41^{+}_{-}0.04$	$7.49^{+}_{-}0.04$	<0.005
HCO_3^- (mmol/L)	$27.6^{+}_{-}4.4$	$31.4^{+}_{-}5.1$	NS
Na (mmol/L)	$137.5^{+}_{-}1.9$	$141.6^{+}_{-}2.3$	<0.005

Inspite of laboratory alkalosis we did not observe any obvious clinical effects.

DISCUSSION

Reducing treatment time has been claimed as one of the advantages of BF treatment (2), not confirmed by all, especially concerning the cardiovascular stability (3). For hours BF appeared to be as adequate as AHD in respect to clinical tolerability, blood pressure and body weight control.

The removing capacity for small molecules and BMG in our group of patients was greater during four hours BF when compared to AHD.

Correction of acid-base parameters was over efficient and metabolic alkalosis was observed in patients without any clinical consequences. The dialytic buffer gain was probably to high due to high dialysis acetate. The amount of administered bicarbonate seems to be of less importance (4).

REFERENCES

1. Zucchelli, P., Santoro,A., Raggiotto,G., Degli Esposti,E., Sturani,A., Capecchi,V. Blood Purification 2: 187-195, 1984.
2. Meloni,C., Taccone-Galluci,T., Morosetti,M., Valentini,G., Tuzzo, C., Mazzarella,V., Elli,M., Marciani,M.G., Rosini,P.M., Casciani, C.U. Int J Artif Organs 9/S-3: 39-42, 1986.
3. Drinovec,J., Močivnik,M., Bren,A., Kandus,A., Ponikvar,R., Kveder, R., Benedik,M., Malovrh,M., Int J Artif Organs 9/5-3,147-148,1986.
4. Feriani,M., Bragantini,L., Dell'Aquila,R. et al. Int J Artif Organs 9/5-3; 1-4, 1986.

IS IT POSSIBLE A MATHEMATICAL VERIFICATION OF Kt/V ?

S. MANDOLFO,T. FIDELIO,C. LICATA,V. CALITRI,G.P. SANCIPRIANO,

G. IACONO,R. RAGNI.

Renal Unit - Ciriè Hospital,Turin,Italy.

INTRODUCTION

The urea kinetic model has been utilized to determine the Kt/V therapy index.This model conceived by Sargent and Gotch is based on the following equation: $Kt/V = \ln(C_i/C_t)$ (a) where K=clearance,t=time,V=urea distribution volume,C_i=pre-dialysis urea,C_t=post-dialysis urea.

The aim of our study was to develop a program that could allow us to: (1) verify mathematically the Kt/V results,(2) evaluate the effects of urea rebound and haemoconcentration on the Kt/V results.

MATHEMATICAL MODEL,MATERIALS AND METHOD

As from the equation (a) and according to the logarithms' properties we can obtain that: $C_t/C_i = e^{-Kt/V}$ (b),where e is Nepero's number.As at each Kt/V value it corresponds a determinated theoretical urea removal, we can derive this removal by using the data of (b) with the formula: $RT\% = 100 - (100/e^{Kt/V})$ (c).If we know V it is possible to calculate the total theoretical urea removal as follow: $RTU = (C_i \times V \times RT\%)/100$ (d). In order to complete the requested parameters for the application of our model it is necessary to determine the real urea removal (RU),in accordance with the following formula: RU= (dialysate urea x dialysate volume) (e).The verification is therefore effected by calculating the ratio between RU and RTU: we consider this verification positive when RU=RTU with a tolerance of ±5%.Our program allows furthermore the calculation of an extraction index of the total pool of urea per minute

&s follow : DRM = (RU/t)/(Ci x V) x 100.

We have studied 60 dialysis with our model: 10 hemofiltration (HF, polyamide,2 1 UF/Kg/wk),13 bicarbonate-dialysis (HDB,cuprophan,240 min),18 two-chamber technique (TCT,polysulfone and cuphrophan on line, 180 min),10 two-chamber technique (TCTP,two polysulfones on line,180 min),9 hemodiafiltrations (HF,polysulfone,UF=9 l,180 min).For each session we have calculated the following indexes: Kt/V,RU,RTU,DRM. The V has been calculated according to: Wosmersley,Watson,Apfelbaum, Bolot-Thomasset,Fixed Volume.In the second stage we have corrected Ct for its rebound (30 min after dialysis) and in the third stage for the plasmatic water.

RESULTS

Kt/V	RT%	Kt/V	RT%	Kt/V	RT%
0.8	54.95	1.1	66.60	1.4	75.23
0.9	59.23	1.2	69.77	1.5	77.58
1.0	63.09	1.3	72.63	1.6	79.71

Table A: corresponding values of theoretical per cent removal of urea for different Kt/V.

	Kt/V	DRM
HF	0.97±0.03	0.19±0.011
HDB	1.21±0.07	0.27±0.016
TCT	1.30±0.05	0.31±0.013
TCTP	1.40±0.03	0.35±0.014
HDF	1.47±0.06	0.33±0.025

Table B : results of Kt/V and the DRM index (mean ± ES).It exist a correlation statistically significant (p<0.0005) between DRM and Kt/V.

Wosmersley	= 59.8±1.4	0	%
Watson	= 54.1±1.9	22	%
Apfelbaum	= 54.0±1.6	0	%
Bolot-Thomasset	= 50.6±1.4	27	%
Fixed volume	= 58	9	%

Table C : results of V,according to the Authors,expressed as percentage of body weight and the percentage of dialysis with positive verification.

For our verification we have taken in account the V obtained by using Watson's formula.The ratio RU/RTU in the first stage was 15.608±2.19 and in the second stage 9.739±3.34 (p<0.05).At the end of the second stage,the percentage of positive verification was of 37%.No statistical change was seen in the third stage with the correction of Ct for the plasmatic water.

DISCUSSION

The Kt/V model is nowdays considered to be a valid guide in the monitorization of the prescriptions and efficiency.Its calculation can nevertheless produce some rather gross valuation errors if it is performed by determing Ci and Ct.In fact it is evident the role of Ct in the solution of Gotch's equation.Furthermore the improvement of efficiency and the shortening of dialysis can influence the sample for the Ct : Haas and Arisi have demonstrated a strict correlation between dialysis effiency and one hour rebound of urea.

Our model allows to verify the results of Kt/V through the ratio real/theoretical urea removal.As the verification is positive only in 22% of the dialysis we have examined,it sets a limit to the Kt/V index,supporting the hypotesis of an overstimation of it.If we correct Ct for its rebound,we have a significant increase (37%) in the number of dialysis for which the verification is positive.These data suggest the importance of correcting the Ct for the rebound,whereas it seems unnecessary the correction for the plasmatic water.Finally the DRM offers another index in the evaluation of dialysis efficiency.

CONCLUSIONS

(1) We can perform a verification of Kt/V through the ratio between real and theoretical urea removal ,
(2) it is important to correct the data of urea post dialysis for its rebound when calculating the Kt/V ,
(3) the DRM supports the Kt/V in the evaluation of the dialysis efficiency.

ADEQUACY OF DIALYSIS AND PROLONGED REUSE

H. PEREZ-GROVAS & J. HERRERA-ACOSTA
Nephrol. Dept., Inst. Nac. Cardiología, 14080 México City, Méx.

INTRODUCTION

Urea kinetic modeling (UKM) has made possible rational prescription of dialysis therapy and has decreased hemodialysis (HD) morbimortality. (1) Elevated costs of HD have prevented its wide use in developing countries. Reuse of dialyzer is safe and extremely cost-effective. (2,) After prolonged reuse, dialyzer urea clearance can change and difficult dialysis adequacy by UKM.
This study was conducted to evaluate the effect of prolonged reuse in dialysis adequacy estimated by a computerized program of UKM calculating KT/V, protein catabolic rate (PCR) and BUN time average concentration (TAC).

MATERIALS AND METHODS

28 chronically uremic adult outpatients were studied during a 4 months period. HD was performed 3 x 4 hs/week in Travenol RSP hemodialyzer system using blood flow of 240 ml/min, 400 ml/min flow rate of commercially available acetate dialysate and 100 mmHg of ultrafiltration pressure by each kg of B.Wt gained in interdialytic period with maximum of 300 mmHg. Cuprophan hollow fiber hemofilter reprocessing was made manually with hypochlorite in reverse pressure and sterilization with 3.0% formaldehyde. (3)
Dialysis equations used for computers program are:

$$G = (V2C2 - V3C3) / Ti$$

generation rate (G) for a post and predialytic product of concentration and volume of distribution (V2C2,V3C3) during interdialytic period (Ti).(4)

$$C2 = C1.e-(KR+KD).TD/V + G/(KR+KD)1-e-(KR+KD).TD/V)$$

postdialytic concentration (C2) for a predialytic concentration (C1), dialyzer clearance (K), dialysis duration (TD) residual renal function (KR) and volume of distribution (V) expressing the intradialytic kinetic relationship.(5)

$$PCR= 9.35 G (mg/min) + 11.04$$

protein catabolic rate as a function of G. (6)

TAC was calculated by the area under the curve C1,C2,C3 vs TD,Ti

RESULTS

To evaluate safety and effectivity of the prolonged reuse dialyzer, as well as adequacy estimated by a computerized program of UKM, the following measurements were made at 1-6, 7-10, 11-14, 15-19 and 20 or more reuses.

Reuse number n	1-6 14	7-10 14	11-14 14	15-19 14	20 or > 14
DIALYZER DATA					
AREA (m²)	0.77±.1	0.59±.1*	0.63±.1*	0.69±.1	0.64±.1*
BUN-K ml/min	123.9±31	94.9±29*	117.9±26	117.1±24	115.0±24
Δ WT/HD kg	1.5±.6	1.4±.5	1.5±.5	1.7±.7	1.8±.8
UFP mmHg	188.0±90	185.7±89	215.4±61	196.8±51	255.7±28*
PATIENTS PREDIALYSIS DATA					
B WT kg	54.7±8	54.9±11	54.8±9	53.3±10	54.3±10
DBP mmHg	85.7±8	87.8±12	80.7±14	82.3±9	87.0±8
BUN mg/dl	64.9±12	72.6±14	70.1±16	70.4±18	66.6±15
CR mg/dl	10.9±3	12.7±3	12.4±3	12.6±4	15.1±5
K mEq/1	5.7±.8	5.7±1	6.2±1	6.1±1	6.0±1
ADEQUACY MEASUREMENTS					
TAC BUN mg/dl	49.1±9	57.4±12	52.4±11	52.6±13	51.8±11
PCR g/kg/d	0.90±.2	0.90±.2	0.96±1	1.00±.2	0.91±.1
KT/V %	0.98±.2	0.87±.2	0.96±.21	1.04±.3	0.97±.3

Values represent mean ± S.D. * $p<.05$ (Bonferroni method) vs 1-6 group. ΔWt/HD=weigth lost during HD. BUN-K=BUN filter clearance.

Dialysis disconfort was present in 14.7 % (172/1168) HD, only one patient required antihypertensive drugs and one patient had a 7 days hospitalization for cardiac failure. In 5 patients HD prescription had to be adjusted.

348

DISCUSSION

Our results show that BUN clearance remained unchanged after 20 or more reuses in spite of decreased surface area suggesting a slight increase in BUN clearance per unit of surface area. This can be attribuited to better biocompatibility (7), to increased convective transfer due to greater ultrafiltration pressure and probably to reduction in membrane wall thickness induced by hypochlorite reprocessing (8). Ultrafiltration ability was unchanged as estimated by the constancy of weight lost after prolonged reuse, although the 20 or more reuse dialyzer group patients required a greater ultrafiltration pressure.

Computerized UKM provided a rapid method to prescribe an adequate dialysis. In individual patients adjusting prescription permitted to achieve adequate dialysis. Stable body weight, diastolic blood pressure and intradialytic weight lost indicate an adequate ultrafiltration. Mean BUN TAC ± 50 mg/dl and KT/V ± 1 indicate adequate dialysis. However, PCR < 1 suggests undernutrition in some patients. In conclusion prolonged reuse did not prevent dialysis adequacy. Reuse has allowed us to extend HD treatment to a greater number of uremic patients.

REFERENCES
1. Gotch F, Sargent J, Keen M, Lam M. Prowitt M & Grady M: Clinical results of dialysis therapy guided by ongoing kinetic analysis of urea metabolism. Trans. Am. Soc. Artif. Intern Organs 22:175, 1976.
2. Pollack V, Kant K Parnell S & Levin N: Repetead use of dialyzers is safe. Nephron 42:217, 1986.
3. Rosete L, Pérez-Grovas H & Herrera-Acosta J: Procedimiento de reuso de filtros de fibra hueca para hemodiálisis por el método de lavado con cloro a presión reversa. Rev. Asoc. Medicina Interna de México 4: 111,1986.
4. Sargent J: Kinetic modeling in the guidance of dialysis therapy. Dialysis & Transplantation 8:1101, 1979.
5. Davidson W & Davidson S: Teaching dialysis kinetics with a minicomputer. Am. J. Nephrol. 4:19, 1984.
6. Sargent J, Gotch F, Henry R & Bennett N: Mass balance, a quantitative guide to clinical nutrition therapy. J. Amer. Dietetic. Assoc. 75:551, 1979.
7. Vanholder R, Pauwels R, Vandenbogaerde J, Lamont H, Van Der Straeten M & Ringoir S: Cuprophan reuse and interdialytic change of lung diffusion capacity and blood gases. Kidney Int. 32:117, 1987.
8. Pérez-Grovas H, Ruiz A, Cerdas M, Romero E & Herrera-Acosta J: Incremento de la dialisancia con el reuso de los filtros para hemodiálisis. Rev. Asoc. Medicina Interna de México 4:78, 1986.

Acid-Base Balance

POSITIVE ACID BALANCE IN PATIENTS UNDERGOING CHRONIC HEMOFILTRATION

G. MIONI, M. GROPUZZO, P. MESSA, G. BOSCUTTI

Servizio di Nefrologia - Ospedale Civile, Udine, Italia

INTRODUCTION

In Hemodialysis, while the kind and rate of Metabolizable Organic Anion (MOA) delivery are well characterized phenomena, the same cannot be said for the kind and rate of MOA dissipation. In fact the usually considered and chemically measured Lactate, BOHB and AcAc are only fractions of all the titratable MOA (1). The aim of the present investigation was to clarify: a) whether the dialysis buffer balance, carried out by measuring all the titratable MOA, still remains positive as when only BOHB and Lactate are considered; b) whether a dialysis net gain of buffer can be found, adequate to offset the interdialytic accumulation of metabolic H ions.

PATIENTS AND METHODS

In 10 anuric fasting patients an arterial blood sample was taken before and 1 hour after the end of 4 consecutive Hemofiltration (HF) treatments, each of 240-300 min. A dialysis solution, containing Lactate 38-44 mEq/l, glucose 1 g/l and standard Electrolytes at standard concentrations, was infused in the average amount of 27 ± 11. Ultrafiltration was 107 ± 11 ml/min and BW decrease 2.8 ± 0.6 kg. ($m \pm sd$). In plasma and ultrafiltrate Na, K, Ca, Mg, Cl, PO_4, SO_4 (mEq), total CO_2 (mmol), PCO_2 (mmHg) and pH were measured with standard Laboratory techniques. Lactate and BOHB were measured with enzymatic methods, while Titr.MOA following the Van Slyke and Palmer technique (2). In plasma Titr.MOA were calculated from BE and Cation-Anion difference (3,4). PCR was calculated according to Sargent et al. (5) and H ion generation from PCR released Sulphuric Acid (0.637 mEq per g of PCR). $HCO_3 = tCO_2 - PCO_2 x0.03$ (mEq/1); ECV (1) = 20% dry BW at the end of dialysis and 20% dry BW at the beginning, plus dial.B.W.loss (kg = 1).

RESULTS

Table 1.   Weekly Dialysis Acid-Base Balances (mEq; $m \pm sd$)

Kind of Balance	Lactate + BOHB	Titr.MOA
Lactate infusion	+ 3111 $\pm$ 189	+ 3111 $\pm$ 189
Bicarbonate Loss	− 1645 $\pm$ 106	− 1645 $\pm$ 106
Lactate Loss	− 734 $\pm$ 77	/
BOHB Loss	− 59 $\pm$ 16	/
Titr. MOA Loss	/	− 1512 $\pm$ 263
Dialysis NBB	+ 650 $\pm$ 78	− 62 $\pm$ 177
Dialysis NAB	− 650 $\pm$ 78	+ 62 $\pm$ 177
GHm	+ 226 $\pm$ 28	+ 226 $\pm$ 28
Total NAB	− 410 $\pm$ 25	+ 288 $\pm$ 155

Table 2.   Plasma Buffer Concentrations (mEq/1; $m \pm sd$)

	Pre Dialysis	1hr Post Dialysis
HCO_3	18.5 $\pm$ 1.6	23.4 $\pm$ 1.8 ...
Titr. MOA	24.7 $\pm$ 2.3	19.6 $\pm$ 2.2 ...
Net Base	42.4 $\pm$ 2.4	44.2 $\pm$ 2.4
pH	7.31 $\pm$ 0.05	7.42 $\pm$ 0.05 ...

Table 3.   ECV Buffer Pools (mEq; $m \pm sd$)

	Pre Dialysis	1hr Post Dialysis
HCO_3	266 $\pm$ 41	267 $\pm$ 39
Titr. MOA	340 $\pm$ 63	223 $\pm$ 57 ...
Net Base	590 $\pm$ 94	491 $\pm$ 81 ...

NBB = Net Base Balance; NAB = Net Acid Balance; NBB = − NAB;
Net Base = HCO_3 + MOA = Na + K + 2Ca + 2Mg − Cl − $1.8PO_4$ − $2SO_4$;
GHm = PCR dependent H ion generation / week
... $p < 0.001$

353

COMMENT

Chemical measuring of only few types of Titr. MOA has led to grossly understimating buffer dispersion during dialysis, as clarly demonstrated in the upper part of table 1. Since a dialysis Net Base balance not different from zero (- 62 mEq) is obtained when Titr. MOA loss is taken into consideration, the interdialytic H^+ion generation from PCR cannot be offset by dialysis buffer donation, as demonstrated in the lower part of Table 1, where positive Net Acid Base Balance results when Titr. MOA loss is considered, but a still positive Net Base Balance (negative Net Acid Balance) is found when BOHB plus Lactate dispersion only is measured. Table 2 shows an increment of post-dialysis HCO_3 concentration, which is considered as an index of buffer restoration. However, owing to the simultaneous decrease of plasma Titr. MOA conc., the total plasma buffer availability (NB concentration) appears to be unchanged by HF. Moreover, Table 3 demonstrates that dialysis, not only is unable to increase the EC pool of HCO_3, but is even able to reduce those of Titr. MOA and NB. As a consequence, the classic model of HF, which controls A-B homeostasis by means of buffer donation can no longer be considered adequate. The post dialysis increase of plasma HCO_3 conc. may be interpreted as a qualitative A-B correction, where plasma non metabolizable anions (SO_4, PO_4, Cl) are replaced by de novo generated HCO_3, during H^+ion consuming processes, due to Lactate oxidation

REFERENCES

1) Gabow, P.A.   Kidney Int. 27: 472-483, 1985
2) Van Slyke, D.D. and Palmer W.W.   J.Biol.Chem. 41: 567-585, 1920
3) Siggaard-Andersen, O.   Scand.J.Clin.Lab.Invest. 37: S146, 15-19, 1977
4) Kildeberg, P., Winters, R.W.   Adv.Pediat. 25: 349-381, 1978
5) Sargent, J., Gotch, F., Borah, M., Piercy, L., Spinozzi, L., Schoenfeld , P., Humphreys, M.   Amer.J.Clin.Nutr. 31: 1696-1702, 1978

TRENDS OF BUN AND ACID-BASE STATUS DURING HIGH EFFICIENCY HEMODIALYSIS

DEPETRI G.C.,BACCHI M.,BRAZZOLI A.,MILETI M.

Renal Unit,Crema,Italy

INTRODUCTION

The observation that post-dialysis rebounds of some solutes (BUN, Creatinine,Uric Acid) might be proportional to the efficiency of dialysis (1) makes this problem a topical subject today,when the so called "High Efficiency Treatments" are winning interest and approbation. The same question can be asked for what concerns Acid-Base status,either for the rapid correction during dialysis or for the trends of blood pH and bicarbonate between a dialysis and the next one. So we have valued the trends of BUN,plasma Creatinine and Acid-Base status in patients treated by High Efficiency Hemodialysis (HEH D) at increasing intervals following the completion of dialysis. As HEHD we intend an adequate dose of dialysis (diffusive,convective or mixed),with a reduction of the time of treatment of,at least,20-25 % in comparison to a Standard Hemodialysis (SHD);in general we could say:in the shortest possible time.

METHODS

Six patients,5 males and 1 female,were treated for six months by HEHD and compared to twelve patients (7 males and 5 females)treated by SHD. The parameters of Paired Filtration Dialysis (PFD) are: QB 300 ml/min,QD 500 ml/min,Dialyzer surface 1.8 m2,Dialysate bicarbonate 37-39 mMol/L,Saline solution infusion of 1.7-2 L/hr (2). The parameters of Rapid High Efficiency Hemodialysis (RHEH) are: QB 500 ml/min,QD 500 ml/min,Dialyzer surface 2.1 m2,Dialysate bicarbonate 35 mMol/L (3). The parameters of SHD:QB 200-300 ml/min,QD 500 ml/min Dialyzer surface 1 m2. The clinical characteristics of patients in HEHD are:Urea distribution volume 35698±3016 ml,KT/V 1.02±0.11,PCR 1.04±0.17 g/Kg,Midweek BUN 85±13 mg%. For patients in SHD:Urea distribution volume 35606±8414 ml,KT/V 0.989±0.262,PCR 1.16±0.26 g/Kg, Midweek BUN 88.8±19.5 mg %. Urea distribution volumes are quite similar and the indexes of adequacy are satisfactory. The mean treatment time is 176 min for HEHD and 229 min for SHD.All patients were in steady state with regard to their body weight and pre-dialysis chemistries. Blood specimens were drawn from the arterial blood line before dialysis and immediately after dialysis,and from A-V fistula at 90 min,150 min,6.5 hrs,24 hrs,44-45 hrs after the end of the dialysis. Patients' serum levels for BUN,Creatinine and Acid-Base status were followed for 48 hrs including dialytic and interdialytic periods. Clinical monitoring of patients in HEHD was performed by nutritional assessment,Evoked potentials and Echocardiography. All data are presented as Mean+1SD and statistical significance of differences between groups was assessed by Student's t test for paired or unpaired data.

RESULTS AND DISCUSSION

Results are summarized in Tables I and II and expressed as mean +SD. First of all we can say that for rebounds of BUN and Creatinine there are not significant differences between the two groups in consequence of the wide standard deviations. However some observations are necessary about the curves of the mean values:it would be possible that by further determinations these differences become significant. This is strongly suggested by the concordant trends of BUN and Creatinine rebounds that are higher in HEHD than in SHD. The explanation for the first part of rebound is the reequilibrium among body compartments.

	HIGH EFFICIENCY HD		STANDARD HD	
TIME	BUN	CREATININE	BUN	CREATININE
Pre HD$_1$	86.7+/-14	13.1+/-1.9	88.82+/-19.5	12.82+/-1.9
Post HD$_1$	36.4+/-8.3	6.5+/-1.1	39.83+/-13.09	6.94+/-1.59
90 min -	40.2+/-7.9 (+11.7 %)	7.5+/-1 (+16.1 %)	41.57+/-14.07 (+4.42 %)	7.6+/-1.73 (+9.9 %)
150 min	41.4+/-8.1 (+14.8 %)	7.89+/-1.1 (+21.3 %)	39.62+/-11.85 (+4.84 %)	7.98+/-1.77 (+16.5 %)
6.5 hrs	46.9+/-7.9 (+44.4 %)	8.6+/-1.2 (+36.9 %)	46.42+/-6.36 (+20.68 %)	8.62+/-1.68 (+27.56 %)
24 hrs	62.4+/-8.5 (+76.8 %)	10.4+/-1 (+64.4 %)	66.59+/-15.9 (+75.36 %)	10.2+/-1.62 (+52.96 %)
Pre HD$_2$ 45 hrs	81+/-11.7 (+127 %)	12.3+/-1.4 (+90.3 %)	86.75+/-18.04 (+131 %)	12.36+/-1.97 (+83.37 %)

Table I: BUN (mg %) and plasma Creatinine (mg%)
at increasing intervals in HEHD and SHD

TIME	HIGH EFFICIENCY HD			STANDARD HD		
	pH	HCO_3^-	PCO_2	pH	HCO_3^-	PCO_2
Pre HD	7.36±0.02	22.2±2.1	37.9±2.8	7.34±0.03	19.2±1.8	34.6±1.7
Post HD	7.47±0.02	27.7±1.8	36.6±2.4	7.42±0.02	19.7±2.1	29.3±3.9
90 min	7.46±0.03	26.8±0.47	37±2.5	7.42±0.02	24.3±2.5	36.3±2.3
150 min	7.45±0.03	28.5±1.5	40±2.5	7.43±0.03	24.6±1.5	36.3±1.7
6.5 hrs	7.44±0.02	28.9±3.1	42.3±4.4	7.43±0.02	26±2	38.4±2
24 hrs	7.39±0.02	26.1±2	41.8±2.4	7.38±0.03	22.8±2.1	37.1±2.8
45 hrs	7.36±0.02	21.5±1.5	36.5±1.37	7.35±0.03	19.5±1.8	34.3±2.6

Table II: Acid-Base status at increasing intervals in HEHD and Acetate SHD

The second part of rebound is probably due to hypercatabolism,induced by dialysis,that generally extends to 8 hrs after dialysis(4). Later we observe that there is a progression of BUN concentration slower in HEHD than in SHD. The clinical consequence of this rebound is an increase of time average concentration of BUN equal to 3.5%. For Acid-Base status, patients in HEHD show a pre-dialysis mild metabolic acidosis and a post-dialysis non compensated metabolic alkalosis:however the compensatory response is evident 90 min after the end of the treatment. They remain in this situation until 18 hrs after dialysis,reaching a situation of normality until 40 hrs after completion of dialysis. So the condition of metabolic acidosis lasts only 3-4 hrs before next dialysis. Of course the good correction of Acid-Base status is obtained paying the price of a postdialytic metabolic alkalosis.

REFERENCES

1. Haas et al. Clin.Nephrol. 19:193,1983
2. Ghezzi P.M. et al. in Bonomini V.,Stefoni S. and Black M.M. Proceedings X Annual Meeting ESAO-Bologna,Italy,1983
3. Keshaviah P. and Collins A. Dial.Transpl. 15:553,1986
4. Borah M.F. et al. Kid.Int. 14:491,1978

CLINICAL RESULTS OF ACETATE FREE BIOFILTRATION (AFB). TWO YEARS EXPE-
RIENCE.

G. BANDIANI, E. CAMAIORA, M.A. NICOLINI, U. PEROTTA.

Divisione di Nefrologia e Dialisi - Ospedale Civile San Andrea - La
Spezia - Italy.

INTRODUCTION
    In order to join the advantages of newer dialysis techniques
(better correction of acid-base status, improvement of cardiovascular
stability, better detoxification, reduction of dialysis time), and to
overcome some drawbacks connected to these methods (special and complex delivery supplies, large amounts of substitution fluid, use of
unsterile bicarbonate solutions and back-filtration problems, postdialytic alkalosis) (1-2), we tested a sort of biofiltration (AFB)
employing a dialysate without any buffer and organic acid and a substitution fluid containing only Na bicarbonate (3).
    In the present study we reported the two years clinical experi-
ence of AFB in a group of 5 patients.

PATIENTS AND METHODS
    The study was carried out during a period of 10-24 months in 5
pts (4 males and 1 female, aged 26-62 years, 4 CGN, 1 PKD) on RDT
from 29 to 50 months. All pts were functionally anephric. The method
was performed using a Monitral modified for AFB (Hospal SpA) and a
dialyzer with a polyacrylonitrile membrane and a surface area of 1.15
sq.m (Hospal Filtral). The schedule of AFB was the following: QBi 350
ml/min; QDi 500 ml/min; dialysate composition: Na 135, K 1.94, Ca 1.7
Mg 0.48, Cl 141 mMol/l; substitution fluid: Na bicarbonate 1/6 M; UF
rate 35-45 ml/min; post-dilution reinfusion rate 26-30 ml/min; treatment time: 3 hrs 3 times a week. Monthly the acid-base balance and
the main biochemical parameters were evaluated in each pts. During
every session the interdialytic weight gain (Δ B.W.), the dry body
weight (D.B.W.), the blood pressure and the incidence of intradialytic symptoms were recorded. Every 6 months the evolution of polyneuro
pathy was evaluated measuring the MNCV of the peroneal nerve. The data were compared to those obtained in the same pts during Ac-HD and
Bic-HD (4-5 hrs 3 times a week, QBi 250-300 ml/min; cuprophan plate
filter 1 sq.M).
    Data are reported as Means $\pm$ SD. Student's t test was employed

for statistical analysis of results.

RESULTS

Pre and post dialysis acid-base balance values are reported in Table 1.

		Ac-HD	Bic-HD	AFB
pH	pre	7.30 ± 0.04	7.35 ± 0.04***	7.37 ± 0.03*
	post°	7.39 ± 0.04	7.43 ± 0.03**	7.44 ± 0.03*
pCO_2	pre	37.0 ± 4.2	36.7 ± 2.4	36.1 ± 4.1
	post°	32.4 ± 4.0	37.3 ± 2.3	35.9 ± 3.9
pO_2	pre	92.0 ± 5.4	84.9 ± 5.7	95.5 ± 9.7
	post°	93.7 ± 5.2	89.8 ± 8.2	101.1 ± 12.3
HCO_3^-	pre	15.5 ± 1.7	19.5 ± 1.8**	20.1 ± 3.3*
	post°	21.6 ± 1.2	25.8 ± 3.2**	24.6 ± 3.3*

* $p < 0.01$ AFB vs Ac-HD ** $p < 0.01$ Bic-HD vs Ac-HD *** $p < 0.05$ Bic-HD vs Ac-HD. ° 2 hrs post dialysis in Ac-HD, end of dialysis in Bic-HD and AFB.

Table 1

During AFB pre dialysis plasma pH and bicarbonate were within the normal range and like those observed during Bic-HD, while during Ac-HD metabolic acidosis was still present, with significant low values of plasma pH and bicarbonate.

Pre-dialysis blood levels of urea, creatinine and uric acid remained stable, without significant differences from previous dialysis treatments. After 24 months of AFB an increase of Hb and Ht occurred. No significant differences were found in the electrolytes and in the anion gap (Table 2).

		Ac-HD	Bic-HD	AFB
Bun	mg/dl	84.4 ± 11.3	76.2 ± 17.3	71.4 ± 10.6
Creat	mg/dl	13.3 ± 1.9	12.8 ± 1.8	12.7 ± 1.7
Ur.Ac.	mg/dl	6.8 ± 0.5	7.1 ± 0.9	6.2 ± 0.4
Hb	mg/dl	8.2 ± 0.7	8.5 ± 1.0	9.8 ± 1.6*
Ht	%	23.6 ± 3.5	24.8 ± 3.7	28.3 ± 5.6*
Na	mEq/l	139.5 ± 4.2	139.4 ± 3.0	139.2 ± 1.4
K	mEq/l	5.5 ± 0.4	5.3 ± 0.9	5.4 ± 0.9
Ca	mg/dl	9.3 ± 0.6	9.3 ± 0.3	9.1 ± 0.7
P	mg/dl	6.2 ± 0.6	6.1 ± 0.7	6.1 ± 1.2
Cl	mEq/l	103.8 ± 6.3	104.1 ± 5.3	101.1 ± 4.9
AG	mEq/l	23.4 ± 2.2	23.7 ± 3.1	22.8 ± 1.5

* $p < 0.01$ AFB vs Ac-HD and Bic-HD

Table 2

No significant changes were observed in the blood pressure, in the Δ B.W. and in the D.B.W. The percentage of symptomatic treatments was significant lower during AFB than during Ac-HD and Bic-HD. MNCV showed a stable trend during the follow-up, rather after 24 months of

AFB a tendency toward an improvement of the neurological parameter
was observed (Table 3).

			Ac-HD	Bic-HD	AFB
B.P.	Syst.	(mm/Hg)	141 ± 12	142 ± 11	143 ± 9
	Dyast.		85 ± 5	84 ± 8	84 ± 7
Δ B.W.		(Kg)	2.4 ± 0.5	2.3 ± 0.4	2.1 ± 0.5
D.B.W.		(Kg)	61.9 ± 8.7	61.2 ± 8.6	61.6 ± 5.5
I.C.S.		(%)	28	12***	3* **
M.N.C.V.		(m/s)	41.8 ± 3.6	41.7 ± 4.4	44.8 ± 4.1°

* $p<0.001$ AFB vs Ac-HD   ** $p<0.005$ AFB vs Bic-HD   *** $p<0.001$ Bic-HD
vs Ac-HD   ° $p<0.01$ AFB vs Ac-HD and Bic-HD

Table 3

DISCUSSION

AFB is a new and feasible dialysis technique, conducted with highly permeable and biocompatible membrane, without any buffer and organic acid in the dialysate. This allows to avoid the drawbacks due to acetate and to overcome the technical problems of Bic-HD and HF. In AFB treatment the buffer is infused directly into the out-flow blood line, as sterile bicarbonate solution, in order to restore the pool of bicarbonate, according to individual needs. In fact, in all pts treated by AFB, an adequate correction of metabolic acidosis was observed without the developement of post-dialytic alkalosis. After 24 months follow-up, despite the reduction in treatment time, the biochemical parameters remained stable, ensued the high efficiency of depuration. The increase of Hb and Ht observed in all pts, is not clearly explained, but it could be ascribed to the better nutritional status, arising from the better well-being and appetite reported by the pts. The reduction of dialysis time did not modify the MNCV in contrast to those observed during conventional HD with cuprophan membrane. The clinical tolerance of treatment was excellent with a significant reduction of intradialytic clinical symptoms, expecially in terms of hypotension episodes. The use of a slightly hypertonic reinfusion fluid, the whole absence of acetate and the improvement of acid-base balance might explain the better intradialytic cardiovascular stability.

REFERENCES
1. Santoro A, Degli Esposti E, Sturani A et Al. Giorn It Nefrol 1: 143-148, 1984.
2. Stiller S, Mann H, Brunner H. Contr Nephrol 46: 23-32, 1985.
3. Buoncristiani U, Ragaiolo M, Petrucci V et Al. Int J Art Organs 9, S3: 9-14, 1986.

SUCCESSFULL TREATMENT WITH BICARBONATE DIALYSIS (BD) OF SEVERE LACTIC
ACIDOSIS IN PHENFORMIN TREATED PATIENTS ON DIALYTIC TREATMENT (DT).

G. FUIANO, P. IMPERATORE, V. SEPE, R. IANDOLO, B. CIANCIARUSO,
G. CONTE*.
Departments of Nephrology, 2nd Faculty of Medicine of Napoli and
Faculty of Medicine of Catanzaro*, Italy.

INTRODUCTION

Phenformin is a well recognized cause of lactic acidosis (1.2) :
for this reason, the health authorities of many Countries have
withdrawn this drug: for istance, in the U.S.A. this is not available
since 1977. Consequently, cases of phenformin related lactic acidosis
are not frequentely reported in the recent literature. In this paper,
we describe a case of severe lactic acidosis in a diabetic patient on
regular dialysis treatment (RDT).

Case presentation

A 49 y.o. lady with chronic renal insufficiency ascribed to
chronic interstitial nephritis and hypertensive state was started on
RDT: at the initiation of RDT, glycemia was sligthly elevated. This
abnormality was treated initially only with dietetic restriction;
despite the diet, however, blood glucose levels continued to rise;
two months after the onset of hyperglycemia, fast glycemic levels
avaraged 200 mg/dl. Insulin therapy was started, obtaining the
normalization of glycemia. In the same period, because of symptoms
of acetate intolerance, the patient was switched on bicarbonate
dialysis, with obvious intradialytic clinical improvement. After one
month of insulin therapy, the patient refused to continue the
prescribed sucutaneous administration and insulin was replaced by
oral therapy with very low dose of phenformin (12.5 mg/day) +
glybenclamide (1.25 mg/day). This therapy resulted in an initially

good control of glycemia. However, after the first seven days of this therapy, she developed progressive weakness, confusional and cloudy state of consciousness and was admitted in our Unit. At the admission time, a state of coma was observed; hyperventilation and sweating were also present; blood pressure was normal. Laboratory investigations showed, besides the values consisting with the uraemic state (plasma urea 157 mg/dl; plasma creatinine 9 mg/dl; mild hyper-phosphatemia and hypocalcemia; anaemia) severe hypoglycemia (32 mg/dl) and acidosis (arterial pH 7.04, pO_2 121 mmHg, blood bicarbonate concentration 2.4 mmol/l). An initial diagnosis of hypoglycemia and severe metabolic acidosis was made; i.v. glucose and bicarbonate infusion was immediately started restoring normal glycemic levels, but with no clinical improvement. So, the observed severe acidosis was considered the most important cause underlying the critical state of the patient and an intensive bicarbonate dialysis program was started (initially 5 hours per day). The main laboratory parameters, including acid base balance, were checked daily; plasma lactate levels wer checked after 2 and 6 days from the admission. Arterial pH, blood bicarbonate and plasma lactate concentrations are depicted in figure 1.

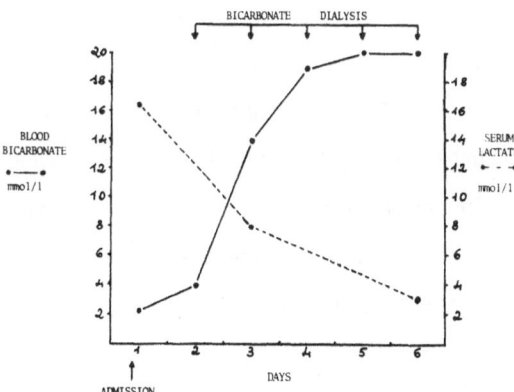

Fig. 1. Behaviour of blood bicarbonate and serum lactate during admission.

As shown in the figure, a striking improvement of acid base balance and a prompt fall of lactic acid levels occurred; a parallel clinical improvement was also seen: the consciousness state rapidly ameliorated since the second day of dialysis and resulted near completely normal after 5 days. Insulin therapy was restarted and after six days the patient was discharged. No relapse occurred in the following 9 months.

CONCLUSIONS

Lactic acidosis is probably the most frequent cause of metabolic acidosis in hospitalized patients(3); among the exogenous factors causing lactic acidosis phenformin is the most frequently reported. This drug causes lactic acidosis by altering the redox state(4). Because of impaired renal excretion, phenformin can accumulate in renal insufficiency; in our patient severe lactic acidosis occurred with a dosage much lower than previously reported in uremic patients . In fact, Ewy et al. described the onset of phenformin related acidosis with a dosage between 75 and 150 mg/day. We observed similar effects with a dosage as low as 12.5 mg/day. This observation confirms once again that phenformin represents a high-risk therapy in renal failure. Also the therapy of lactic acidosis secondary to phenformin is not well estabilished. In particular the use of bicarbonate infusion is controversed. We treated our patient with intensive bicarbonate dialysis obtaining a prompt and progressive improvement, probably by correcting the severe acidosis and by removing the drug. In conclusion, this report emphasizes that phenformin is highly toxic ij renal failure also at very low dose and that intensive bicarbonate dialysis is a safe and effective way of treating lactic acidosis.

REFERENCES
1. Kreisberg RA. Am. Rev. Med. 35: 181-193, 1984.
2. Seltzer HS. Am. Rev. Med. 31: 261-272, 1980.
3. Madias NE Kidney Int. 29: 752-774, 1986.
4. Lloyd MH. Diabetes 24: 618-624, 1975.

METABOLIC ASSESSMENT OF ACETATE-FREE BIOFILTRATION (AFBF).

V. La Milia, S. Di Filippo, R. Ponti, A. Citterio, G. Pontoriero,
F. Tentori, S. Andrulli, F. Locatelli.
Divisione di Nefrologia - Ospedale di Lecco - Lecco, Italy.

INTRODUCTION.

AFBF is an hemodiafiltration which utilizes a buffer-free dialysate and hypertonic sodium bicarbonate as replacement fluid (1). It
allows to overcome the side effects of acetate-dialysis as well as
the clinical and technical problems of bicarbonate-dialysis such as
bacterial contamination of dialysate and toilsome maintenance.
The aim of this study is to evaluate the "adequacy" of AFBF as regards depuration and electrolytes balance.

PATIENTS AND METHODS.

10 AFBF sessions were studied in 3 uremic patients stabilized
in maintenance hemodialysis whose pre-dialysis body weight was $53.5 \pm$
7.7 kg. AFBF was performed utilizing a modified Monitral BSM/2 monitor and AN 69, 1.2 sqm dialyzer. The foreseen buffer-free dialysate
compositions was: Na 139, Ca 1.75, K 2, Mg 0.5, Cl 145.5 mmol/l.
The replacement fluid contained 167 mmol/l of sodium bicarbonate.
Blood flow was 350 ml/min and dialysate flow 469.7 ± 40.4 ml/min; the
mean duration of the sessions was 177.0 ± 4.2 min. An ultrafiltration
rate of 46.5 ± 1.2 ml/min was applied to allow a body weight loss of
2.9 ± 0.2 kg and a replacement rate of 28.3 ml/min. A specimen of the
influent dialysate was obtained by utilizing a suction pump throughout the session and checked for Na^+, K^+, Cl^-, Ca, Ca^{++}. All the ef-
fluent dialysate was collected and checked for urea, creatinine, Na^+,

K^+, Cl^-, Ca, Ca^{++}, PO_4^{--}, TCO_2 and gas-analysis. At the start and at the end of each AFBF session blood samples were drawn from the patients and checked for urea, creatinine, Na^+, K^+, Cl^-, Ca, Ca^{++}, PO_4^{--} and gas-analysis. The depuration parameters and the mass balances were evaluated. The protein catabolic rate (PCR) and the intersession hydrogen-ions generations (gH^+) were also calculated.

RESULTS.

The electrolytes concentrations and the mass balances are shown in Table I.

TABLE I: Electrolytes plasma concentrations (mmol/l) at the start (PCi) and at the end (PCf) and mass balances (MB, mmol) in AFBF.

	PCi	PCf	MB
Na^+	142.5+2.8	146.7+1.2	-330.8+70.9*
K^+	4.5+0.4	3.1+0.2	-45.5+12.2
HCO_3^-	21.9+2.3	26.6+2.6	+185.2+85.3
Ca	2.4+0.1	2.7+0.1	-5.8+1.5
Ca^{++}	1.2+0.0	1.3+0.0	-4.8+6.5
PO_4^{--}	1.5+0.4	0.7+0.1	-20.3+3.9

*Total Na.

The depurative parameters, PCR and gH^+ are shown in Table II.

TABLE II: Depurative parameters, PCR and gH^+ in AFBF.

Urea i (mg/dl)	Urea f (mg/dl)	Creat. i (mg/dl)	Creat. f (mg/dl)
175.7+26.6	66.5+10.4	13.5+2.9	5.6+1.7
Vb (1)	Kd (ml/min)	KT/V	PCR (gr/kg/day)	gH^+ (mmol/week)
31.7+4.0	173.6+14.4	0.96+0.09	1.1+0.1	345.7+51.3

Urea i, Urea f: plasma urea concentration at the start and at the end of AFBF; Creat. i, Creat. f: plasma creatinine concentration at the start and at the end of AFBF; Vb: urea distribution volume (2); Kd: urea dialytic clearance; KT/V: dialysis adequacy index (3).

DISCUSSION.

In our patients AFBF provided an adequate depuration levels. The resulted Kd can provide a KT/V of 1, for 180 min of treatment, in patients with Vb of 31.5 1 (i.e. body weight = 54.3 kg). For patients over 54.3 kg or with Vb > 31.5 1 the treatment time should be adequately increased.

In spite of hypertonic sodium bicarbonate infusion the sodium mass balance is acceptable. Some problems could arise when the intratreatment weight loss or the plasma sodium concentration are low or when the sodium intake is higher than 100 mmol per liter of water: to avoid sodium balance being little negative or even positive the dialysate sodium concentration should be reduced.

The metabolic acidosis correction and the bicarbonate mass balance resulted satisfyng, considering the calculated gH^+.

The calcium balance is negative. This is due to the high ultrafiltration rates replaced with calcium-free fluid.

CONCLUSIONS.

In our patients, with mean body weight 53.5 kg, mean plasma sodium 142.5 mmol/1 and mean intratreatment body weight loss 2.9 kg, AFBF allowed to obtain adequate depurations indexes and satisfyng electrolytes handling except for a negative calcium balance.

REFERENCES.

1) U. Buoncristiani et al. International Journal Of Artificial Organs 9, S-3:9-14, 1986.
2) P. S. Malchesky et al. Dialysis & Transplantation 11:42-49, 1982.
3) F. A. Gotch, J. A. Sargent. Kidney International 28:526-534, 1983.

BICARBONATE AND CALCIUM BALANCE IN POSTDILUTIONAL HEMODIAFILTRATION.

B. Memoli, R.M. Gazzotti, C. Libetta, A. Dello Russo° and V.E. Andreucci.
Dept. of Nephrology and °Dept. of "Scienze Biochimico-Fisiche" II Faculty of Medicine, Univ. of Naples, Italy.

INTRODUCTION

During Hemodiafiltration (HDF) the kinetics of bicarbonate and calcium involves both a convective loss through the filter into the dialysate and a diffusive uptake from the dialysate (1). A careful study of these phenomena is, therefore, necessary to avoid acid-base and calcium imbalance. Aim of this study was to evaluate the balance of both bicarbonate and calcium through the filter during postdilutional HDF.

MATERIALS AND METHODS.

The study was carried out in 4 patients on regular dialysis treatment with HDF. A capillary polysulfone hemofilter, $1.0\ m^2$ filtering surface was used (Bellco, Italy). Blood flow rate (Qbi) was 300 ml/min, dialysate contained 35 mmol/L of bicarbonate and 1.75 mmol/L of calcium. Mean ultrafiltration flow rate was 70 ml/min. The substituting fluid was a bicarbonate saline solution (HCO_3^- 40 mmol/L, Na^+ 144 mmol/L and Cl^- 104 mmol/L.

The study was carried out by measuring bicarbonate and calcium balance through the filter at different ultrafiltrate flow rate (range 0 - 82.5 ml/min) which were obtained by modifying the transmembrane pressure without changing Qbi. For each ultrafiltrate value two blood samples were simultaneously drawn at the hemofilter inlet and outlet. On each sample blood pH, pCO_2 and plasma total CO_2 (TCO_2), total calcium and total proteins concentrations were measured. Plasma bicarbonate was calculated by direct measurement of plasma TCO_2, as suggested by Santoro et al. (2): since $TCO_2 = 0.03pCO_2 + HCO_3^-$,

$$HCO_3^- = TCO_2 - 0.03pCO_2.$$

Bicarbonate and total calcium balance through the filter was calculated as the difference between the amount of the solute at the filter outlet minus the amount of the solute at the filter inlet. The calculations were performed by using plasma solute concentrations and plasma volumetric flow rates.

RESULTS AND CONCLUSIONS.

The relationships between ultrafiltrate flow rates and bicarbonate balance and total calcium balance are depic-

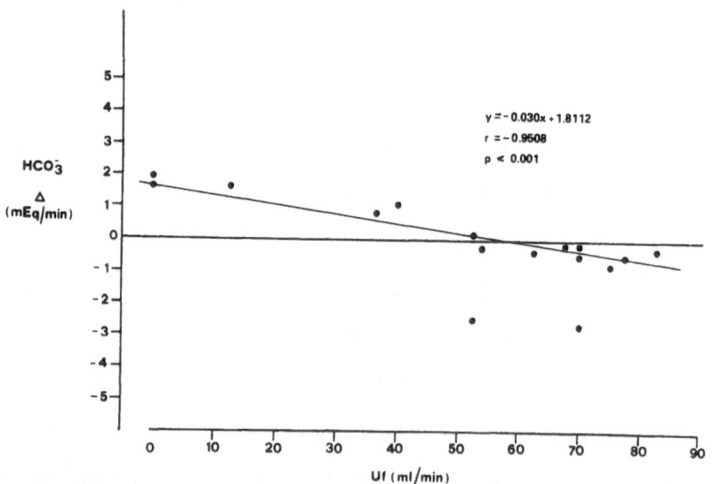

Fig.1. Relationship between ultrafiltration flow rate(Uf) and bicarbonate balance through the filter during HDF.

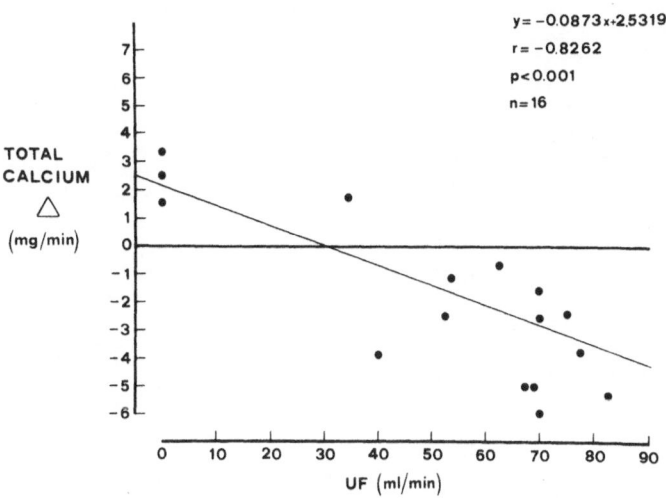

Fig.2. Relationship between ultrafiltration flow rate(Uf) and total calcium balance through the filter during HDF.

ted respectively in Figs. 1 and 2. Analysis of these Figures shows that, in postdilutional HDF, both bicarbonate balance and total calcium balance through the filter become negative at ultrafiltration flow rates greater than 50 ml/min. Such effects results from the convective removal of both HCO_3^- and calcium in spite of a diffusive solutes transport from dialysate to plasma. The reduction of plasma flow, induced by the ultrafiltration process, however, may also play some role (3).

REFERENCES.
1) Feriani M, Biasioli S, Bragantini L, Dell'Aquila R et al. Trans Am Soc Artif Intern Organs, XXXII: 422-424,1986.

2) Santoro A, Ferrari G, Spongano M, Cavalli F and Zucchelli P. Artif Organs 11:491-495, 1987.

3) Goldsmith RS, Furszyfer J, Johnson WJ, Beeler GW and Taylor WF. Nephron 20:132-140, 1978.

Vascular Access

INTRA-ARTERIAL DIGITAL SUBTRACTION ANGIOGRAPHY (aDSA) FOR EVALUATION OF AV-FISTULAS IN HEMODIALYSIS PATIENTS

P. KURZ, H.J. HERMANN, J. VLACHOJANNIS

St. Markus Hospital, Frankfurt/Main, FRG

INTRODUCTION:

Despite all progress achieved in technique of dialysis, vascular access remains the most vulnerable point of chronic hemodialysis treatment. The subcutaneous arterio-venous (av) fistula, as introduced by Brescia and Cimino in 1966, is still the fistula of choice. Problems arising from fistula account for 20 to 25% of the complications seen in patients on chronic hemodialysis. Conventional angiography and sonography, as well as clinical investigation are well established methods for diagnosis of fistula problems. To evaluate digital subtraction angiography (DSA) for diagnosis of fistula complications we investigated 35 patients by intra-arterial DSA (aDSA).

MATERIALS AND METHODS:

Thirty-five hemodialysis patients with vascular access complications (diminished graft pulsation, signs of stenosis, difficulties in cannulation, diminished flow during hemodialysis) were investigated by aDSA. Puncturing of the arteria brachialis was performed with a 21 G needle and approx. 6 ml (maximum 10 ml) of contrast media were injected by hand. A non-ionic contrast media (Iopamidol) was chosen to reduce irritation of the vessel wall. Digital angiography was performed by Siemens Angiotron (matrix 512 x 256, 2 images per sec). Sonography scanning of the fistula was carried out in 20 patients prior to angiographic visualization, performed by a real-time scanner (Picker microview) equipped with a 7.5 and 10 MHz transducer.

RESULTS:

35 patients on maintenance hemodialysis treatment and with clinical signs of fistula malfunction were examined by aDSA. Thrombi in the venous part of the fistula could be found in 20 patients (complete occlusion in 12 and partial thrombosis in 8 patients). Stenoses were seen in 11 cases. The stenoses occured proximal to the anastomosis in 8 out of 11 patients (Fig. 1a). Multiple stenoses were found in 2 patients, in 1 case having a length of 10 cm. In 3 patients a normal vascular pattern was seen. aDSA was performed on an out-patient basis and complication (small hematoma) was seen in 1 patient only , when puncture of the A. brachialis did not succeed.

Sonographic evaluation of the vascular access site was performed in 20 out of these 35 patients. Thrombi as the cause of fistula malfunction were seen in 11 patients. In 2 of these 11 patients partial thrombosis of the fistula vein, as demonstrated by aDSA, were sonographically interpreted as total occlusion. In 2 other cases with multiple thrombi more proximal thrombi did not show up. Stenoses were demonstrated sonographically in 7 patients. In 1 patient with multiple stenoses these could not all be visualized. In 3 patients with angiographically proven stenotic lesions sonography revealed fistula occlusion (Fig. 1b). However a small aneurysm filled with thrombotic material could be visualized by sonography only. In comparison to angiography sonography yielded a correct diagnosis in about 60% only.

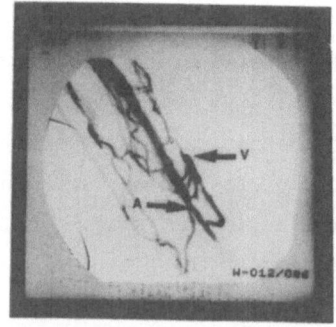
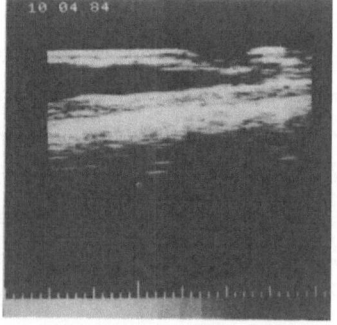

Fig. 1. a) aDSA revealed a long stenosis of the fistula vein (V) and the development of a collateral circulation. b) Sonography did not convey the differentiation between stenosis and total occlusion. (A = artery)

375

DISCUSSION:

Angiography is the standard for the visualization of vessels. Conventional angiography requires a high flow rate of contrast media, achieved by a 16 or 18 gauge needle, and a relatively high amount of contrast media, which both can lead to unwarranted side effects especially in uremic patients (1). Sonography has been recommended for the diagnosis of vascular access complications as a non-invasive, simple and accurate diagnostic procedure (2,3). Especially extra-vascular complications (hematoma, abscess) can easily be imaged by sonography and may be missed by angiography (4). However, stenotic lesions with a caliber of 3 mm or less and more complicated lesions (multiple thrombi or stenoses) cannot be easily imaged by sonography.

With the development of digital subtraction angiography (DSA) some side effects of conventional angiography could be reduced (5). As the vessel of interest is punctered with aDSA a low flow rate of diluted contrast media is sufficient to obtain high-quality vascular images at very low intra-vascular iodine concentration. This allows the use of a very thin needle (21 G). Thus the danger of causing da-mage to the vessel wall is minimized. Compared with sonography aDSA enables the visualization of the whole vessel tree and of stenotic lesions with a diameter of 3 mm or less. In addition a hemodynamic evaluation is possible by evaluating blood flow speed and flow di-rection. aDSA is superior to sonography and is only a minor invasive procedure with a very low complication rate. aDSA should be perfor-med prior to surgical fistula revision.

REFERENCES:

1. Glanz, S., Bashist, B., Gordon, D.H., Butt, K., Adamsons, R.
    Radiology 143: 45-52, 1982.
2. Scheible, W., Skram, C., Leopold, G.R.
    AJR 134: 1173-1176, 1980.
3. Weber, M., Kuhn F.P., Quintes, W., Keidl, E., Köhler, H.
    Clin. Neph. 22: 258-261, 1984.
4. Kottle, S.P., Gonzalez, A.C., Macon, E.J., Fellner, S.K.
    Radiology 129: 751-754, 1978.
5. Meaney, T.F., In: Contrast Media in Digital Radiography (Eds. R. Felix, W. Frommhold, J. Lissner, T.F. Meaney, H.P. Niendorf, E.Zeitler), Exerpta Medica, Amsterdam, 1983, pp. 83-86.

Miscellany

OXALATE CLEARANCE BY HIGH FLUX HAEMODIALYSIS USING POLYACRYLONITRILE MEMBRANES

D SETHI[1], SH MORGAN[2], P PURKISS[2], JR CURTIS[1], RWE WATTS[2].

[1] Charing Cross Hospital London and [2] MRC Clinical Research Centre Harrow, UK.

INTRODUCTION

Hyperoxalaemia is of importance because it may cause significant morbidity and mortality due to the tissue deposition of calcium oxalate crystals. It has been most extensively studied in the primary hyperoxalurias but oxalate retention and raised serum levels also occur late in renal failure and hyperoxalaemia is well documented in patients on treatment with haemodialysis and continuous ambulatory peritoneal dialysis (CAPD). There have been no studies however on the clearance of oxalate in patients treated with high flux dialysers. We therefore measured the clearance of oxalate in 6 patients on treatment with polyacrylonitrile dialysers (AN69HF). This was compared to the oxalate clearance in 5 patients on treatment with cuprophane dialysers, reported in a previous study (1).

PATIENTS AND METHODS

The 5 patients treated by cuprophane haemodialysis (Gambro flat plate 1.1 m^2) had been on haemodialysis for a mean of 28 months (range 15-43 months). The 6 patients studied during high flux haemodialysis (Hospal AN69HF 1.15 m^2) had been on conventional heamodialysis for a mean of 11 years (range 7 months - 17 years) and were changed to high flux dialysis for a mean of 4 months (range 0.5-6 months) prior to the study. All patients were dialysed for 6 hours twice weekly with comparable extracorporeal blood flows (250-300 ml/min). No patient suffered from primary hyperoxaluria, the age and sex distribution was similar in both groups and they had all been taking ascorbic acid 100 mg daily as routine supplementation.

Pre and post dialysis plasma oxalate was measured by a continuous flow assay using immobilised oxalate oxidase (2). The dialyser clearance of oxalate (DCOx) was studied using [^{14}C]oxalate (3). Statistical analysis was by the student's t test.

RESULTS

The results of the study are shown in the table. The mean DCOx during high flux haemodialysis was 121 ml/min (range 82-152) and was significantly higher than the DCOx during conventional haemodialysis using cuprophane (mean 85 ml/min, range 56-119). There was no significant difference between the pre-dialysis plasma oxalate concentration. Although the post dialysis plasma oxalate concentration was lower in patients treated by high flux haemodialysis, this difference was not statistically significant when compared to the patients on conventional haemodialysis.

Table

Comparison of plasma oxalate (POx) (umol/L) and dialyser oxalate clearance (DCOx) (ml/min) in patients treated with cuprophane (HD) versus AN69HF (HFD) haemodialysis. Results are represented as means (range).

	n	age	POx		DCOx
			pre	post	
HD	5	56	27	12	85
		(35-75)	(12-63)	(4-33)	(56-119)
HFD	6	50	23	6.8	121
		(25-60)	(18-32)	(2.8-14)	(82-152)
normal			1.3	-	3.1

DISCUSSION

The overall retention of oxalate despite its partial removal by dialysis may result in tissue accummulation in end stage renal failure with deposition in the myocardium, synovium, kidneys and peripheral blood vessels. This may cause myocardial conductive and functional abnormalities, erosive arthritis, kidney stone formation and peripheral vascular disease leading to ischaemic ulcers, shunt and fistula failure. Deposition may be enhanced by the development of hyperparathyroidism, the prescription of inappropriately high doses of ascorbic acid and may be related to the duration of dialysis. The increased efficiency of haemodialysis over CAPD has been previously shown. Although haemodialysis reduces the plasma oxalate and the clearance is only half that in normal subjects studied using similar techniques, pre-dialysis plasma oxalate levels remain elevated. The performance of high flux dialysers has not previously been described.

This study has shown that DCOx is greater using high flux AN69HF haemodialysis in comparison to conventional cuprophane haemodialysis. The mean DCOx was 121 ml/min which is 67% of oxalate clearance by the normal kidney. Although the pre and post dialysis plasma oxalate levels were lower in patients studied with high flux dialysers than in patients on cuprophane dialysis, the difference was not of statistical significance. The study group however was small, and we suggest that the preferential use of high flux dialysers may avoid the complications of chronic hyperoxalaemia. Long term prospective studies are needed to see if the use of high flux dialysis leads to decreased morbidity from hyperoxalaemia.

REFERENCES

1.   Morgan, S.H., Maher, E.R., Purkiss, P., Watts, R.W.E., Curtis, J.R. Nephrol. Dial. Transplant. 3: 28-32, 1988.
2.   Kasidas, G.P., Rose, G.A. Clin. Chim. Acta. 154: 49-58, 1986.
3.   Watts, R.W.E., Veall, N., Purkiss, P. Clin. Sci. 66: 591-597, 1984.

TECHNICAL AND CLINICAL EVALUATION OF A NEW LOW FLUX POLY-SULPHON MEMBRANE.

C.Ronco, A.Fabris, M.Feriani, S.Chiaramonte, A.Brendolan, G.Emiliani*,L.Bragantini,M.Milan,R.Dell'Aquila,G.La Greca
Depts. of Nephrology, Vicenza and Ravenna*, Italy.

INTRODUCTION

In recent years, the clinical use of highly permeable membranes has permitted the application of treatments with high convective transport thus overcoming the limitations imposed by the classic cellulosic membranes. However the introduction of these membranes has also created a new series of problems linked to their high permeability such as the need for ultrafiltration control machines, the requirement for replacement solutions and the high risk of backfiltration.In an attempt to overcome these problems while maintaining the advanta-ges of synthetic membranes ,a new low flux polysulphon membrane has been recently developed. The aim of this study is to evaluate the characteristics of this membrane in terms of solute and water transport in vitro and in vivo.

METHODS

In vitro experiments have been carried out on a pool of FRESENIUS F6 hollow fiber dialyzers(1.250 m2) in order to test hydraulic properties and permeability characteristics of the membrane.The tests were devoted to establish flow-dynamic resistance of the device,obligate filtration rates and pressure profiles in response to different blood flows and finally, membrane ultrafiltration coefficient and solute sievings under different operational conditions. The in vitro studies were performed with human blood taken from voluntary donors. The blood was diluted with plasma to achieve an average hematocrit of 28% and a mean plasma protein concentration of 5 g/dl. Blood was maintained at 37 degrees centigrade by a thermostating system. In vivo studies were also performed to evaluate the performances of the filter during dialysis at various blood flows and transmembrane pressures. Solute sieving and device ultrafiltration coefficient were measured during sessions of isolated UF.

RESULTS

The blood flows allo-wed by the device at dif-ferent hydrostatic pressu res generated by gravity, are remarkably high (2.05 ml/mmHg).This observation demonstrates the good de-sign of the blood ports and the geometry of the blood compartment that are confirmed also by the pres-

Fig.1

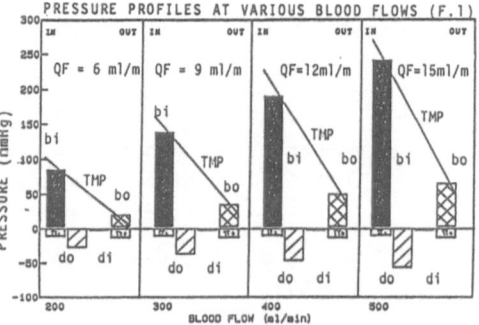

PRESSURE PROFILES AT VARIOUS BLOOD FLOWS (F.1)

sure profiles inside the
filter at different blood
flows.In detail the inlet
pressure averages 250 mmHg
at 500 ml/min of blood flow
being this value obtained
with a mean hematocrit of
28%. The pressure drop is
comparable to the one pre-
dictable on the basis of
the Hagen-Poiseuille law
and averages 100 mmHg at

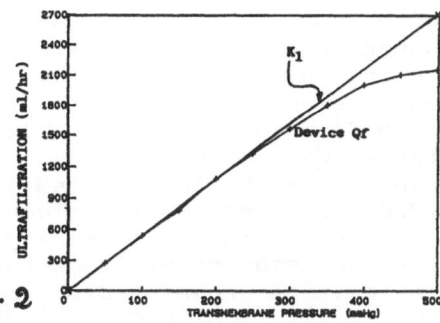

Fig. 2

300 ml/min of blood flow.   The low resistance of the
device and the low hydraulic permeability of the membrane
allow for a significant reduction of the obligate ultrafiltration as a function of the blood flow in comparison
with other devices with highly permeable membranes (8.5
ml/min of Qf at 300 ml/min of Qb). This behaviour is critical when the device is used for techniques requiring
high blood flows. Under those conditions one of the main
problems is the excessive ultrafiltration that must be
counterbalanced by reinfusion of substitution fluids, or
by the use of a positive pressure of the dialysate. This
may complicate the treatment and enhances the risk of
backfiltration. Whith F6 device the low spontaneous
obligate filtration permits a better control of the
dialysis session and reduces the risk of backfiltration.
This point is confirmed in Figure 1, where the pressure
profiles recorded at different blood flows are reported.
The obligate filtration influences the changes of the
oncotic pressure (π) and the pressure drop inside the
fibres because of a change in blood viscosity. It can be
observed that despite a higher pressure drop at high
blood flows in the blood compartment, transmembrane
pressure (TMP) remains always positive thus avoiding the
risk of backfiltration. The ultrafiltration coefficient
appears to be stable and reproducible. For TMP ranging
between 250 and 350 mmHg, ultrafiltration rates range
between 22 and 30 ml/min.   This permits to calculate an
average Device ultrafiltration coefficient K1 of 5.4
ml/hr/mmHg (Figure 2).   The plateau of the curve is
reached at 500 mmHg with an ultrafiltration rate of 2300
ml/hr; this value is mostly determined by the surface

area of the device (1.25 m2).
When the ultrafiltration coef
ficient is considered per m2
of surface area, it offers the
real membrane UF coefficient
(Ko) which in our experiments
averaged 4.32 ml/hr/mmHg/m2.
Ko has a very low value consi
dering the values presented by
other polysulphon membranes.
This demonstrates that the goal

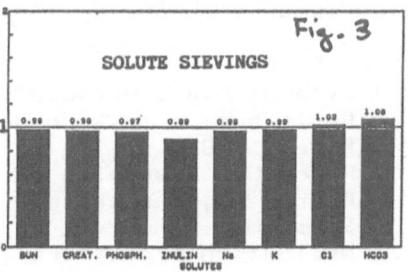

Fig. 3

384

of a low flux membrane has been successfully achieved\The
other point of a good solute permeability has also been
reached as demonstrated by figure 3.It must be noted that
while sieving coefficient for small non charged solutes
such as urea is near 1, slight differences can be noted
for charged solutes probably due to Donnan's effect.
Finally it should be noted that sieving values for inulin
(0.89) and beta-2-microglobulin (0.55) are remarkably
high confirming that despite its low hydraulic permeability F6 membrane still represents an open membrane.

The clinical results confirmed
the observations recorded in vi
tro. The solute clearances are
quite good reaching values near
300 ml/min for BUN at 500 ml/min
of Qb (fig. 4). The values re
mains stable for the entire dura
tion of the session although a
wide variability from one patient
to another can be observed. The
membrane presents a good biocompa
tibility as demonstrated by the
stability of the white cell and
platelet count during dialysis

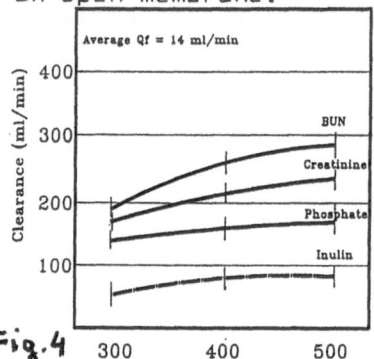

Fig.4

and by the extremely low complement activation. Beta-2-
microglobulin clearances differ significantly when
measured from the blood and dialysate side, being the
latter remarkably lower.This phenomenon can be explained
by the adsorbitive capacity of the membrane that may trap
large amounts of globulins in the polysulphonic structure
as demonstrated by immunofluorescent studies.

CONCLUSIONS

In conclusion, the F6 device seems to maintain the
advantages of a classic polysulphonic membrane overcoming
at least in part the above mentioned problems. The low
hydraulic permeability and the good blood path geometry
allow for a marked reduction of obligate filtration rates
and therefore for a significant reduction of the risk of
backfiltration. The good biocompatibility and the excellent solute sieving together with the relative low cost
will probably widen the clinical application of this
membrane and will make it as a modern alternative to
cuprophan membrane.

REFERENCES

1) Lysaght M.J.: Hemodialysis membranes in transition.
   Contribution to Nephrology, Vol. 61, pp. 1-17, Karger
   Basel, 1988.
2) Ronco C., Brendolan A., Bragantini L., Chiaramonte S.,
   Fabris A., Feriani M., Dell'Aquila R., Milan M., Sca-
   Bardi M., Pinna V., La Greca G.:Technical and clinical
   evaluation of different short, highly efficient dialy-
   sis techniques, Contr. Nephrol. Vol.61, pp.46-68,1988.

ULTRAFILTRATION CONTROL IN SHORT TIME DIALYSIS

S. Stiller, U. Schallenberg*, E. Ernst*, H. Mann,*

Dept. of Medicine III (*: II), Technical University
of Aachen, Pauwelsstr., D-5100 Aachen, FRG

INTRODUCTION

Further shortening of dialysis time to less than
3 hrs requires not only considerable increase of
solute clearance but also increase of ultrafiltration
rate (UFR) to remove the same amount of fluid within a
shorter time. Therefore, a method has been developed
by us to control UFR according to changes in blood
volume [1].

The method: Blood is continuously drawn from the
extracorporeal circuit at a rate of 0,1 ml/h,
thereafter diluted and hemolyzed. Absorbance of the
hemoglobin solution is measured at 415 nm. The
response time of the measured value is 2 min.

Changes in hemoglobin concentration as a measure
of relative blood volume are in good agreement with
conventional measurements of blood volume like
hematocrit, protein concentration, blood conductivity
[2], and labelled erythrocytes.

RESULTS

From measurements of blood volume during
conventional ultrafiltration (UF) it has been found
that a decrease of blood volume of about 20% usually
is tolerated by patients without drop in blood
pressure. We tried to optimize UF by obtaining a

decrease of blood volume up to -20% as quick as possible with high initial UFR up to 3000 ml/h. Thereafter UFR was reduced to maintain a hemoconcentration of 20%. In Fig. 1 this is shown compared with dialysis treatment of the same patient with constant UFR throughout a 5 hr dialysis run.

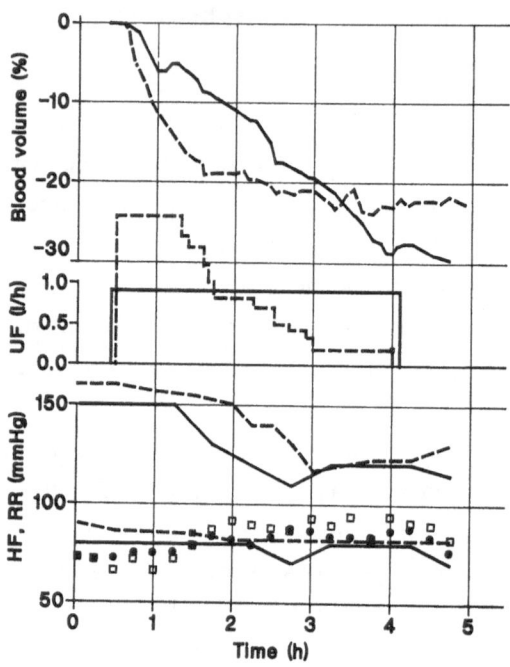

Fig. 1: Two different modes of ultrafiltration in the same patient. Dotted line: blood volume controlled UF. As can be shown with high initial and subsequent decreasing UFR the same amount of fluid can be removed within about half the time than with constant UFR.

To provide a blood volume dependent control system we then tried to conduct UFR with a high rate in an on-off manner. Blood volume was allowed to vary between -13% and -17% (mean -15%). When the upper or the lower limit was exceeded UF was stopped or initiated to the same amount.

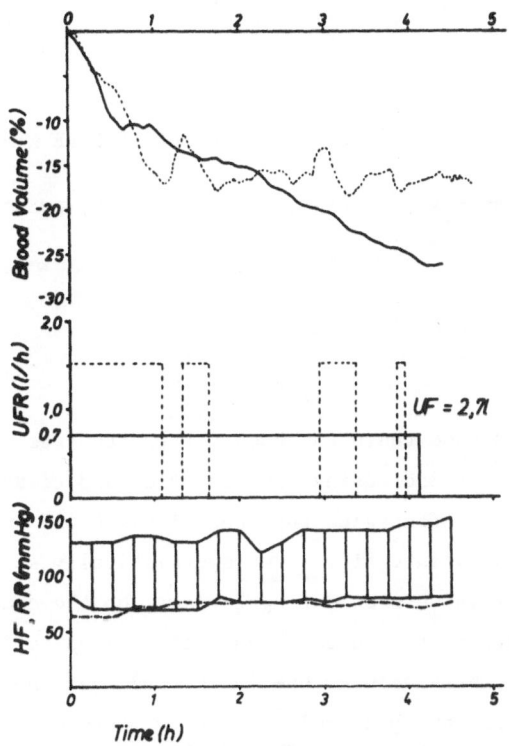

Fig. 2: On-off-control of UFR maintaining a decrease in blood volume of about 15%. Blood volume can be easily maintained at about -15% and most part of UF can be done within the first two hours.

CONCLUSIONS

Continuous hemoglobinometric measurement of blood volume during dialysis is a reasonable method to optimize UF of fluid. Using this method UF can be adapted to the refilling of the intravascular compartment. Using high UFR which are controlled by a definite amount of hemoconcentration, fluid can be removed in about 2-3 hrs. Blood volume controlled UF seems to be a useful tool for further shortening dialysis time.

REFERENCES
1. Schallenberg, U., Stiller, S., and Mann, H. Life Support Systems 5: 293-305, 1987.
2. Stiller, S., Mann, H., Byrne T. Proc. Europ. Soc. Artif. Intern. Organs (ESAO) 7: 167-171, 1980.

RED CELL FRAGMENTATION (RCF) SYNDROME IN CHRONIC SINGLE NEEDLE
DIALYSIS.

R. HOMBROUCKX, A.M. BOGAERT, F. LEROY, L. LARNO, J.Y. DE VOS.
Dialysis Unit, Kliniek Hogerlucht, Ronse, Belgium.

INTRODUCTION

Since the last decade there has been a trend towards a decrease
in dialysis duration (by increasing the bloodflow)and towards single
needle techniques - two strategies that negatively could influence
the red blood cell (RBC) integrity -, we systematically screened for
RCF during each dialysis session during 2 years, on the double head
pump (DHP) unipuncture system in 30 chronic stabilised patients(pts).

Other causes of intravascular hemolysis (HL) than the mechanical destruction of RBC have been ruled out (e.g. serological factors, hemoglobinopathies, RBC-membrane defects, enzymatic deficiencies, micro-angiopathic factors, infectious agents, drug induced
hemolysis, etc.).

MATERIAL AND METHODS

After an initial period of broad screening for HL, we selected
as practical hemolysis index (HLI) the increase of lactic acid de-
hydrogenase (LDH) in the serum during dialysis.

$$HLI = \frac{\text{LDH concentration postdialysis}}{\text{LDH concentration predialysis}}$$

(Beware of artificial HL during blood sample taking and laboratory
processing).

RESULTS

It appeared that the HLI per pt remained practically unchanged
over several dialyses (more or less a constant factor per pt)(Fig.1)
Only a few pts showed a HLI of 1 (= no HL).

Type of HL :
- A broad hematological screening showed no differences between severe and less hemolytic pts (no known genetic or acquired factors
responsable for differences in HLI between pts). We had to conclude
for mechanical RCF by exclusion of other causes of HL and by the
appearance of fragmentocytes or schistocytes.
- Then we looked for the site of HL in single needle dialysis : the
observation that no central catheter dialysis pt showed any degree
of HL, proved the needle tip to be the origin of the RCF. This was
also proven by different needle-central catheter combinations for
dialysis.
Tests with different needle types were performed.
We also tried to influence the degree of HL by adding O2, Vit. C,
glucose and ATP (pure or in combinations) to the dialysate,but this
proved unsuccessful. A very limited benefit was encountered for
Vit. E as chronic p.o. medication.

DISCUSSION

1/ The symptoms during the dialysis session attributed to RCF
were, with increasing degree of HL: nervousness, anxiety, epigastric
malaise, nausea, headache, epigastric or retrosternal pain, vomitus,
hypotension, cyanosis of lips and nailbeds, oesophagal spasms after
dialysis, interdialytic hypotension, flushing, angina, shock, cyanosis, icterus.

2/ We remarked the coïncidence of several parameters, namely
the predialysis level of LDH and bilirubin, a macrocytosis and a reticulocytosis, but also a severe hyperferritinemia in high grade HLI
pts.(In contrast to RCF in normal individuals, there is an important
iron overload in hemolytic dialysis pts)(Fig. 2); this was liver-
biopsy proven in several pts. Previously unexplained liver test disturbances and splenomegalies proved to be due to chronic RCF, and
disappeared after HL reduction.

CONCLUSION

Think about RCF in cases of :
- bad dialysis tolerance (hypotension, nausea, anxiety), recurrent

angina or even "infarction" during dialysis, interdialytic hypotension or oesophagal spasms.

- anemia, reticulocytosis, macrocytosis, hyperbilirubinemia.

- iron overload,"unexplained" liver test disturbances ("non A - non
B" - hepatitis) and splenomegaly,

especially in chronic single needle dialysis on peripheral needles
or catheter needles (too high shear stress in needle or catheter
tip).

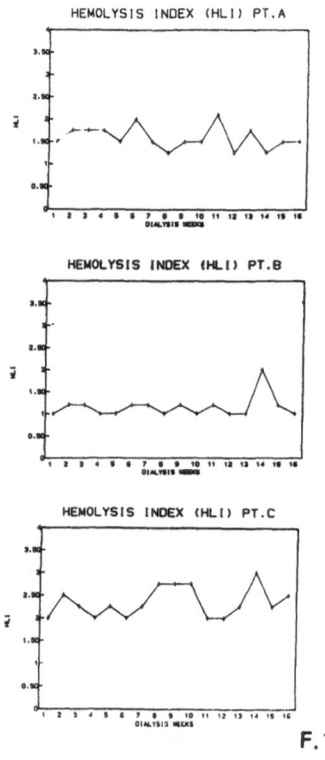

F.1

PTs. MORE THAN 5 YEARS ON DIALYSIS.

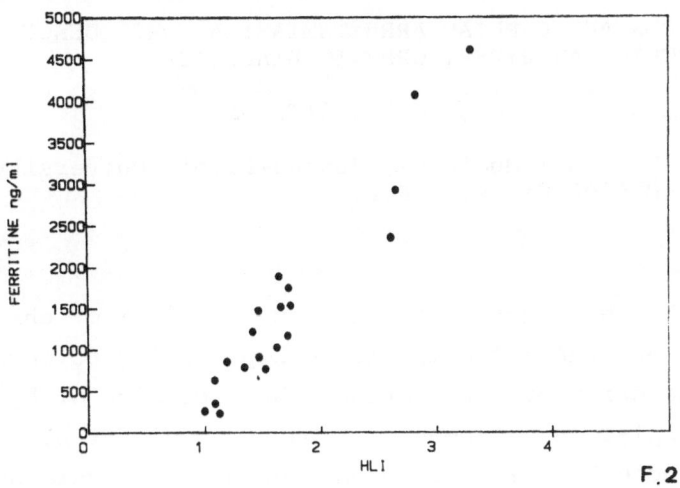

F.2

HYPOTENSION AND CARDIAC ARRHYTHMIAS: A CONSEQUENCE OF LEFT VENTRICULAR HYPERTROPHY IN DIALYSIS

V. WIZEMANN, W. KRAMER, G. SCHÜTTERLE

Dept. of Internal Medicine, Justus-Liebig-University of Giessen, D-6300 Giessen, F.R.G.

It has been estimated that in 25 - 30 % of chronic dialyses episodes of symptomatic hypotension do occur. In the majority of publications the incidence of hypertensive episodes has been attributed to differences in the choice of renal replacement methods. However, hypotension is a late symptom of a chain of physiologic and pathophysiologic processes which vary largely dependent on the cardiovascular status of the patients. Thus, to prevent or treat hypotension adequately, the individual status of the cardiovascular system has to be evaluated before a potentially dangerous therapy is commenced. Cardiovascular events are the most common causes of death in chronic dialysis patients (1) and sudden death is a non-rare fatal complication in this patient population (1, 2). In this paper we tried to characterize the cardiac status of dialysis patients in order to identify patients of risk. Furthermore, we want to address the issue whether sudden death or other significant cardiac arrhythmias are typical complications in dialysis patients with hypertrophied left ventricles. In non-renal patients with left ventricular hypertrophy sudden death has been described following changes of cardiac pre- and afterload as well as inotropism. It has been well established that during dialysis all these three parameters are influenced.

Echocardiographic findings.

209 pts on RDT were evaluated by M-Mode echocardiograms and 57 by Doppler-sonocardiography. Only 15 % had normal echocardiograms. 12 % had calcifications of angulus mitralis, 15 % a sclerosis of aortic valve, 14 % thickening of the pericardium. The main finding was the presence of left ventricular hypertrophy (57 %) (LVH) and dilatation of the left artrium (40 %). Presence of LVH was associated with a 8.3 higher incidence of dialysis hypotension as compared to dialysis pts with echocardiologically normal

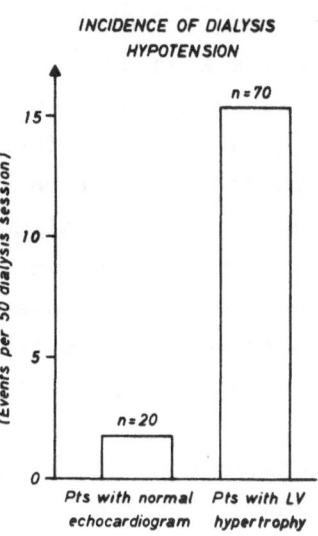

INCIDENCE OF DIALYSIS HYPOTENSION

hearts (Fig. 1). Invasive measurements and pharmacological stress testing of left ventricles revealed the presence of secondary hypertrophic cardiomyopathy in approximately 30 % of chronic dialysis pts (3), which occured in about one half of pts with LVH. Reduced diastolic compliance is common in that subgroup. It can be suspected that dialysis, where underfilling of the left ventricle is the final consequence of a series of counterregulatory events during ultrafiltration, leads to hypotension (4). In a first step pts with LVH should be identified and short dialysis resp. rapid ultrafiltration should be avoided in order to prevent dialysis hypotension (5).

Cardiac arrhythmias.

Since cardiac ectopies are a symptom but no disease the problem of arrhythmias in dialysis pts is interrelated to the presence of coronary artery disease and/or LVH. Studying a large number of dialysis patients (n = 105) we could show that occurrance of significant

ventricular arrythmias is not dependent on dialyis or on
the mode of dialysis therapy (6). However, by careful
analysis we could demonstrate that significant premature
ventricular beats were present in two thirds of pts with
LVH and in three fourth of pts with confirmed CAD. Thus,
detection of arrythmias asks for further cardiological
evaluation to dialyze a pt safely.

In summary, pts on chronic dialysis have a high
prevalence of cardiac disease. Presence of left ventricular hypertrophy is associated with dialysis hypotension on the basis of left ventriccular underfilling
during ultrafiltration. It appears that dialysis hypotension and sudden death are both sequelae of the same
events occurring during dialysis. Hearts with LVH are
sensible to reduction of cardiac pre-load, afterload and
increase in inotropisms. Dialysis is associated to a
considerable extent with all these unfavourable
conditions. To prevent complications a careful
cardiologic characterization has to be performed before
regular dialysis is being commenced. In pts at risk the
less aggressive renal replacement method is the most
adequate.

REFERENCES
1. Wing, A.J., Brunner F.P., Brynger, H., Jacobs, C.,
    Kramer, P., Selwood, N.H. and Gretz, N. Contr.
    Nephrol. 41: 306-311, 1984.
2. Chazan, A. Dialysis and Transplantation 16: 447-
    448, 1987.
3. Kramer, W., Wizemann, V., Lämmlein, G., Thormann, J.,
    Kindler, M., Schlepper and Schütterle, G. Contr.
    Nephrol. 52: 110-124, 1986.
4. Ruffmann, K., Mandelbaum, A., Bommer, i., Kübler,
    W. and Ritz, E. 23rd EDTA congress 1986, abstract
    148.
5. Wizemann, V. and Kramer, W. Blood Purification 5:
    193-201, 1987.
6. Wizemann, V., Kramer, W., Thormann, J., Kindler, M.
    and Schütterle, G. Contr. Nephrol. 52: 42-53, 1985.

ONE YEAR EXPERIENCE WITH SHORT DIALISYS USING A HIGH EFFICIENCY DIALYZER.

J. ARTEAGA, M.J. SORBET, M. ASIRON
Servicio de Nefrologia, Hospital de Navarra, 31008 - Pamplona, Spain.

INTRODUCTION

The treatment of IRC by Dialisys has been a technical process subjected to continuous changes.

In the last ten years, average dialysis treatment time has decreased more than 50% (1), but in spite of the progress made in recent years we still have incomplete knowledge of the nature and biological importance of substances that pass through the membrane.

At this moment, the new membranes give the possibility of assay a new protocol.

We decided to short the time of dialysis and use a high surface dialyzer, high blood flow and bicarbonate bath.

MATERIALS AND METHODS

Eighteen patients (6 males and 12 females), with a mean age of 50 years (range 19-73) and a period of time on hemodialysis longer than 12 months, were included in this study. All patients had a stable hemodinamic situation, a vascular access able to deliver over 350 ml/min, an interdialytic gain weight lees than 3 kg and the patient's weight was less than 70 kg.

We make a comparison between the old protocol using a cuprophan dialyzer of 1.3 square meters, 11 microns,

12 hours/week and a new protocol of short dialysis, 9
hours/week using a dialyzer of cellulose acetate of 2.1
square meters. Open circuit with precise volumetric control monitor was used always.

In the control period the blood flow was nearly 250
ml/min and the dialysate flow was 500 ml/min. The dialysate bath was bicarbonate in 75% and acetate in 25%. In
the short dialysis blood flow was kept over 350 ml/min
and dialysate flow 500 ml/min. The bath was in all cases
bicarbonate.

Clinical and analytical controls were made at monthly intervals. The blood samples were drawn after the
longest interdialytic period.

All patients were their own control.

Table 1.   Clinical and biochemicals parameters.

Parameter	9h	12h	p
Hematocrite	26.9	25.4	0.024
Hemoglobin	9.2	8.6	0.054
T. protein	6.7	6.3	0.000
Sist. Press.	141	150	0.009
Dias. Press.	79	83	0.011
Body weight	59.7	62.4	0.001
Calcium	9.4	9.5	0.096
Phosphorus	4.8	5.1	0.039
Uric Acid	8.7	8.7	0.947
Urea	1.9	1.8	0.613
Creatinine	12.9	13.1	0.535
Potassium	5.5	5.2	0.022
Acceptance	94%		
Muscle cramps	15%		
Hipotensive episodies	8%		

RESULTS

Table 1 gives the main clinical and biochemical parameters.

It can be seen that there is no difference for serum uric acid, urea or creatinine. The hematocrite, hemoglobine and total proteins are slightly higher in the short dialysis schedule, while sistolic and diastolic pressure are lower. The phosphorus and potasium are less controlled with the short dialysis.

When we analyze the non numeric parameters we can see that there is a good acceptance to this form of treatment. Only one patient was removed because of into lerance.

DISCUSSION

A dialysis schedule requires at least four conditions: 1.- Adequate clearence of small and middle molecules. The NCDS (2) suggest that dialysis associated morbidity was related to a high midweek blood urea and a low protein catabolic rate. 2.- A good control of ultrafiltration and Acid-Base equilibrium. 3.- A good patient's tolerance. 4.- A competitive cost.

Dialysis time can be shortened with membranes which are hightly permeable to middle molecules or increasing the active surface area of conventional membranes.

We choose the second possibility because of economical advantages. At one year the results are satisfactory. The use of bicarbonate bath and monitor with volumetrically controlled ultrafiltration increase the cost per session 20% but this could be counterbalanced by a minor personal cost per session.

REFERENCES
1. Gotch, F.A. Kidney Int 33:s-100-s-104, 1988
2. Gotch, F.A., Sargent, J.A. Kidney Int 28:526-537, 1985.

THE INFLUENCE OF NIFEDIPINE ON SERUM LIPIDS IN ELDERLY CHRONIC
DIALYSIS PATIENTS

M.BENEDIK, R.KVEDER, J.DRINOVEC, J.VARL, A.GUČEK, M.MALOVRH

University Medical Center, Department of Nephrology, 61000 Ljubljana,
Yugoslavia

INTRODUCTION

Hypertension is one of the most important factors for the
development of atherosclerosis in patients with chronic renal
failure (CRF). Nifedipine, a calcium antagonist, has recently been
reported to be a useful drug for the treatment of arterial hypertension in patients with CRF (1). Preliminary reports show that the
use of Nifedipine may reduce total cholesterol in serum of patients
with mild hypertension (2). Little information exists in literature
on its influence on serum lipids in patients with CRF.

PATIENTS AND METHODS

In this study, 10 stable patients with CRF on chronic kidney
replacement program older than 60 years with arterial hypertension
were included. This group consisted of 5 women and 5 men, with
average age 63.5 ± 2.3 years who were on chronic kidney replacement
program for 50 ± 36 months (7 patients were on hemodialysis, and
one each on CAPD, biofiltration and hemofiltration). For the
treatment of hypertension the patients were given Nifedipine
retard as a monotherapy. Average daily dose per patient was $34 \pm$
21 mg (range 20-80 mg). The study lasted 9 months. During the
study, systolic and diastolic blood pressures were measured every
3 months by a mercury sphygmomanometer; after a 30-minute rest,
smoking was not permited before the measurement. Mean arterial
pressure (MAP) was estimated as follows:
MAP= pulse pressure/3 + diastolic blood pressure.
At the beginning and in the end of the study, that is, after

9 months, serum lipids were measured in the morning on an empty
stomach after 12 hours of fasting. Standard methods of our
laboratory were used for the determination of serum lipids.

RESULTS

At the beginning of the study the average systolic blood
pressure was 159 $\pm$ 24 mm Hg, after 3 months 158 $\pm$ 19 mm Hg, after
6 months 168 $\pm$ 16 mm Hg and after 9 months 159 $\pm$ 9 mm Hg. At the
beginning of the study the average diastolic blood pressure was
91 $\pm$ 10 mm Hg, after 3 months 89 $\pm$ 8 mm Hg, after 6 months 93 $\pm$ 9
mm Hg and after 9 months 88 $\pm$ 5 mm Hg. At the beginning of the
study the average MAP was 115 $\pm$ 11 mm Hg, after 3 months 112 $\pm$ 11
mm Hg, after 6 months 118 $\pm$ 10 mm Hg and after 9 months 112 $\pm$ 6
mm Hg. These differences in blood pressures were not statistically
significant (Student's t-test).

Total serum cholesterol at the beginning of the study was
5.68 $\pm$ 1.23 mmol/L and in the end dropped to 5.45 $\pm$ 0.91 mmol/L.
LDL cholesterol decreased from 3.2 $\pm$ 1.09 mmol/L at the beginning
to 3.12 $\pm$ 1.13 mmol/L in the end of the study. Triglycerides
decreased from 2.2 $\pm$ 1.2 mmol/L to 2.07 $\pm$ 1.13 mmol/L, while HDL
cholesterol rose from 1.15 $\pm$ 0.44 mmol/L to 1.3 $\pm$ 0.50 mmol/L. All
these differences were not statistically significant (Student's
t-test).

The concentrations of total cholesterol, HDL cholesterol, and
LDL cholesterol were within the normal range of our laboratory,
while the concentrations of triglicerydes were about the upper
limit of our laboratory.

CONCLUSION

It can be concluded from our data that Nifedipine retard has
a favorable influence on serum lipids in elderly patients with
CRF. In the future longer study must be conducted to study the
beneficial influence of Nifedipine on serum lipids.

REFERENCES

1. Kusano,E., Asano, Y., Takeda, K., Matsumoto,Y., Ebihara,A. and Hosoda,S. Arzneim.-Forsch/Drug.Res. 32: 1575-1580, 1982.
2. Weinberger,M.H., Arch. Intern. Med. 145: 1102-1105, 1985

EFFECT OF DIALYSATE CALCIUM CONCENTRATION CHANGES ON PLASMA CALCIUM
AND PTH IN DIALYSIS PATIENTS TREATED WITH CALCIUM CARBONATE AS A PHO-
SPHATE BINDER

F.Malberti,M.Surian,A.Montoli,F.Barbisoni,F.Mercantini[*],M.Marchini[*],
M.Ciscato[*].
Dialysis and biochemical units[*],Ospedale Maggiore,LODI,Italy

Even though the efficacy of calcium carbonate($CaCO_3$)as a phosphate bin

der has been documented since 1966(1),only recently its use in substi

tution of Aluminum containing phosphate binders has been recommended

in uremic patients in order to avoid the risk of aluminum accumulation

and toxicity(2-5').An extensive clinical use of $CaCO_3$ has been limited

by frequent occurrence of hypercalcemia(2,4-6).Thus,the reduction of

dialysate calcium concentration(DCa)to 1.5 mmol/l or less has been sug

gested to decrease the potential risk of hypercalcemia(3,4).The aim of

our study was to evaluate whether the decrease of DCa from 1.75 to 1.5

mmol/l was associated with a lower incidence of hypercalcemia and

equal control of secondary hyperparathyroidism in hemodialysis patie

nts treated with $CaCO_3$, as a phoshate binder.

MATERIALS AND METHODS

   Twenty patients(20-62 yr old)with a biopsy proven mild osteophaty

associated with negative aluminum staining,on chronic hemodialysis for

6-156(49+52)months were studied.Hemodialysis was performed for 4-5 hrs

thrice weekly using 1-1.3 m^2 capillary flow cuprophan dializer at $Q_B$of
                                     the
300 ml/min in order to satisfy criteria of adequacy based upon urea

kinetics analysis(urea Kt/V≥ 1,dietary protein intake ranging between

0.9-1.4 g/Kg/day).All the patients were treated with $CaCO_3$ to control

plasma phosphorus(PP).In 16 patients aluminum-containing phosphate bin

ders had been discontinued 8-12 months prior to the initiation of the

study;4 patients had never taken aluminum gels.The duration of the
study was 24 mos:during the first period(12 mos)the pts continued to
be treated with the usual DCa(1.75 mmol/l,H-Ca),while during the seco
nd period(12 mos)DCa was lowered to 1.5 mmol/l(L-DCa).Intradialytic Ca
balances(determined collecting all the dialysate in a big tank)and cha
nges of serum proteins and total(PCa)and ultrafiltrable(UFCa)plasma Ca
were evaluated in 20 dialysis sessions during both H-DCa ahd L-Ca.UF
Ca was measured in the ultrafiltrate obtained by disconnetting the di
alysate supply from the dialyzer and applying a negative pressure of
300 mmHg by a suction pump.Throughout the study the dose of $CaCO_3$ was
adjusted in order to maintaing PP $<$ 6 mg/dl.Also the dose of calcitriol
was modified in order to maintain PCa between 9.5 and 10.5 mg/dl.Besi
des $CaCO_3$,no other P binders was prescribed.PP and PCa were checked
montly;alkaline phosphatase(AP,normal range:85-220 IU/l)and PTH(COOH,
Immunonuclear,normal:0.1-0.7 ng/ml)were measured at the beginning of
the study and at the end of 1st and 2nd period.The frequency of hyper
calcemic($\geq$ 11 mg/dl)and hyperphosphatemic($\geq$ 6mg/dl)episodes during the
2 periods was compared.

RESULTS

Net ultrafiltrate rate was 2.5+0.5 lduring the dialysis sessions in
which Ca balances studies were performed.PCa and UFCa incresed and Ca

Table 1.Intradialytic Ca balance and pre to postdialysis changes of
serum proteins and PCa and UFCa in relation to DCa.

DCa(mmol/l)	PCa mg/dl		UFCa mg/dl		Protein g/l		Ca balance
	PRE	POST	PRE	POST	PRE	POST	mg/session
H-DCa	9.8+	11.6+*	6.0+	6.6+*	65.7+	75.5+*	+ 110+
(1.75+0.1)	0.6	0.7	0.5	0.6	4.0	7.7	180
L-DCa	9.4+	10.2+§•6.0+		5.9+§	64.4+	73.3+*	− 98+§
(1.53+0.05) 0.7		0.7	0.3	0.3	3.1	7.0	61

*=p $<$ 0.001 and • p$<$0.02 vs PRE; § =p$<$ 0.001 vs H-DCa

was gained by the patients when H-DCa was used;on the contrary intra
dialytic Ca balance was negative and UFCa unchanged,using L-DCa(Tab.
1). Over 1 yr follow up on H-DCa,the frequency of hypercalcemia was

6.5% and unchanged(6.8%)during the successive 12 mos on L+DCa.Also the
frequency of hyperphosphatemia was similar using H-DCa(13.5%)or L-DCa
(16.5%).The daily dose of $CaCO_3$ ranged between 1 and 6 g throughout the
study.The average dose of $CaCO_3$ was similar at the end of the two periods in which a similar and sactisfatary control of PP was achieved(Tab.2).
PCa at the end of the study was higher than at the end if first period
in spite of a lower average daily dose of calcitriol(Tab.2).Hypercalce-
mia ,detected in 9 of 20 patients, was severe($>$ 12 mg/dl)only in 1 pts.
No pts developed permanent hypercalcemia,because all the hypercalcemic
episodes were promptly reversible with adjustment of calcitriol dose,
Without the necessity of $CaCO_3$ withdrawal.Over 1 yr of follow-up using
H-DCa no change of AP(baseline:169$\pm$50 IU/l;after 12 mos:166$\pm$38)and PTH
(2.9$\pm$1.8 ng/ml and 3.1$\pm$1.9 ng/ml)was detected.On the contrary,AP and
PTH significantly increased during the successive treatment with L-DCa
(Tab.2).

Table 2. Biochemical parameters at the end of 1st and 2nd period

	PCa mg/dl	PP mg/dl	AP IU/l	PTH ng/ml	$CaCO_3$ g/day	Calcitriol dose µg/day
H-DCa	9.7$\pm$ 0.4	4.86$\pm$ 0.70	166$\pm$ 38	3.1$\pm$ 1.9	2.4$\pm$ 1.0	0.21$\pm$ 0.13
L-DCa	9.9$\pm$* 0.4	4.76$\pm$ 0.91	208$\pm$* 59	5.1$\pm$* 2.9	2.4$\pm$ 0.9	0.14$\pm$* 0.09

*=p $<$0.02 vs H-DCa

CONCLUSIONS

The frequency of hypercalcemia in our pts treated with $CaCO_3$ is lower than that reported in other study(2,4-6),due to the use of lower doses of $CaCO_3$ and the selection of
pts with less severe osteophaty.Indeed,the occurence of hypercalcemia was noted most
frequently in pts with bone biopsy proven Al-related osteophathy(5).The reduction of
dialysate Ca content from 1.75 to 1.5 mmol/l gives negative intradialytic Ca balances
but does not decrease the incidence of hypercalcemia.Moreover,AP and PTH levels increase
suggesting an aggravation of secondary hyperparathyroidism in our pts.

REFERENCES

1)Clarkson,E.M.,McDonald,S.J.,De Wardener H.E.Clin.Sci.30:425-438,1966.
2)Moriniere P.H.,Russel,A.,Tahiri, Y. et al. Proc. Eur. Dialysis Transplant Ass.
19: 784-787, 1982.
3)Slatopolsky,E.,Weerts,C.,Lopez-Hilker,J.,et al.N.Engl.J.Med.315:157-161,1986.
4)Fournier,A.,Moriniere,P.,Sebert,J.L.,et al.Kidney Int.29:S114-S119,1986.
5)Hercz,G.,Kraut,A.,Andress,D.A.,et al.Mineral Electrolyte Metab.12:314-319,1986.
6)Raine,A.E.G.,Oliver D.O.Lancet I:633-634,1987.

CEREBRAL ATROPHY IN LONG-TERM HAEMODIALYZED PATIENTS

R. MUSOLINO, V. SAVICA*, G. TROILO, P. DE DOMENICO, L. MARABELLO, A. BLANDINO**, L. SALVI**, G. BELLINGHIERI* and R. DI PERRI

Clinica Neurologica I, *Clinica Medica I, **Istituto di Oncologia - University of Messina, Italy

INTRODUCTION

In adult young patients on long-term regular haemodialytic treatment cerebral computed tomography (CT) scans have often revealed a high incidence of cerebral atrophy (CA), even in the absence of clear neurologic or psychiatric symptoms [1]. On this basis we performed a CT investigation on a group of asymptomatic selected haemodialyzed outpatients, distinguishing between geriatric and adult subjects, in order to detect the possible incidence and severity of CA.

PATIENTS AND METHODS

Our study was performed on 18 chronic haemodialyzed (11 adults, mean age 48.00 ± 8.77 yrs and 7 geriatrics, mean age 70.14 ± 4.67 yrs), dialyzed three times a wk for more than 12 mos (average 40.14 ± 20.24 mos).

All subjects underwent the following: - Neurological examination; - Laboratory blood tests including aluminium level (Perkin-Elmer 410) and acid-base balance; - Neuropsychological assessment including a battery of tests able to evaluate memory, attention and psychomotor performance; - CT of the brain. All the CT scans were performed according to Huckman et al's criteria [2], in order to evaluate indexes of cortical and subcortical atrophy. The control group consisted of 60 healthy subjects (40 adults and 20 geriatrics) matched by age and sex. Statistical evaluation was performed using Wilcoxon's test and regression line analysis.

RESULTS

On neurological examination our selected patients did not show nervous central system impairment, but 13 did have peripheral nervous system involvement. On specific cognitive tests, a significant difference between the adult patients and their controls was found for memory quotient (MQ), short-term memory and attention. On MQ adult uremics significantly differed also respect to the geriatric controls (p < 0.05). CT scans revealed CA in 77.7% of patients. 3 (1 adult and 2 geriatric) had cortical, 5 (4 adult and 1 geriatric) subcortical and 6 (4 adult and 2 geriatric) diffuse atrophy. Considering cortical sulci width, adult uremic patients significantly differed respect to their controls (p < 0.001), while they did not show any difference respect to the geriatric controls. Furthermore significant cortical sulci differences were not found between geriatric dialyzed and geriatric controls. Cortical sulci width was higher in geriatric dialyzed respect to adult dialyzed (p < 0.05). Ventricular width appeared to be higher in adult uremics respect to their control group (p < 0.002). As regards this parameter no difference was found between adult dialyzed, geriatric dialyzed and geriatric controls. Geriatric dialyzed significantly differed when compared to their control group (p < 0.002). No correlations were found between CT and neuropsychological data.

DISCUSSION

In 77.7% of our patients CA was found, in agreement with Savazzi et al. (1). Adult patients appeared to be significantly more altered respect to their controls as regards cortical and subcortical atrophy, while did not differ respect to geriatric patients and geriatric controls. CT findings seem to follow a parallel behaviour to memory data: adult uremics presented with values similar to those of geriatric controls. CT alterations did not show any correlation with neuropsychological parameters, in agreement with Earnest et al. (3) and Gonzales et al. (4). On the contrary, other authors (5) found an important relationship between CA and cognitive impairment. These contradictory reports and the discrepancy between clinical picture and CT data could lead us to doubt the significance of CA, since it has been also ascertained that widening of cortical sulci and enlargment of the ventricles can be present in normal aging adults (6). However it is important to note, according to Willanger et al. (7) that, even if intellectual damage does not depend on the cortical atrophy, subcortical damage should really be considered, since the ventricular cavities enlargment has shown a more specific correlation with the decay of higher brain functions.

In our study the parallel behaviour of memory impairment and CT alterations suggests that chronic toxaemia, even in absence of aluminium toxication, could determine a praecox decay of mental functions, together with morphological and structural alterations, i.e. CA. These findings could be explained by different concomitant mechanisms, such as chronic anemia (1), PTH effect (8), sudden pressure variations (9), modifications of brain density caused by the dialytic session (10). All these factors could act in uremic patients to determine CA and intellectual impairment.

REFERENCES

1. Savazzi, G.M., Cusmano, F., Degasperi, T. Clin. Nephrol. 23: 89-95, 1985.
2. Huckman, M.S., Fox, J.C., Topel, J.L. Radiology 116: 85-92, 1975
3. Earnest, M.P., Heaton, R.K., Wilkinson, W.E., Manke, W.F. Neurology 29: 1138-1143, 1979
4. Gonzales, C.F., Lantieri, R.L., Nathan, R.J. Neuroradiology 16: 120-122, 1978
5. Soininen, H., Puranen, M., Riekkinen, P.J. J. Neurol. Neurosurg. Psychiat. 451: 50-54, 1982
6. Baron, S.A., Jacobs, L. Neurology (Minneap) 26: 1011-1013, 1976
7. Willanger, R., Thygesen, P., Nielsen, R., Peterson, O. Dan. Med. Bull. 15: 65-93, 1968
8. Massry, S.G. Nephron. 19: 125-130, 1977
9. Skimboi, E., Strandgaards, S. Lancet 1: 461-462, 1973
10. Ronco, C., Biasioli, S., Borin, D., Brendolan, A., Chiaramonte, S., Fabris, A., Feriani, M., Pisani, E., La Greca, G. Min. Nefrol. 29: 185-193, 1982

BENEFICIAL EFFECT OF DESFERRIOXAMINE ON THE ANAEMIA OF A HAEMODIALYSIS PATIENT WITHOUT ALUMINIUM OR IRON OVERLAOD.

R. CUVELIER, P. DECEUNINCK, G. MOULIGNEAU

Department of Medecine, Clinique du Refuge, MOUSCRON
7700, BELGIUM.

INTRODUCTION

Desferrioxamine (DFO) has been proved to be effective in
the traetment of the anaemia of haemodialysis (HD) patients with aluminium (Al) (1) or iron (2) overload.
We report the beneficial effect of DFO (Desferal , Ciba)
on the anaemia of a 62-year-old woman treated for 3
years by HD in whom we found no evidence of Al or iron
overload.

CASE REPORT : see figure

After her first two packed red cell transfusions near the start of
HD, we were unable to find any compatible packed cell preparation
for further transfusions for this patient.

Blood studies revealed that after the transfusions she had developed antibodies towards a high-frequency red blood cell antigen
(public antigen), namely Er (3). The life-span of transfused labelled homologous red cells Er(a+) was demonstrated to be very shortened (t 1/2 of   Cr red blood cell : 7 h   N : 25 - 33 days) as the
result of the anti-public antibodies.

Before DFO therapy, anaemia was severe, normochromic (mean
cellular haemoglobin concentration : 33.3 g/dl), normocytic (mean
cell volume : 89 fl) and unchanged after three courses of parente-
ral iron therapy.

Two courses of DFO of 17 and 11 weeks were administered. DFO was infused weekly during the last hour of a routine HD with a polyacrylonitrile (AN69-S) membrane (Biospal 2400 S, 1 m², Hospal) in a dose of 40 mg/Kg body wt, associated with a daily dose of 125 – 250 mg of oral ferrous sulfate. The two courses of DFO therapy induced a progressive increase of haemoglobin which rapidly return to baseline after DFO withdrawal. Serum ferritin and Al concentrations before and during DFO therapy are indicated as well as the values of the DFO infusion test (serum Al before and 48 hours after the first DFO dose).

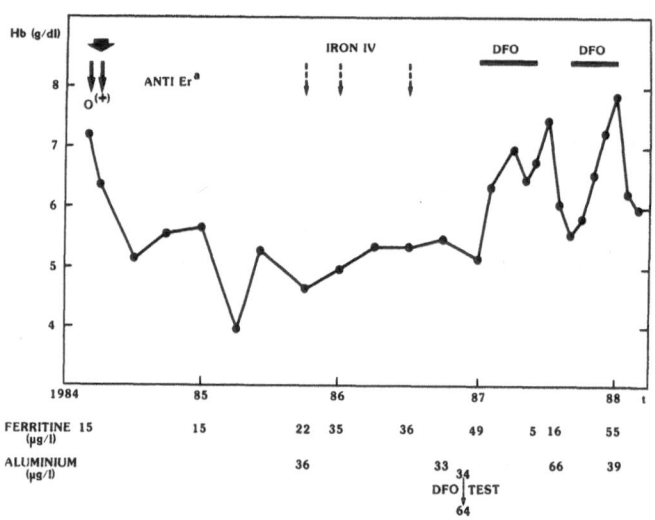

COMMENT

Al and/or iron accumulation in this patient is unlikely :
- water used to prepare dialysate is desionised resulting in a water Al concentration lower than 0,5 µg/l.
- the patient uses moderate doses of Al-containing phosphate binders.
- serum Al levels are consistenly lower than 100 µg/l with no rise of serum Al during DFO therapy.

- serum ferritin a reliable indicator of iron body stores is
  normal in this non-polytransfused patient.
- anaemia is non microcytic as in Al intoxication.

Mechanisms of improvement of anaemia of this patient
during DFO therapy are speculative :

- mean cell volume remain unchanged at variance with patients
  with Al-induced microcytic anaemia treated with DFO (4).
- despite concommitant oral iron supplement, serum ferritin
  decreases beyond normal values; this may indicate beyond the
  expected iron-chelating effect of DFO, better ferrous iron
  utilisation for heme biosynthesis. Iron supplement in association with DFO may be relevant for therapeutic efficacy.
- Hosokawa and al(5) demonstrated in chronic HD patients a significant correlation between corpuscular zinc levels and the
  severity of anaemia. The mechanism of action of DFO in anaemia
  of this patient could be the result of chelation of toxic
  trace metals other than Al or iron.

References :
1. Tielemans, C., Collaert, F., Wens, R., et al. Clin. Nephrol.
    24 :
    237 - 241, 1985.
2. Praga, M., Andres, A., de la Serra, J., et al. Nephrol.
    Dial. Transplant. 2 : 243 - 247, 1987.
3. Daniels, G.L., Judd, W.L., Moore, P.L., et al. Transfusion
    22 : 189 - 193, 1982.
4. Abreo, K., Brown, S.T., Sella, M.L., Kidney Int 33 : 215,
    1988 (abstract).
5. Hosokawa, S., Nishitani, H., Tomoyoshi, T. et al In : Blood
    purification in perspective : New insights and future trends
    (Eds. N-K Man, C. Mion, L.W. Henderson), ISAO Press N° 308,
    Cleveland, 1987, pp. 115-117.

TRANSIENT ERYTHROCYTE VOLUME (MCV) INCREASE IN HEMODIALYSIS

R. Gellert., Z. Billip-Tomecka
Department of Medicine, Warsaw Medical School, Warsaw, Poland

Blood volume changes during hemodialysis can be computed using simple laboratory blood tests (1, 2, 3). These methods do not take into account the possible water shifts between plasma and blood cells, a phenomenon reflected by MCV changes. The aim of this study was to reinvestigate the MCV changes due to dialysis, both in vessels and in blood passing the dialyser.

Material and Methods

125 uncomplicated dialysis treatments were performed in 25 adult, stable, chronically hemodialysed men and women. Gambro's AK-10 artificial kidney and 1.0 m^2 hollow fiber dialysers were used. The acetate, glucose-free dialysis fluid contained 137 mmol/l of sodium. Transmembrane pressure (TMP) was adjusted to reduce body weight by 1kg in 60, 120 or 180 minutes of observation (groups A, B and C respectively), or was 90, 40 or 300 mmHg throughout the fifteen-minutes sessions performed at the initial of treatment (groups D, E and F respectively). In groups E and F the dialyser did not contain any dialysis fluid. Blood samples were taken from the A-V fistula at the beginning of each session and from the arterial and venous part of dialysis tubing at the end of each observation. Hematocrite (Hct) was determined by microhematocrite method, hemoglobin (Hb) by cyanomethemoglobine method and erythrocyte count (E) by a semiautomatic counter (Picoscale, Hungary). The mean corpuscular volume (MCV), mean corpuscular hemoglobine (MCH) and mean corpuscular hemoglobine concentration (MCHC) were computed using the routine

formulas (Hct/E, Hb/E and Hb/Hct respectively). Student's t-test for paired data and analysis of variance were used for statistics. All data are presented as mean±SD.

Results

The changes of MCV are presented in Table 1 and Table 2 for intravascular and intradialyser data respectively.

Table 1
Intravascular MCV, MCH and MCHC during hemodialysis (percent of predialysis value)

Group	Duration of obs.	MCV [%]	MCH [%]	MCHC [%]
D	15'	100.34±5.80	99.82±7.49	99.49±4.90
A	60'	99.49±4.57	100.38±7.57	100.91±6.26
B	120'	100.28±2.60	102.80±9.29	100.62±4.85
C	180'	97.34±6.85	99.50±7.06	97.61±6.35

Table 2
MCV changes due to bypassing the dialyser

Group	Time from start	TMP [mmHg]	Dial. fluid	Δ MCV[a] [fl]	n[b]
D	15'	90	+	4.61±6.31*	20
A	60'	200	+	3.14±3.74#	30
B	120'	90	+	2.94±6.22*	20
C	180'	50	+	2.10±4.47	15
E	15'	40	−	3.95±7.68	15
F	15'	300	−	2.17±4.50	15

[a] value next-to-dialyser minus prior-to-dialyser
[b] n=number of dialysis sessions
# $p < 0.05$; * $p < 0.001$;

The intradialyser erythrocyte swelling significantly decreased along with the time of treatment ($F < 0.05$).

The mean diameter of erythrocytes entering the dialyser was 8.5±0.8μ and 9.8±0.8μ when leaving the dialyser ($p < 0.01$).

412

Discussion

     No change of erythrocyte indices could be observed for blood taken prior to the dialyser regardless of duration of observation and TMP. This is in agreement with data reported by others (1-5).

     Passing the dialyser caused significant increase in MCV and erythrocyte diameter. The erythrocyte swelling decreased along with the time, disappeared in the third hour of hemodialysis and was observed only at the presence of dialysis fluid within the dialyser. These data suggest that osmotic shifts occurring in the dialyser can result in water influx into erythrocytes. The similar finding within the vessels was demonstrated by Fleming et al., when 126 and 154 mmol/l of sodium concentration dialysate was used (6).

     In every minute erythrocyte entering the dialyser swelled. At the same time no change in MCV was observed in blood taken from the A-V fistula. Thus the cell swelling was only transient, and disappeared quickly.

     We conclude that erythrocyte volume can change very easy and quickly. This should be taken into account in nondirect-method-determinations of blood volume changes during dialysis.

ACKNOWLEDGEMENTS
Support by Grant MZ-XIII from Polish Ministry Of Health and Welfare. Dr. Gellert received financial support from Gambro AB (Sweden)

Literature
1. Fleming S. J., J. S. Wilkinson, C. Aldridge, R. N. Greenwood, S. D. Mugglestone, L. R. I. Baker, W. R. Catell, Clin. Nephrol., 1988, 29, 63.
2. Hsu C. H., R. D. Swartz, M. G. Somermeyer, A. Raj, Nephron, 1984, 38, 202
3. Van Beaumont W., J. Appl. Physiol., 1972, 33, 55.
4. Rodriguez M., J. A. Pederson, F. Llach, Kidney Int., 1985, 28, 808
5. Shimamoto K., I. Watari, M. Miyahara, J. Clin. Endocrinol. Metab., 1977, 45, 714.
6. Fleming J. S., J. S. Wilkinson, R. N. Greenwood, C. Aldridge, L. R. I. Baker, W. R. Catel, Kidney Int., 1987, 32, 267

ASSESSMENT OF LIVER ABILITY TO BIOTRANSFORMATION OF ANTIPYRINE IN URAEMIC PATIENTS ON REGULAR PERITONEAL DIALYSIS TREATMENT

A. Grzegorzewska, Z. Łowicki, E. Chmara, A. Mrozikie-wicz, K. Bączyk

Departments of Nephrology and Clinical Pharmacology, K. Marcinkowski's Academy of Medicine, Poznań – Poland

INTRODUCTION

Data on hepatic elimination of drugs in experimental uraemia and in uraemic patients indicate either the induction of hepatic enzymes or their inhibition /1-6/. Our paper concentrates on the evaluation of liver ability to biotransformation of drugs expressed by antipyrine elimination in uraemic patients regularly treated with peritoneal dialyses.

MATERIALS AND METHODS

Examinations were performed in 10 HBs-negative patients with end-stage renal disease treated with intermittent peritoneal dialyses during 2 - 14 months. In all patients gamma-glutamyltranspeptidase activity as well as glutamic pyruvic oxaloacetic aminotransferases activities were normal. The control group in examinations of antipyrine elimination consisted of 13 healthy physicians.

Antipyrine was given orally at the dosis of 18 mg//kg b.w. The blood samples were taken before antipyrine administration and after 3, 6, 9, 12, 18 and 24 hours from its ingestion. Antipyrine was quantitated by the method of Brodie et al. /7/. The elimination constant rate /k/, biologic plasma half-life /$t_{0,5}$/, distribution volume /V_d/ and plasma clearance /Cl_p/ of the drug

were calculated using one-compartment model. The results
were statistically analysed with Spearman tests.

RESULTS
    Pharmacokinetic parameters of antipyrine, shown in
Table 1, did not differ significantly in both examined
groups. There was no significant correlation between
antipyrine pharmacokinetics and duration of dialysis
treatment in uraemic patients as well as between the
drug pharmacokinetics and body weight of these patients
and healthy persons.

Table 1. Antipyrine pharmacokinetics in peritoneally
dialysed uraemic patients and healthy persons /$\bar{x} \pm$ SD/.

	Uraemic patients n = 10	Healthy persons n = 13
k /hr^{-1}/	$0,069 \pm 0,043$	$0,084 \pm 0,057$
t$_{0,5}$ /hr/	$13,2 \pm 6,8$	$11,8 \pm 8,1$
V$_d$ /l/	$44,9 \pm 9,3$	$34,3 \pm 24,8$
Cl$_p$ /ml/min/	$50,2 \pm 30,2$	$33,6 \pm 30,2$

DISCUSSION AND CONCLUSIONS
    HBs-negative patients with end-stage renal disease
regularly treated with peritoneal dialyses do not show
the delayed antipyrine elimination. It indicates that in
dialysed patients the cytochrome P-450 content in hepatic microsomes is not significantly decreased, so the
liver ability to the oxidative metabolism of other drugs
can be also not deteriorated.
    In nondialysed uraemic patients the liver elimina-
tion of some drugs is delayed /3,6/, but during regular
dialysis treatment the oxidative metabolism can be even
enhanced /5/. Fine et al. /1/ observed an acceleration
of the conjugation of sulphadimidine when some patients
were reinvestigated after regular dialysis therapy had

been started and Held et al. /2/ showed an accelerated
phenylbutazone conversion in dialysed patients. Single
haemodialysis, however, does not influence antipyrine
pharmacokinetics /4/; our data indicate that values of
these parameters do not depend on the duration of regular
dialysis treatment.

A great dispersion of antipyrine pharmacokinetics
observed in healthy persons as well as in dialysed patients must, however, be mentioned. This individual variability indicates either the great interpersonal differences in this drug metabolism or the influence of extra-
hepatic factors /8/. Our examinations did not reveal
a significant correlation between antipyrine pharmacokinetics and body weight of uraemic and healthy persons
but Fraser et al. /8/ observed higher values of antipyrine biologic half-life in patients with greater body
weight. Because of this variability, the assesssment of
hepatic oxidative metabolism by antipyrine test in individual patients we regard as helpful only in recognizing
of more pronounced deviations from normal hepatic status.

REFERENCES
1. Fine, A. and Summer, D. Proc. Eur. Dial. Transplant.
   Assoc. 11:433-439, 1975.
2. Held, H. and Enderle, C. Clin. Nephrol. 6:388-393,
   1976.
3. Leber, H.W., Harders, A. and Schütterle, G. Klin.
   Wschr. 50:1092-1096, 1972.
4. Lichter, M., Black, M. and Arias, I.M. J. Pharmacol.
   Exp. Ther. 187:612-619, 1973.
5. Maddocks, J.L. Proc. Eur. Dial. Transplant. Assoc.
   13:624-631, 1976.
6. Reidenberg, M.M., Kostenbauder, H. and Adams, W.P.
   Metabolism 18:209-212, 1969.
7. Brodie, B., Axelrod, J., Soberman, R. and Levy, B.
   J. Biol. Chem. 179:25-30, 1949.
8. Fraser, H.S., Mucklow, J.C., Bulpitt, C.J., Khan,
   C., Mould, G. and Dollery, C.T. Clin. Pharmacol.
   Ther. 22:799-808, 1977.

CLINICAL PITFALLS OF SHORT-TERM DIALYSIS

STEPHEN SANDRONI, ROBERT PATTON, GREGORY BEALE, BETTY DILLMAN

Division of Nephrology, University Hospital, Jacksonville, Florida, USA

INTRODUCTION

The initial evaluation of recently introduced modalities such as short-term high efficiency dialysis has concentrated appropriately on two areas: morbidity and adequacy of dialysis (1). Such data allow comparisons with conventional hemodialysis, but give little guidance as to the actual practical implementation of the newer modalities. Our phased implementation of short-term dialysis in a large hemodialysis population has revealed several problem areas. We have learned that these problems are not unique to our center.

The program which we implemented consisted of these factors: QB=350 ml/minute or greater, QD=500 ml/minute, 15 gauge needles, a large surface area high efficiency membrane, bicarbonate dialysate, and ultrafiltration monitoring. A morbidity study performed prior to initiation of the program served as a baseline for acute morbidity observations made during the initial implementation of the short-term program. During our initial experience the mean reduction in treatment time was one hour (from 4 to 3 hours). Subsequently shorter times have been achieved for many patients. Currently there are 115 patients in the short-term program.

We identified problems in five areas: compression of morbidity, water quality and machine rinsing technique, local evaluation of performance of equipment, logistics of increased patient and equipment turnover, and increased need for patient counseling.

PROBLEM AREAS

COMPRESSION OF MORBIDITY. Morbidity will vary with the patient pop-

ulation, skill of the staff, and experience with the equipment. We
examined two parameters of acute morbidity: hypotension requiring
saline infusion and morbid events requiring a physician's intervention. Observations of 34 patients during our initial six-month
short-term experience revealed no significant difference in these
parameters compared to the baseline period (2). This means that the
frequency of morbid events was actually increased per unit time,
and patient observation became more important.

WATER QUALITY AND MACHINE RINSING TECHNIQUE. De-ionization water
treatment with downstream charcoal filtration had provided us with
good quality water for three years prior to the short-term program.
Informal discussions with manufacturers and other centers indicate
that at this time many users believe that reverse osmosis systems
provide more consistent water quality, and it has been recommended
that reverse osmosis systems be employed for high volume needs (3).
We mix our own bicarbonate solution using commercial powder. This
method led to several episodes of precipitation of the bicarbonate
bath within the dialysate pathway. Use of an in-line pH meter revealed episodic pH variation of our water supply prior to preparation of bicarbonate bath; subsequent preparation of bicarbonate
solution was done only within strict pH limits and has prevented
recurrence of this problem. Bicarbonate solution is now prepared
daily. Discussions with other centers reveals that this problem has
occurred also in the setting of failure to provide periodic rinsing
of machines with citric acid -- a procedure unknown initially to
ourselves and others which has only recently become widely recommended by manufacturers. In addition to rinsing of the dialysate
pathway, a bleaching technique is necessary for proper maintenance
of some ultrafiltration modules. Lack of standardization of the
newer equipment results in the need for different rinsing and
bleaching requirements for machines from different manufacturers.

LOCAL EVALUATION OF PERFORMANCE OF EQUIPMENT. Centers wishing to do
short-term dialysis generally need to acquire bicarbonate dialysate
capability and some form of ulfiltration monitoring. This can be
accomplished either by acquiring new machines or by adding modules
to existing equipment. Performance in-situ cannot be inferred.
Despite the manufacturer's claims, add-on modules were not immedi-

ately compatible with existing machines and required repeated visits
by the manufacturer before the performance approximated that which
was advertised. Recurrent electrical problems involving up-graded
and new machines caused us to investigate power requirements. Our
engineers estimate that some of the equipment requires 4 times as
much electricity as our conventional equipment.

LOGISTICS OF INCREASED PATIENT AND MACHINE TURNOVER. We could theo-
retically perform 33% more treatments with the same staff in the
same space and same length day with short-term methodology. In
reality we have achieved only a 12% increase to date. The more
varied treatment times have complicated the scheduling of patients,
many of whom are elderly and require assistance with transportation.
Preparation time for the extra treatments subtracts from available
time for the treatment itself. It appears that the increased
patient and staff traffic caused by the additional treatments also
causes delays; better results may be possible by utilizing a larger
and more open area; this would be an additional expense.

INCREASED NEED FOR PATIENT COUNSELING. In our two year experience
we have noted improved chemistries and stable inter-dialytic fluid
gains for 85% of the patients. In addition we have noted a reduction in the number of missed treatments. However 15% of the patients
have had deterioration in chemistries and marked increases in interdialytic fluid gains. Dietary histories and kinetic modeling support the view that some patients view short-term dialysis as an
opportunity to eat and drink in an uncontrolled fashion. Counseling
has been effective with some of these patients; but for now about
half of them or 7% of our total population have been returned to
conventional dialysis.

REFERENCES

1. Gotch, F. Kidney International 33: S100-104, 1988.
2. Sandroni, S., Dillman, B. Kidney International 33: 237, 1988.
3. Ahmad, S., Blagg, C., Scribner, B. In: Diseases of the Kidney
   (Eds. R. Schrier and C. Gottschalk), Little Brown, Boston,
   1988, p. 3294.

FARMACOKINETICS OF CHLORDESMETHYLDIAZEPAM IN PATIENTS ON REGULAR HEMODIALYSIS.

J. Sennesael*, D. Verbeelen*, L. Vanhaelst** and SR Bareggi***
Department of Nephrology(*) and Pharmacology(**), Academisch
Ziekenhuis - Vrije Universiteit Brussel, Belgium. Department of
Pharmacology, Chemiotherapy and Medical Toxicology(***), Univer-
sita degli Studi, Milano, Italy.

Introduction

Chlordesmethyldiazepam (CDDZ) is a 1,4-benzodiazepine. Farmaco-

kinetic data in humans after single- and multiple-dose oral and

intravenous administration showed a long half-life, extensive

biotransformation and low clearance (1). Only one brief report

(2) shows that diazepam has shorter half-life and higher clear-

ance in patients with renal failure. It seemed therefore worth-

while to study in patients with renal failure the pharmacokine-

tics of CDDZ both after intravenous and oral administration.

Materials and methods

Nine patients on regular hemodialysis treatment (RHD) with

uncomplicated renal failure, 33 - 76 years old, weighing 36 - 89

kg were studied. None of the patients received drugs affecting

liver metabolism. Six healthy volunteers, described elsewhere

(1), served as controls.

CDDZ, 2 mg was given orally as tablet or intravenously at 8 a.m.

after an overnight fast. Nine patients received an intravenous

dose of the drug, four patients received both formulations following a crossover randomized sequence with an interval of four weeks between doses. Venous blood was drawn into heparinized tubes 5 minutes before drug administration and 10, 20, 30 minutes and 1, 2, 3, 4, 6, 8, 12, 24, 48, 72, 96, 168, 216, 264, 312, 360 and 512 hours afterwards.

Plasma CDDZ was determined by electron-capture GLC after extraction into toluene (3). Plasma concentrations of CDDZ were analysed by iterative nonlinear least-squares regression analysis (4). One or two compartment models with first order absorption were used as appropriate. The following relevant kinetic parameters were determined : peak plasma concentrations (CMax), time for achievement of peak levels (TMax), elemination half-life (T1/2), area under the plasma concentration-time curve (AUC 0 - ∞), clearance (Cl), apparent volume of distribution (Vd).

Results

Mean (± SEM) kinetic parameters for intravenous CDDZ in patients and controls, respectively, were as follows : T1/2, 116 (±21) vs 112 (±28) h.(NS); Cl, 0.29 (±0.06) vs 0.21 (±0.03) $ml.min^{-1}.kg^{-1}$ (NS); Vd, 3.86 (±0.34) vs 1.7 (±0.19) $l.kg^{-1}$ ($p < 0.01$).

Mean (± SEM) values of kinetic parameters in the four patients who received both intravenous and oral formulations of the drug, respectively, were as follows : T1/2, 177 (±30) vs 207 (±51) h. (NS); AUC, 2154 (±873) vs 1757 (±432) $ng.h.ml^{-1}$ (N.S.); Tmax, 0.2 (±0.0) vs 3.5 (±1.0) h.($p < 0.01$); Cl, 0.23 (± 0.08) vs 0.26 (± 0.03) $ml.min^{-1}.kg^{-1}$ (NS); Vd, 2.9 (± 1.3) vs 4.9 (± 1.7)

$1.kg^{-1}$ (NS).

None of the patients showed any significant modification of cardiovascular and respiratory function. Patients complained for only few and slight side effects (mostly sleepiness).

Discussion

The results of this farmacokinetic study show that patients on regular hemodialysis have clearance and elimination half-life similar to healthy subjects but a slightly larger volume of distribution (1). In renal failure, an increase of volume of distribution has been reported for several drugs such as antibiotics, phenytoin, naproxen and is generally explained as being a consequence of a decrease of plasma protein binding (5).

As previously shown in healthy subjects (1), there were no significant differences in the AUC values between intravenous and oral administration, indicating a good systemic bioavailability of the drug after oral dosing.

References

1. SR Bareggi, G Truci, S Leva, L Zecca, R Pirola and S Smirne. Pharmacokinetics and bioavailability of intravenous and oral chlordesmethyldiazepam in humans.
Eur J Clin Pharmacol 34 : 109 - 112 (1988).

2. HR Ochs, DJ Greenblatt, DR Abernethy, M Divoll. Diazepam kinetics in chronic renal failure. Clin Pharmacol Ther 29 : 270 (1981).

3. L Zecca, P. Ferrario, R Pirola, SR Bareggi. Analysis of chlordesmethyldiazepam and its metabolites in plasma and urine. J

Chromatogr Biomed App 420 : 417 - 429 (1987).

4. G Sacchi Landiani, V Guardabasso, M Rochetti. NL - FIT : A microcomputer program for non-linear fitting. Comput Progr Biomed 16 : 35 - 42 (1983).

5. JG Gambertoglio. Effects of renal disease : altered pharmaco-kinetics. In LZ Benet et al : Pharmacokinetic basis for drug treatment. Raven Press, New York, 149 - 171 (1984).

EFFECT OF POLYACRYLONITRILE MEMBRANE UPON PLASMA OSTEOCALCIN AND iPTH LEVELS IN PATIENTS ON MAINTENANCE HEMODIALYSIS

V.STEFANOVIĆ, S.KOSTIĆ, S.STRAHINJIĆ

Institute of Nephrology and Hemodialysis, Faculty of Medicine, Niš, Yugoslavia

INTRODUCTION

Renal osteodistrophy is a major complication of end-stage kidney disease. Determinations of iPTH in chronic renal failure patients with assays directed toward the middle and C-terminal portion of PTH have provided a reliable index of the progression of secondary hyperparathyroidism (1). Osteocalcin, a noncollagenous protein, has also been implicated in the regulation of skeletal metabolism (2). It is cleared by glomerular filtration and accumulates in renal insufficiency (3).

The aim of this investigation in end-stage kidney disease patients on maintenance hemodialysis (HD) was to study acute and chronic effects of dialysis membrane upon plasma osteocalcin and iPTH levels.

MATERIALS AND METHODS

Twenty-four patients on HD from 18 to 103 months, mean 51 ± 23, were studied. HD was performed for 4 hours on 1 sq.m dialyser, three times a week. Dialysate was made from deionized water and contained 1.75 mmol/l calcium and 0.75 mmol/l magnesium. None of the patients received vitamin D metabolites or glucocorticoid therapy.

Immunoreactive C-terminal and middle region PTH were determined in heparinised plasma by commercial radioimmunoassays (RIA) from Mallincrodt (W.Germany). Osteocalcin was determined by a competitive, double antibody RIA kit from CIS, France. Means $\pm$ SD are given throughout. Statistical significance was estimated by the Student's t-test for unpaired samples.

RESULTS

Acute effects.

In 6 patients blood samples were obtained before, 1 h,
2 h, and 4 h after HD on cuprophan plate dialysers (Zdravlje-
Travenol) or PAN plate dialysers (AN69, Hospal) of 1 sq.m.
In patients dialysed with PAN membrane a significant decrease
of plasma osteocalcin (p<0.01) and both midregion (p<0.001)
and C-terminal (p<0.01)iPTH was demonstrated (Fig.1).

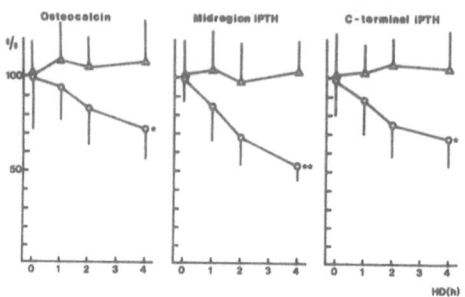

Fig.1. Plasma osteocalcin and iPTH levels during HD with
a cuprophan(△–△) and PAN(O–O)dialyser.*p<0.01,**p<0.001

Chronic effects.

Patients were transfered from the usual HD treatment
with cuprophan to PAN dialysers of 1 sq.m. Lower plasma
osteocalcin and midregion iPTH levels were found after a
three month treatment on AN69 membrane, however, the difference was not significant (Fig.2).

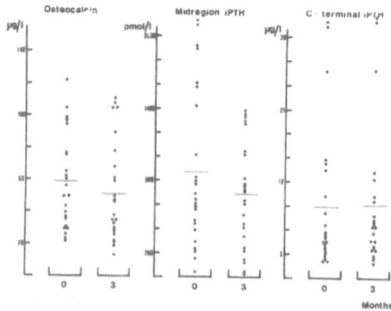

Fig.2. Pre-dialysis osteocalcin and iPTH levels in HD
patients treated for 3 months with cuprophan and PAN membrane.

DISCUSSION

Our results demonstrate a strong correlation between post-treatment plasma osteocalcin and iPTH fragments and the membrane (cuprophan, PAN) characteristics of the dialyser. In accordance with this observation, removal of β_2-microglobulin has previously been described during dialysis with PAN, not with cuprophan membrane (4).A slight increase of the immuno-reactivity during dialysis on cuprophan membrane, representing less than 8.6 of the circulating level, could be explained by ultrafiltration reduction of the circulating volume.

We have demonstrated in 1985 that serum β_2-microglobulin level was lower in end-stage kidney disease patients dialysed with PAN membrane (5). Our present study shows lower plasma osteocalcin and midregion iPTH levels in patients dialysed for 3 months with PAN membrane than when dialysed with cuprophan membrane, however, the difference was not significant. This could be explained, at least partly, by the fact that dialysis of small molecules including phosphate is not dif-ferent in the two dialysis schedules (cuprophan and PAN) and that factors governing PTH secretion are not much influenced by dialysis on a highly permeable membrane. Much effective removal of the midregion and C-terminal iPTH fragments by PAN membrane could possibly be balanced by the increased secretion and/or decreased degradation.

REFERENCES

1. Slatopolsky, E., Martin, K.J., Morrissey, J.J. and Hruska, K.A. In: Nephrology II (Ed.R.R.Robinson),Springer-Verlag, New York, 1984, pp.1292-1304.

2. Price, P.A., Parthemore, J.G. and Deftos, L.J. J.Clin. Invest. 66: 878-883, 1980.

3. Delmas, P.D., Wilson, D.M., Mann, K.G. and Riggs, B.L. J.Clin. Endocrinol.Metab. 57:1028-1030, 1983.

4. Vincent, C., Revillard, J.P., Galland, R. and Traeger, J. Nephron 21: 260-268, 1978.

5. Kostić, S., Djordjević, V., Lečić, N. and Stefanović V. Kidney Int. 28: 338, 1985.

ABDOMINAL HERNIAS AS COMPLICATION OF C.A.P.D.:IMPORTANCE OF THE
EARLY DIAGNOSE AND SURGERY

P.STRIPPOLI,*M.R.BASILE,ORBELLO G.,COVIELLO F.,MINGRONE G.,A.SCATIZZI
Renal Unit,*Surgery Department,Reg.Hospital"SS.Annunziata"
U.S.L.TA\5 Taranto Italy.

Chronic peritoneal dialysis effectively maintains life in patients
with end-stage renal disease (ESRD).In particular,children,the elderly and patients with compromised cardiovascular system may benefit from the simplicity of the technique,the easier insertion
and maintenance of an access route,and the more gentle fluid
shifts as compared to hemodialysis.With the advent of continuous
ambulatory peritoneal dialysis (CAPD),this therapy has been extended to a larger ERSD population.

Abdominal hernias are frequent complication of CAPD with a mean
incidence of 12%;bibliography reports a high variability concerning the effective incidence,the interval of appearance after the
start of dialysis and the facilitating risk factors.(1-2).
On the contrary the little influence of hernias as causes of dropout is generally confirmed.

PATIENT MATERIAL
Between February 1982 and December 1987,31 patients (15 men $52.5^{\pm}$
$12.1(\bar{x}^{\pm}S.D.)$years old,and 16 women $58^{\pm}13$ years old)were trained
for CAPD at our center .All patients were dialysed through a
curled double-cuff Tenckhoff peritoneal catheter (CPC) inserted by
an infra-umbilical midline incision.The number of the daily exchan
ges and the volume of dialysate used were related to the individual's age,body size and the level of serum creatinine;most of the
patients were on four,two-litre exchanges per day.
Catheter Implantation:
The CPC was implanted under local anaestesia using the Tenckhoff
technique.The CPC is reinforced by a longer obturator to be put
into a straight position during implantation through the trocar.
The catheter is advanced gently and should slide in easily until
resistance is met in the deeper pelvic area.When the patient no-
tes discomfort in the rectal area,it can be assumed that the ca-

theter tip is in its proper position;the obturator is withdrawn
slowly and the catheter is pushed downwards to keep its curled
section in the pelvis.There should be no resistance to fluid as-
piration.The implantation procedure is terminated to Tenchkoff's
specifications.

Results:

After the first year of CAPD,8 patients (27.5%)developed abdominal
hernias (6 umbilical,1 incisional,1 inguinal).The hernia presented
as a painless swelling in four episodes.Only two patients had a
previous history of repaired hernia,umbilical hernia 1 and iguinal
hernia 1.

Management and outcome:

All the hernias were repaired surgically;nobody presented complication after surgery and nobody needed discontinuation of CAPD
(one litre four times a day).

Discussion:

Digenis (3) reported that 11.4% of their patients developed hernias and proposed that the main cause in the pathogenesis is related to the intrinsic weakness in the abdominal wall aggravated by
increased intra-abdominal pressure due to the input of the dialytic peritoneal fluid.Therefore,it is not surprising that patients
on this treatment are prone to develop abdominal hernias,particu-
larly those with weak areas in their abdominal wall from previous
pregnancies or old age.

In our study :

-among the women,previous pre-gnancies and among the men,old age
seem to be the principal predisposing factors;

-catheter survival is lower (in 2 cases,surgery correction requested catheter change);

-peritonitis is significantly greater in patients with abdominal
hernias;

-none of the following factors affected the incidence of hernias:
activity,prior surgery,steroid therapy,hypoalbuminemia,type of catheter implanted;

-early diagnose and surgical treatment(4-5)prevent herniary compli
cations.Abdominal-wall hernias should be repaired promptly but
electively to prevent the distressing,intermittently massive di-
stention of the hernial sac and more importantly to avoid the disa-

strous sequelae of incarceration and strangulation.Incision for
insertion of dialysis catheters must be closed with careful technique to prevent ventral hernias.
—no eventration are reported from our experience.

AGE ,SEX OF PATIENTS ON CAPD WHO DEVELOPED HERNIAS
TYPE OF HERNIA AND DURATION OF CAPD BEFORE THE
DEVELOPMENT OF HERNIAS

	All patient on CAPD	
	Men	Women
Patients	15	16
Age (years $\bar{x} \pm SD$)	$52.5^{\pm} 12.1$	$58^{\pm} 13$

	Patients with hernias	
	Men	Women
Patients	3	5
Age (years $\bar{x} \pm SD$)	$49.3^{\pm} 10.1$	$60^{\pm} 10$
Type of hernia		
—umbilical	1	3
—incisional	1	2
—inguinal	1	
Months of CAPD <6	1	4
6—12	2	1

REFERENCES

1. Chan MK,Bailloid Ra,Tanner A. et al.   BR.MED.J.1981,282:826
2. Rocco MV,Stone WJ   PERIT.DIAL.BULL.1985,3:171-174.
3. Digenis GE,Khanna R,Mathews R,et al.   PERIT.DIAL.BULL.1982,2:
   115-117.
4. O'Connor JP,Rigby RJ,Hardie IR et al.   AM.J.NEPHROL.1986,6:
   271-274.
5. Valenti GN,Cresseri D,Bianchi ML,Corghi E,Lorenz M and Buccian
   ti G.   PERIT.DIAL.BULL.1985,1:39-42.

HEMODIALYSIS IN THE ELDERLY

A. Capuano, V. Sepe, P. Cianfrone, T. Castellano, V. Ter
racciano, R. Gallo, V.E. Andreucci.

Dpt of Nephrology, 2nd Faculty of Medicine, University of
Naples, Italy.

INTRODUCTION
Most nephrologists believe that hemodialysis (HD) mana
gement in elder uremic patients may be adversely influen
ced by poor dialytic tolerance due to impaired cardiovas
cular conditions (1). This study has been carried out to
evaluate HD tolerance and strategy in patients aging 65y
or more. HD "young" patients (45y or less) were selected
as control subjects since it is reasonable to expect good
cardiovascular conditions and HD tolerance below this age
limit.

PATIENTS AND METHODS
HD patients aging 65y or more and 45y or less at the
moment of investigation were included in the study. Both
elder patients (EP, n.77) and young patients (YP, n.57)
underwent in-centre HD which was performed by cuphropan
dialyzers in single-pass. Sodium and glucose concentrati
on and temperature of dialysis bath were similar for all
patients (sodium 138-142 mEq/lt, glucose 100 mg/dl) and
kept constant during each treatment. Blood samples for la
boratory investigation were obtained at the end of the
longest inter dialytic interval. Body Weight (BW) was the
mean of the post-dialysis weights of the last 2 months.
Body Mass Index (BMI) was calculated by weight and height.
Interdialytic BW gain was the mean of the values observed
in the last 2 months. All data were collected by the ne
phrologists taking care of the dialysis unit who included
in the study all the patients who satisfied the age crite
rion. Statistical analysis was performed by student t te
st and X^2 test. All data are means and SD.

RESULTS
Incidence of chr.g.nephritis was higher in YP than EP

(65% vs 18%, p 0.01). Diabetic nephroph. and hypert. Nephroscerosis were more frequently cause of Renal Failure in EP than YP (19% vs 3% and 23% vs 2% respectively, p 0.01). Duration of treatment was lower in E males than Y males (11.8±0.9 vs 12.4±0.9, hours/week, p 0.01) but not in females (11.7±1.3 vs 12.2±0.8, NS). Blood flow rate was lower in EP than YP both in males (243±43 vs 279±41, ml/min, p 0.01) and females (244±47 vs 279±38, p 0.01). Dialyzer surface area and potassium concentr. in dialysate were similar in EP and YP (1.1±0.1 vs 1.2±0.1,males,m2, 1.0±0.2 vs 1.1±0.2, females,NS)(1.8±0.4 vs 1.8±0.3, mEq/l NS). Bicarbonate dialysis was performed in 18% EP and 9% YP (NS). Arrhythmias independent from HD treatment (in the most of cases atrial fibrillation) were present in 12 % EP and no YP (p 0.05). HD related arrhythmias were present in 15% EP and 9% YP (NS). Habitual HD related hypotension was present in 44% EP and 31% YP (NS), amount of saline infused per each treatment was similar in the two groups (537±533 vs 523±499, ml,NS). Intradialytic incidence of headache, nausea, vomiting, muscle cramps and angor was not different in the two groups. HD related arterial pressure fall was higher in EP than YP for systolic (21± 13 vs 15±15, mmHg, p 0.001) but not diastolic (7±8 vs 8±8 NS). HD strategy in EP with habitual hypotension (HH) relied on the wider use of bicarbonate dialysis (29% in EP with HH vs 9% in EP not HH, p 0.05) rather than reduction of blood flow and dialyzer surface area or increase of saline infusion. BW and BMI were significantly higher in E than Y females (60±15 vs 53±9, Kg, p 0.05) (24±9 vs 21±3, p 0.05) and a higher % of Y than E females had a BMI below the acceptable range (44% vs 15%, p 0.01). Interdialytic BW gain was lower in E than Y males (2.5±0.9 vs 3.5± 1.1, p 0.01) but not in females (2.6±1.0 vs 3.2±0.7, NS). Serum urea and phosphate were lower in EP than YP (148± 38 vs 163±46, 4.1±1.3 vs 5.3±1.3, mg/dl, p 0.05 and p 0.01 respectively). Hypercholesterolemia was present in 52% EP and 28% YP (p 0.05). Serum albumin was similar in the two groups (3.9±0.5 vs 4.0±0.4, g/dl, NS), values below 3.5 g/dl were present in 17% EP and 10% YP (NS). Duration of hypertension before HD institution was 9.2±7.7 y in EP and 3.5±2.8 y in YP (p 0.01). A cardiovascular disease (myocard. infarction, ischemic heart dis., cerebrovasc. accidents, heart failure) occurred in 27% EP and 10% YP before HD institution (p 0.01). Incidence of syst. hypert. at the moment of investigation was 45% in EP and 20% YP (p 0.01). Incidence of diast. hypert. was similar in the two groups (8% vs 15%, NS). Digoxin and nitrates were more frequently prescribed in EP than YP (36% vs 5% and 19% vs 2%, respectively, p 0.05).

CONCLUSIONS

Our data show that HD strategy was not strikingly dif_ ferent between E and Y patients since only a moderate re_ duction of blood flow and duration of treatment was appli_ ed to EP although these showed a significantly higher com_ promision of cardiovascular apparatus (as expected) than YP.The approach to EP with habitual hypot. seemed to be the most judicious since it relied on the wider use of bi_ carbonate HD rather than manipulation of parameters which can compromise the efficaciousness of treatment. HD tole_ rance was satisfactory in our EP and the relative low inci_ dence of dangerous intra-dialytic complications (namely ar_ rhythmias) probably relied on the judicious use of digita_ lis (36% EP treated in our study vs about 60% in other se_ ries) (2) rather than elevation of potassium in dialysate as suggested by others (1). Laboratory findings showed lo_ wer levels of pre-dialysis urea and phosphate in EP than YP. Together with the finding of a lower interdialytic BW gain in EP than YP these data could rise the suspicion of lower nutrient intake in E than Y patients and this has been related to mortality and morbidity in elder uremic pa_ tients (3). Although it is not possible to exclude that nutrient intake was lower in EP than YP, the data of Albu_ min and BMI seem to suggest that it was at least sufficie_ nt to avoid overt malnutrition.

REFERENCES

1 Ponticelli C., Graziani G., Cantaluppi A., Moore R.. In: Renal Function and Disease in the Elderly (Eds Nunez JF and Cameron JS), Butterworths Publ., London, pp. 509-528.
2 Shaefer K., Asmus G., Quellhorst E., Pauls A., Von Herrath D., Jahnke J.. Proc EDTA-ERA, 21: 510-517, 1984.
3 Chester A.C., Rakowski T.A., Argy W.P., Giacalone A., Schreiner G.E.. Arch Intern Med, 139: 1001-1005, 1979.

IV. TRANSPLANTATION

Age and Renal Transplantation

AGE AND RENAL TRANSPLANTATION

H. BRYNGER MD

Transplant Unit, Sahlgrenska Hospital, University of Göteborg,
Göteborg, Sweden

Throughout the relatively short history of renal transplantation
high age of the recipient has been considered a major risk factor,
negatively influencing the outcome of the procedure. However, there
is no general consensus regarding the definition of age in this context. Frequently, chronological age has been used quite arbitrarily.
Upper age limits of 50, 55 and 60 years have been used in an unsys-
tematic fashion. Rarely account is taken into the biological age
of the recipient, thus, some old patients might be in a very good
mental and physical health, while young persons not necessarily are
in the same situation. Therefore the biological age must be the most
pertinent parameter in renal transplant patients.
In Europe today, policies differ greatly regarding acceptance of
elderly patients for transplantation, despite the fact that an increasing number of old patients are accepted for dialysis treatment.

There are of course several reasons for the reluctance to transplant
elderly patients, such as depressing historical experiences, un-
certainty on the long term benefit for an old patient, with a much
shorter life expectancy that in a young individual.

The major problem in renal transplantation is certainly the lack of
organs. At present some 25 000 patients await a cadaver renal transplant in Europe, while approximately 9 000 such grafts are obtained
per year. It is selfevident that this inbalance leads to younger
patients having priority when a cadaver kidney becomes available.
However, this difficult situation creates ethical problems. Is it

really justified, to deny a person a treatment that could lead to a dramatically improved quality of life, just because he/she has reached a certain age? In my opinion it is not justified, and therefore the problems have to be solved. All efforts must be put into this task, with the aim to be able to offer the best treatment modality to all patients irrespective of age.

Old recipients

In a historical perspective, the outcome of renal transplantation in old patients, defined as over 55 years of age, used to be rather depressing. The major concern was a high mortality, frequently occuring in patients with functioning grafts. The main causes of death were infections and cardiovascular diseases. The main contributing factor to these events was the high steroid doses used during that time when Cyclosporine was not available. However, with increasing experience the results improved, to a large extent depending on better knowledge of selection criteria. With the introduction of Cyclosporine on a large scale in 1982, the results have further improved, probably due to the fact that the need of steroids was substantially reduced. At the present time, the patient survival after first cadaver grafts in this group is around 90%, the graft survival around 70%. With these results, it seems justified to state that the outcome is acceptable and the treatment could be offered to this patient group without great hesitation.

It must be pointed out, that the selection of these patients is of great importance. In our unit the policy has been to bring in patients over 55 years of age for special evaluation and information: thus, some biologically aged patients have not been accepted for transplantation. The selection principles have been focused on the general physical and mental health of patients with special reference to serious heart ailments considered contraindications for transplantation. We have also found it important to evaluate the patient's own desire to undergo transplantation, and that he/she is well informed regarding the pros and cons of the treatment. If dialysis problems exists, such as accessproblems or very long distances between the patients home and the dialysis unit (this is a common situation in the northern part of Scandinavia), we tend to take a liberal attitude in accepting such patients for transplantation.

Old donors

With increasing numbers of elderly patients accepted for active renal replacement therapy, it seems obvious that kidney transplantation must be considered for a larger number of these patients, as otherwise the pressure on the limited resources of dialysis will create serious problems. One main limiting factor for transplantation is, as mentioned above, the availibility of donor organs. To a certain extent however, this might be improved if similar age limits for donors are used as for recipients. It seems selfevident that when transplanting old patients we will also have to use old healthy donors. This means that the upper age limit for a kidney donor could well be 75 years. The present experience of using kidneys from old donors is positive, there might be a slightly inferior outcome of the old kidneys compared to young ones, but the difference is modest, and in some reports no such difference has been found. The function of an old kidney graft, in our experience, is not statistically different from younger kidneys at two years post transplantation.

We also are of the opinion, that use of live donors, when available should be actively considered also for this group of patients. From obvious reasons, potential live donors are not very frequent in the old patient category, but if there is a volontary healthy relative in the same age group as the recipient, this individual should be considered for kidney donation. The experience with the use of elderly live donors has been positive, the morbidity of the donor has not differed from that seen in younger donors and the quality of the kidneys has been adequate and remained so for periods over 10 years.

Comments

As renal transplantation today is an important part of the total treatment of the uremic population, it is necessary to try to solve the specific problems regarding the old patients.

Today, satisfactory results are obtained with cyclosporine as basis

for immunosuppression. Needless to say adequate selection principles
must be followed, basically those aimed at the biological, not
chronological age of the patients.

As many of the patients could be successfully treated with renal
transplantation, the donor pool must be increased by accepting
cadaver and live donors of an equal age as the recipients'. In many
cases, it could be proper to use old kidneys in old recipients, although it does not seem necessary to introduce strict age matching
for available grafts. With the present inbalance between available
grafts and waiting patients, it is a long way to go until we reach
a situation when an old individual could be offered a kidney graft
on the same conditions as a young one. However, the rather quick increase of the transplantation rate gives a basis for cautious opti-
mism. It must be a duty of all individuals involved in treatment of
end-stage renal disease, to be able to provide alternative treatments
to patient on equal grounds irrespective of age. Personally I find it
highly inproper to exclude any patient from treatment due to a date
on a birth certificate.

INFLUENCE OF RECIPIENT AGE ON THE OUTCOME OF CADAVER KIDNEY TRANSPLAN-
TATION IN PATIENTS TREATED WITH CYCLOSPORINE (CyA)

G. LUNDGREN, H. PERSSON, D. ALBRECHTSEN, H. BRYNGER, A. FLATMARK, L.
FRØDIN, C.G. GROTH, A. LINDHOLM, H. WEIBULL

Huddinge Hospital, Stockholm; Sahlgrenska Hospital, Gothenburg; University Hospital, Uppsala; Malmø General Hospital, Malmø, Sweden;
and National Hospital, Oslo, Norway

INTRODUCTION

When renal transplantation was started in the beginning of the
60-ies it was mainly offered to young patients, and an upper age limit of 45 years was often practised. However, with the introduction
of less toxic immunosuppressive protocols, this age limit was successively increased, and today a recipient age as high as 70 years is no
longer looked upon as an absolute contraindication by several groups.

In the Scandinavian countries, we have for many years taken a
rather liberal approach towards transplantation in the elderly, and
this presentation summarizes the experience from two Scandinavian
multicenter studies undertaken between 1982 and 1987. All first cadaveric renal transplantations performed in Sweden and Norway during
that period are included, and all patients were treated with CyA.
When a low dose CyA protocol was used and the cold ischemia times
(CIT) were kept short, recipient age turned out to be the most important factor affecting graft survival (GS) and patient survival (PS)
rates.

MATERIAL AND METHODS

The first study was designed to evaluate the effect of pretrans-
plant blood transfusions and HLA matching in patients treated with
CyA (1), and the second study was a randomized study comparing a
double drug protocol (CyA + prednisolone) with a triple drug protocol (CyA + azathioprine (Aza) + prednisolone) (2).

The first study comprized 488 recipients of first cadaveric kidneys. The mean age was 47.8 years, 33% of the patients were above 55

years of age and 18% were above 60 years. They received a high-dose
CyA protocol. On the day of transplantation, 10-15 mg/kg was given by
IV infusion, and on day 1, 7.5-10 mg/kg was given. On day 2 an oral
dose of 15 mg/kg was started which was gradually decreased. The mean
dose at 3 months was 7.0 mg/kg and at 6 months 5.9 mg/kg. Prednisolone was started on the day of transplantation at 100 mg/day and was
gradually tapered to 20 mg/day at day 9. At 3 months a maintenance dose of 10 mg/day was reached. Rejections were treated with IV bolus doses of methylprednisolone. The details about the immunosuppressive
treatment, HLA matching, transfusions etc. were given earlier (2).

The second study included 463 patients, 229 randomized to the
double drug protocol (Group 1) and 234 to the triple drug protocol
(Group 2). The mean age was 51.0 years for all patients and was the
same in the two groups. 44% were over 55 years and 29% over 60 years.
On the day of transplantation, patients in Group 1 received 7.5 mg/kg
of CyA IV divided in three doses, while patients in Group 2 received
no CyA at all but instead Aza 2 mg/kg. The following day Group 1 patients received CyA orally, 12 mg/kg, and Group 2 patients an oral
dose of 8 mg/kg in combination with Aza 1 mg/kg. The CyA doses were
gradually reduced according to the blood levels. The mean dose at 3
and 6 months were 5.3 mg/kg and 4.3 mg/kg, respectively, for Group 1
and 4.2 mg/kg and 4.0 mg/kg, respectively, for Group 2. Prednisolone
was given as in study 1, and the same was true for methylprednisolone.
Again, the details have been reported earlier (2).

Graft and patient survival probabilities and the probability of
being free from rejection were estimated by the Kaplan-Meier method.
The log rank test (Mantel-Cox) was used to test the equality of the
curves. The Chi-square method with Yate's correction was used to compare portions of patients in different groups, and Student's t-test
to compare mean values between groups. Patient death, if it occurred,
was registered until 3 months after graft loss. After that period the
patient was considered as lost to follow up.

RESULTS AND DISCUSSION

Study 1.

In order to get a comprehensive view of the effect of recipient
age on the survival rates, the patient material was divided into two

groups, young and old, using every year between 25 and 65 as the cut off point between young and old. When GS was analysed, the highest difference between young and old was obtained at a cut off point of 55 years ($p<0.001$). Significant differences were, however, also obtained at other cut off points, but not all, between 29 and 59 years.

When PS was analysed, a statistically significant difference ($p<0.05$) between young and old was obtained at all cut off points between 25 and 65 years, and the difference was very strong ($p<0.001$) at cut off points between 33 and 59 years.

This study represents a learning period regarding CyA treatment. High doses were used and long CITs were accepted resulting in a high frequency of never functioning kidneys (9.3%). A CIT above 27 hours and the presence of panel reactive antibodies in a recent recipient serum were shown to strongly ($p<0.001$) influence the GS rate (1). An uneven distribution of these factors among the various age groups might well explain why significant differences in GS were obtained between young and old patients at some, but not all, cut off points between 33 and 59 years. In general terms, however, recipient age had a strong effect on the PS rate and also seemed to have an important influence on the GS rate. Of special interest also was the finding that a cut off point as low as 35-45 years, between young and old, gave highly significant differences in survival rates.

Study 2.

The age distribution and the number of graft losses and mortality in the various age groups are illustrated in Fig. 1. The numbers represent the accumulated graft losses and deaths during 1-3 years follow up. The highest graft loss frequency was found in patients 50-69 years of age (32-34%), and the mortality increased successively with age until the 60-64 year age group (21%). There was no mortality in patients below 35 years of age.

When the material was divided into young and old with various cut off points (Fig. 2), a statistically significant difference in GS was demonstrated at all cut off points between 28 and 58 years. The strongest differences ($p<0.001$) were recorded at cut off points between 45 and 51 years. In patients below 45 years of age the 1 year GS rate was 87% and in patients above 45 years it was 71% ($p=0.0002$). The 1 year GS rates for patients above 55, 60 and 65 years

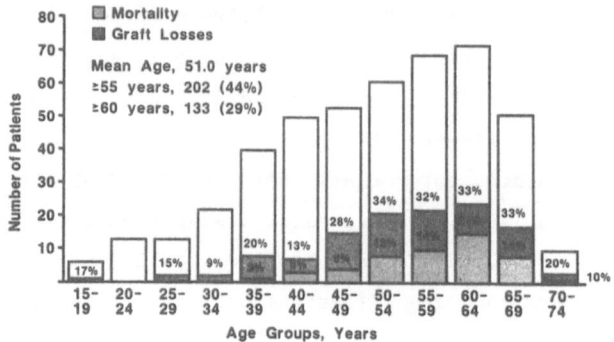

Figure 1. Study 2. Age distribution and mortality and graft loss rates within the various age groups. Figures in bars indicate per cent mortality and graft failures of all transplanted patients in that age group.

of age were 71%, 70% and 73%, respectively. When the differences in PS rates were analysed in the same way, a significant difference (p<0.05) between young and old was obtained at all cut off points between 30 and 63 years, and it was highly significant (p<0.001) at cut off points between 40 and 60 years.

Rejection (47.5%) and graft loss due to the death of the patient (26.7%) were the most common causes of graft failure. Other causes were vascular thrombosis (9.2%), never functioning kidneys for unknown reasons (7.5%), wound infection (2.5%) and other (6.7%). There was no tendency towards a reduced frequency of graft loss due to rejection with increasing age. On the contrary, graft failure due to rejection occurred more frequently among patients above 45 years of age than in

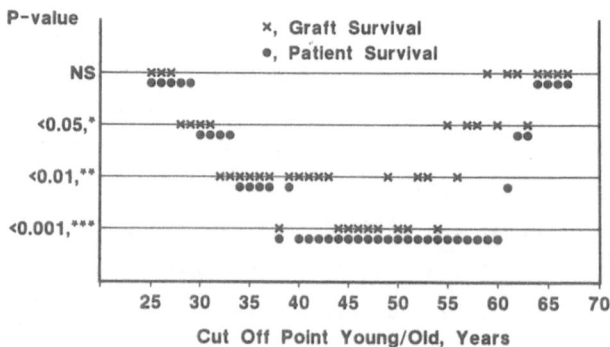

Figure 2. Study 2. Statistical significance of difference in survival between young and old patients with different cut off points.

patients below this age (p=0.016). The same was true for graft loss due to the death of the patient (p=0.009).

Cardio-cerebro-vascular disease (50%) and infections (44%) were the most common causes of death and occurred more frequently among patients above 45 years of age (p=0.049 and p=0.010, respectively).

In spite of the finding that more patients above 45 years of age lost their grafts due to rejection compared to patients below 45 years, there was a tendency towards a reduced rejection frequency with increasing recipient age. These seemingly contradictory findings may be explained by the fact that patients above 45 years of age received significantly lower doses of CyA throughout the first year and also were treated less vigorously at third rejection episodes. At 1, 3, 6 and 12 months, the mean CyA dose among patients below 45 years was 471, 342, 297 and 265 mg/day, respectively, and among patients above 45 years the CyA dose was 388 (p<0.001), 292 (p<0.001), 256 (p<0.001) and 229 (p=0.005), respectively. The mean methylprednisolone dose given at third rejections to patients below 45 years of age was 1204 mg and to patients above 45 years 881 mg (p<0.05). The oral prednisolone doses were the same in patients below and above 45 years of age.

The survival figures reported here justify that elderly patients are offered the possibility of kidney transplantation. With an efficient organ retrieval program, a maximal use of living related donors, and a willingness to accept donors up to the age of 65-70 years, the number of available organs will be sufficient for also accepting the elderly for transplantation. A careful selection of suitable recipients with regard to cardio-vascular disease and an individualized immunosuppressive treatment in order to avoid lethal infections seem to be advocated already in patients at the 40-45 years age level.

REFERENCES
1. Lundgren, G., Groth, C.G., Albrechtsen, D., et al. Lancet 2:66-69, 1986.
2. Persson, H., Andersson, C., Lundgren, G., et al. Transplant. Proc. 19:3586-3588, 1987.

RENAL REPLACEMENT THERAPY(RRT) IN PATIENTS OVER 60 YEARS
OF AGE AND THE USE OF ELDERLY LIVING DONORS.

P.FAUCHALD,D.ALBRECHTSEN,T.LEIVESTAD,T.TALSETH,A.FLATMARK
Department of Medicine and Surgery,University Hospital, .
Rikshospitalet,0027 Oslo 1,Norway.

INTRODUCTION.

The acceptance rates of elderly patients for RRT have
increased the last years,but show great variations(1,2).
Opinions differ regarding the optimal choice of treatment
modality;long-term dialysis or renal transplantation(3,4).
Also the use of elderly living donors is controversial.

The purpose of this study was to evaluate the mode and
the results of RRT in elderly patients within a defined
population.In the second part of the paper we describe
the extent and the results of using elderly living donors.

METHODS.

All patients in Norway(population 4.1 mill.) 60 years
or older when starting RRT during a five years period(81-
85) were included.No exclusions were made and they were
followed til 15.02.87.Transplant patients received Prednisolone and Azathioprine until 1982.From 1983 low-dose
Prednisolone and Cyclosporine A were used.

The living donor material consists of all living donor
transplantations performed in Norway from 01.03.85 till
31.12.87.They were followed till 01.03.88 and donors over
the age of 60 years at uninephrectomy are compared to
those under 60 years.

RESULTS.

During the five years period 368 patients(18 per mill.
inhabitants per year) with chronic renal failure were 60
years or older when starting RRT.They represented 39% of

all patients accepted for RRT during that period.Mean age
was 66.7 years(range 60-83 years) and 98 patients were 70
years or older.Hemodialysis was the initial treatment in
335 patients,while 21 patients were started on CAPD and
12 patients were predialytic grafted.None were lost to
follow-up.

Due to cardio/cerebrovascular or malignant disease and/
or patients preference 119 patients(32.3%) were allocated
to long-term dialysis.Transplantation was planned for the
remaining 249 patients(67.7%).Out of them 127 patients
were not grafted,either because they died while waiting,
or because they were still at the waiting list at follow-
up.Transplantation was performed in 122 patients.The mean
age at start of treatment is given in Table 1.The actuarial patient survival for all patients from start of RRT
was 81% at 3 months,67% at 1 year,50% at 2 years and 31%
at 4 years.The survival in the 3 treatment groups is given
in Table 1.

Treatment group	Mean age at start of RRT years(range)	Actuarial survival(%) from start of RRT(months)				
		3	6	12	24	48
Long-term dialysis	70.3(60-83)	74	63	48(58)	29(29)	13(2)
Tx planned	65.9(60-80)	72	63	44(57)	30(27)	7(1)
Tx perfor-ed	65.9(60-83)	96	93	87(78)	73(44)	62(15)

Table 1.Age at start of treatment and actuarial patient
survival.Number at risk in parenthesis.

Cadaveric donor grafts(CD) were used in 96 patients,whi-
le 26 patients received living donor(LD) grafts.Mean time
on dialysis before transplantation was 10.5 months(range
0-39 months).Actuarial graft survival is given in Tbale 2.
Retransplantation was performed in 6 patients(all CD) with
a patient survival of 83% at 1 year.

	Actuarial graft survival(%)				
	3	6	12	24	48 months
All first transplants (n=122)	74	70	67(70)	63(41)	48(12)
Recipients of CD-grafts(n=96)	71	69	67	61	49
Recipients of LD-grafts(n=26)	85	77	73	73	

Table 2.Actuarial graft survival.Number in parenthesis: patients at risk.

Out of 235 living donor transplantations in Norway between 01.03.85 and 31.12.87 70 donors(30%) were 60 years or older at nephrectomy.The mean age in these elderly donors was 66.2 years(range 60-81 years).Eight donors were HLA-identical siblings,49 were one haplotype mismatch and 13 donors were two haplotypes mismatches.There was no postoperatively or short-term complications,except for a non-fatal myocardial infarction in one donor.This was a father who had concealed for us that he suffered from angina pectoris,knowing that this would have excluded him as a donor. Taking the recipients age into consideration,graft survival(GS) at one year in the recipients of grafts from donors above and below 60 years was not different(Table 3).

Recipients age	Donors age(years)		Total
	Below 60	Over 60	
Below 55 years	91(84)	91(37)	91(121)
Over 55 "	86(17)	79(12)	83(29)
Total	90(101)	89(49)	90(150

Table 3.GS at one year for 1 haplotype mismatched grafts. Number at risk in parenthesis.

This was also the case in the smaller groups of HLA-identical and 2 haplotypes mismatched grafts.
Mean serum creatinine at one year in the recipients of grafts from elderly donors was higher in the group of 1 haplotype mismatched grafts(Table 4),but not different in the two other groups.

	Donors age(years)	
	Below 60	Over 60
HLA-identical grafts	$121.6^{\pm}27.8$(n=25)	$143.5^{\pm}5.3$(n=4)
1 haplotype mismatch	$153.7^{\pm}69.4$(n=62)	$218.8^{\pm}66.2$(n=27)
2 haplotypes mismatch	$169.3^{\pm}49.0$(n=17)	$167.7^{\pm}41.2$(n=7)

Table 4.Serum creatinine(umol/l)$^{\pm}$SD at one year after transplantation.

DISCUSSION.

The survival of the total group of elderly patients(67, 50 and 31% at 1,2 and 4 years,respectively) is fairly similar to that reported as over-all results in treatment programs based mainly on dialysis(1,5).The patient survival is heavily dependent on the selection criterias for accepting patients.In this study approximately 18 patients per mill.inhabitants per year aged over 60 years were accepted for RRT,which is a relatively high number compared to other European countries(6).Also the high mortality in the groups treated only with dialysis may reflect that liberal selection criterias have been practised.We therefore conclude that our results are representative for a treatment program offered to the elderly uremic population according to liberal selection criterias.

Patient and graft survival rates were satisfactory,as also reported in smaller series of elderly transplant patients(4,7).Results of dialysis and transplantation can not be compared in this study due to selection of high risk patients to long-term dialysis.However,the results suggest that early transplantation is the treatment of choice for most elderly patients requiering RRT.

The living donors over the age of 60 years constituted nearly one-third of all living donors.No serious short-term complications were seen.In a long-term study we have shown that donors age is not related to increase in blood-pressure or protein excretion at follow-up(8).However,the compensatory increase in the creatinine clearance of the remaining kidney is inversly related to donors age,but this did not result in clinical significant reduction of renal function(8).The graft survival rates at one year were not related to donors age.However,in the group of 1 haplotype mismatch the creatinine level at one year was higher in the group receiving grafts from donors above 60 years of age.

Elderly living donors are an important source for grafts and they are often well motivated.Provided they are in good health,the risk of donor nephrectomy is not different from younger donors.The results concerning the recipients of these elderly kidneys are satisfactory.

REFERENCES.
1.Kjellstrand,C.M.,Koppy,K.,Umen,A.,Nestrud,S.,Westlie,L. In:Geriatric nephrology(Eds.Oreopoulos,D.G.),Martinus Nijhoff publ.,Dordrecht,1986,pp.135-145.
2.Kramer,P.,Broyer,M.,Brunner,F.P.,Brynger,H.,Challah,S., Oules,R.,Rizzoni,G.,Selwood,N.H.,Wing,A.J.,Balas,E.A.Proc. EDTA-ERA 21:5-65,1984.
3.Westlie,L.,Umen,A.,Nestrud,S.,Kjellstrand,C.M.,Trans.Am. Soc.Artif.Organs 30:21-30,1984.
4.Øst,L.,Lundgren,G.,Groth,C.G. Progress in Transplantation 2:1-15,1985.
5.Held,P.J.,Pauley,M.V.,Diamond,L. JAMA 257:645-650,1987.
6.Wing,A.J.In:Geriatric nephrology(Eds.Oreopoulos,D.G.), Martinus Nijhoff publ.,Dordrecht,1986,pp.227-239.
7.Taube,D.H.,Winder,E.A.,Ogg,C.S.,Bewick,M.,Cameron,J.S., Rudge,C.J.,Williams,D.G. Br.Med.J.286:2018-2020,1983.
8.Talseth,T.,Fauchald,P.,Skrede,S.,Djøseland,O.,Berg,K.J., Stenstrøm,J.,Heilo,A.,Brodwall,E.K.,Flatmark,A. Kidney Int. 29:1072-1076,1986.

IMPACT OF DONOR AGE IN RELATION WITH GRAFT SURVIVAL AND QUALITY OF REMAINING KIDNEY OF DONOR.

G.SAKELLARIOU, E.ALEXOPOULOS, E.KOKOLINA, M.DANIILIDIS, D.GAKIS, M.PAPADIMITRIOU.

Departement of Nephrology Hippokratio General Hospital, Aristotelian University of Thessaloniki-Greece.

INTRODUCTION

Kidney donation remains an important decision from ethical point of view for both the donor and the physician. Living related donors have been utilised for kidney transplantation since 1955 and in some countries up to 5% of the transplanted kidneys come from living related donors (LRD)[1,2]. This procedure is preferred if cadaveric organs are not readily available. On the other hand the superiority of graft survival from LRD is undoubted. Controversy exists regarding the quality of function achieved and the graft survival obtained after transplantation with "aging kidneys"[3,4]. Also it has been reported that the renal function of the remaining kidney of LRD shows a variable degree of deterioration after donation[5]. In view of these important points we studied the role of donor age on graft survival and the consequences of donor nephrectomy in the late renal function of the remaining kidney.

PATIENTS AND METHODS

From January 1968 to December 1987, 195 kidney grafts from related donors (177 parents, 18 siblings) were transplanted in 190 patients with end-stage renal disease. The mean age of the donors at the time of donation was 57 ± 10 years (M ± SD) and of the recipients 32.2 ± 9.8 years.Two groups of recipients were reviewed according to the age of the donor. Those who received the grafts from 118 "young" donors aged <60 yrs (49.8 ± 5.9 yrs) (Group A) and those who received the kidneys from 77 "elderly" donors aged ≥ 60 yrs (68.4 ± 6.5) (Group B).

The HLA-A,B,C,and DR antigens were equally distributed in both groups except for six cases from group A which had full house idently with their sibling donors. Also, no differences were observed between the two groups in the number of preoperative blood transfusions. To analyse the functional and anatomic changes of the remaining kidney we studied 86 donors who had available follow up. The mean time of follow-up after nephrectomy was 55.19 ± 42.9 months (range 3-140 months). Clinical examination, routine blood and urine tests, plasma creatinine and 24 hurine protein exerction were used for the evaluation of the patients.

RESULTS

Study I. The cumulative graft survival in both groups at the end of the first and the fifth year after transplantation was 90% and 70% for Group A and 86% and 52% for Group B.

The differences between the two groups were not statistically significant. The mean plasma creatinine at the end of the first 6 and 12 months after transplantation were 2.0 ± 1.3 mg/dl and 1.86 ± 0.18 mg/dl respectively for group A and 1.92 ± 0.79 mg/dl and 1.99 ± 0.70 mg/dl for group B (P = NS) The incidence of arterial hypertension did not differ significantly at 3 and 12 months between the 2 groups. Concerning the long term results 58.4% of the recipient of group A had functioning grafts, while in group B was 54.5% (p = NS). Study II. The mean age of the 86 donors ($\pm$ SD) at the time of nephrectomy was 59.1 ± 7 yrs and at the time of the last follow-up 65 ± 9.0 yrs. Pcr ($\pm$ SD) rose from 1.16 ± 0.11 to 1.38 ± 0.23 after nephrectomy (p<0.001). Twenty five of 86 donors showed a Pcr greater than 1.4mg/dl at reexamination (range 1.5 ± 2.2 mg/dl). Also Pcr values at follow up did not differ significantly between the donors and it was irrespective of the period of follow up.

Proteinuria was present in 12 donors at reexamination. Nine of them had minimal proteinuria; in the remaining three, the 24 hour protein excretion was 1600 mg, 900 mg and 750mg respectively. No significant changes in BP were observed before and after donation. Seventeen out of 86 donors (19,7%) had a mild arterial hypertension .At the time of last follow up 28 donors (32,5%) had a systolic BP > 150mmHg and/or a diastolic BP > 90 mmHg.

DISCUSSION

In clinical practice, variable results have been reported after transplantation from elderly renal graft donors. Darmady[6] reviewed data from the United States Organ Transplant Registry and observed a diminished patient survival for those who received the grafts from older donors. Also the 5 yr patient survival with kidneys from donors between 21 and 30 year old was surerior compared that obtained with donors between 61 and 84 years old. However, patient data from that study were pooled from multiple centers and the results were not controlled for recipient age. Also Morling et al[7] analysed the influence of donor age on the outcome of 355 cadaver transplants from a single center and found that the cumulative graft survival decreased with increasing donor age. In contrast we did not find a significant decrease in graft survival for the so- called aging kidney (>60 yrs of age)[4]. The long term results were similar in the two groups of donors. Also mean plasma creatinine and the incidence of hypertension were equal in the two groups. Similar results were reported by other investigators[7,8,9]. On the other hand, the survival of cadaveric kidneys has been improved in recent years after the introduction of CyA; in addition, glomerulosclerosis after partial nephrectomy is a well known complication in experimental and clinical transplantation. Thus, our policy in the kidney donation should be reconsidered[10]. In our study we found a significant increase in plasma creatinine at the time of last follow-up, although the mean values were within the normal range. From clinical point of view in countries where the cadaveric organ transplantation is not expanded, a balance between immunological advantages of the relative kidneys and possible disadvantages from changes in the remaining kidney of the donor should be taken into condideration[11]. On the other hand despite claimes to the contrary elderly donors should be accepted for transplantation especially in countries such as Greece where the sources for cadaveric kidneys are limited.

REFERENCES
1. Chavers, B.M. Michael, A.F. Weiland, D. Am J Surg 149:343-346, 1985
2. Sakellariou, G. Memmos, D. Alexopoulos, E. et al: Transplant Proc 17:191-193, 1985
3 Mallas, A.J. Simmons, R.L. Kjellstrad, C.M. et al: Transplantation 21:160-163, 1976
4. Sakellariou, G. Daniilidis, M. Alexopoulos, E. et al: Trnasplant Proc 1:2071-2074, 1987
5. Goldszez, R.C. Hakin, R.M. Brenner, B.M: Kidney Int 23:124-127, 1984.
6. Darmady, Em: Lancet 2:1046-1049, 1974
7. Morling, N. Ladefoge, J. Lange, P. et al: Tissue Antigens 6:163-165, 1975
8. Askari, A. Novick, A.C. Brown, W.E. et al: J Urol 124:779-781, 1980
9. Solheim, B.H. Thorsby, E. Ossbakk, T.A. et al: Tissue Antigens 7:251-254, 1976
10. Brenner, M.B. Meyer, T.N. Hosteffer, T.H: N Engl J Med 307:652-655, 1982
11. Sakellariou, G. in: Transplantation and clinical Immunology (Eds. Touraine, J.L. Traeger, J. Betuel, H. Brochier, J. Dubernard, J.M. Revillard, J.P. Triau, R.). Exerpta Medica Amsterdam 1985, pp. 23-30.

IS AGE OVER 55 YEARS RISK FACTOR FOR KIDNEY DONOR AND FOR GRAFT FUNCTION IN LIVING RELATED RENAL TRANSPLANTATION?

M.MALOVRH, J.DRINOVEC, A.KANDUS, R.PONIKVAR, R.KVEDER

University Medical Center, Department of Nephrology,
Ljubljana, Yugoslavia

INTRODUCTION

The role of the renal transplantation program in the management of end-stage renal disease is well established. Living related donor (LRD) renal transplantation is a common and safe procedure (1,2). In some centers, up to 75 % of grafts come from LRDs. The main reasons are the inadequate supply of cadaveric kidneys and the higher success rate (1-6). In situations of extreme recipient needs kidneys from LRDs older than 55 years can be used (5). The renal transplantation from elderly LRD may represent a possible risk for the donor and also for the renal allograft function immediately after transplantation. A retrospective study was performed to evaluate changes in renal function, proteinuria, and hypertension in LRD older than 55 years and to examine function of renal allograft from elderly LRD in first few days.

PATIENTS AND METHODS

82 LRD renal transplantations were carried out at the University Medical Center, Ljubljana. 31 (38 %) LRDs were older than 55 years. There were 21 (68 %) women and 10 (32 %) men, all parents. Ages ranged from 55 to 79 years, the average $\pm$ SD was 63 $\pm$ 6 years. 11 (35 %) LRDs had borderline hypertension before nephrectomy. Follow up was from 1 month to 51 months. One LRD

was not available for follow up. We evaluated short and
long-term complications, blood pressure (BP), kidney
function, and proteinuria. Among recipients there were
9 (29 %) women and 22 (71 %) men, aged between 22 and 49
years. In insufficient allograft function, the percutaneous renal allograft biopsies were performed from 3 to
7 days after transplantation.

RESULTS
There were a significant differences between pre-
and post nephrectomy values of serum creatinine (p $<$ .001)
(Table 1). The serum creatinine levels tended to decrease with time after nephrectomy.

Table 1. Mean Serum Creatinine Levels in 30 LRDs Over
55 Years Before and After Nephrectomy

Nephrectomy	Serum creatinine level (μmol/l)
before	83.7 ± 15.5 (40 - 109)
1 month after	111.8 ± 20.4 (77 - 160)*
6 months after	101.3 ± 31 (74 - 161)*
1 year after	100.9 ± 15.3 (80 - 135)

*p $<$ .001

Only 1 (3 %) LRD developed hypertension after kidney
donation, 11 LRDs had the same BP as before nephrectomy.
No proteinuria was detected in any LRD. Short-term complications were found in 5 (16.6 %) LRDs (Table 2).

Table 2. Short-term complications in LRD Over 55 years
of Age (n=30)

Complications	n	percentage
Pneumonia	1	3.3
Urinary infection	2	6.7
Wound infection	1	3.3
Urine retention	1	3.3
Total	5	16.6

Signs of acute ischemic damage of renal allograft
with histological patterns of acute tubular necrosis
were found in 6 (19 %) recipients (Table 3).

Table 3. Characteristics of Recipients with Signs of
Acute Ishemic Damage of Kidney Allograft
Immediately After Transplantation (n=6)

Recipient	Age of LRD	Hypertension in LRD before nephrectomy	Warm ischemia	Histology
1	76	Y	31 min	ATN
2	59	No	22 min	ATN
3	73	Y	26 min	ATN
4 *	72	Y	16 min	ATN
5	79	Y	16 min	ATN
6	66	Y	25 min	ATN

* transient hemodialysis treatment

DISCUSSION

Many studies of long term renal function in LRDs
have demonstrated a variable incidence of hypertension,
and proteinuria with well preserved renal function (1,3,
4). In our study, we found a 3 % incidence of hypertension after kidney donation. Our evaluations indicated
that there was an elevation of the serum creatinine
level which tended to decrease with time after nephrectomy. On the basis of this study, it seems that age of
LRD and also hypertension in LRD before nephrectomy has
some influence of immediately graft function, but further
studies are required to evaluate such adverse effects.
We can conclude that age over 55 years is no risk factor
for LRD, and may be a little risk for allograft function
immediately after transplantation.

REFERENCES

1. Drinovec,J.,Malovrh,M.,Kandus,A.,at al. Transplant
   Proc 19:3645-3646,1987
2. Prandini,R.,Bonomini,V.,Vangelista,A.,et al.Transplant
   Proc 19:1498-1499,1987
3. Sakellariou,G.,Memmos,D.,Alexopoulos,E.,et al.
   Transplant Proc 17: 191-194,1985
4. Fehrman,I.,Widstam,U.,Lundgren,G. Transplant Proc 18:
   102-105,1986
5. Bay,W.H.,Herbert,L.E.Ann Intern Med 106:719-727,1987
6. Mendoza,A.,Gabilondo,R.,Odor,A.et al.Transplant Proc
   19:1500-1502,1987

RENAL TRANSPLANTATION IN PATIENTS AGED OVER 50 YEARS

Segoloni G.P., Messina M., Piccoli G.B., Triolo G., Vercellone A.
Chair of Nephrology, University of Turin
Division of Nephrology and Dialysis, Kidney Transplant Unit
Ospedale S.Giovanni Battista - Molinette - Turin

INTRODUCTION

Mean age of dialysis patients is increasing; in our region 25% of new entries, in the years 1981-1987, were 50 to 60 yrs old.

At the transplantation Center of Turin, since the beginning of the activity, the age bias was not an a priori selection criterion.

MATERIALS AND METHODS

From November 1981 to April 1988, 279 kidney transplants have been performed in our center; 4 were from a living donor; 16 patients (pts) received a second graft. 60 pts (24%) were over 50 yrs at time of transplantation. 92 pts, before May 1984, were treated with Azathioprine (Aza), 3 mg/kg, and low doses prednisone (P); 187 pts, transplanted after May 1984, were treated with P and Cyclosporine A (CyA) according to different protocols, as published elsewhere [1]. In his report two age groups, older than 50 yrs (n=17 in Aza; n=45 in CyA regimen) and younger (n=75 in Aza; n=138 in CyA), are compared.

RESULTS

On CyA regimen patients' survival rates in the elderly were superimposable to those of the younger population; at 1,2,3 yrs: 95-89-89% vs 98-96.5-91.5%. On Aza regimen, survival rates were lower in the aged: 82-82-82% vs 97-97-96%. Graft survival rates were

83-70-64% vs 85-73-61% in CyA schedule, and 82-82-76% vs 75-65-60% in
Aza schedule. Infections are analyzed in detail in table 1. The
overall rate of infections was higher in the aged in Aza than in CyA

Table 1 - Infectious complications in patients ≥50 vs < 50 years old

	AZA		CyA	
	≥50 yrs	< 50 yrs	≥50 yrs	< 50 yrs
	%	%	%	%
UTI	16	16	10	12
BPN	10.5	5	8	11
CMV SEROCONVERSION	42	34	36	30.5
WOUND INFECTIONS	0	7	2	3
SEPTICEMIA	0	11	4	6
OTHER	26	9.5	6	2
TOTAL N° OF EPISODES	18 --	p < 0.01	-- 33	

(p<0.01). Notably, no wound infection or septicemia occurred in the
elderly in Aza regimen.

Incidence of non infectious complications is reported in table 2;
statistical difference (p<0.02) was reached only for cardiovascular

Table 2 - Non Infectious complications in pts ≥50 vs < 50 years old

	AZA ≥50	<50yrs	CyA ≥50	< 50 yrs	AZA vs CyA ≥ 50
	%	%	%	%	
DIABETES	10.5	12	12	5	p = NS
LIVER DISEASE	10.5	12	2	7	p = NS
CARDIOVASCULAR	21	5	4	0	p < 0.02
UROLOGICAL	10.5	18	12	13	p = NS
R.ARTERY STENOSIS	5	7	10	9	p = NS
TENDON RUPTURE	5	0	6	1	p = NS
CATARACT	5	3	6	3	p = NS
AVASCULAR NECROSIS	5	4	8	5	p = NS
GN.	0	8	8	7	p = NS
MALIGNANCIES	10.5	0	2	2	p = NS
OTHER	7	3	24	9	p = NS

complications, more frequent in the aged (in Aza vs CyA). Remarkably,
for malignancies no significant difference was found. 5 deaths were
reported in the elderly in Aza regimen: cerebrovascular 1,cardio-
vascular 1, liver disease 1, malignancy 2. In CyA regimen 2 pts died
for cardiovascular disease and 1 for pneumonia.As for graft survival,

rejection cumulative rates and mean serum creatinine (sCr) values were compared at 3 months, 1,2,3 yrs. No statistical difference was found between the two age groups, at any time interval. At 3 mo and 3 yrs rejection rates and sCr were respectively 0,54-0,61 pts/mo and 2±1-1.7±0.5 mg%. As for the causes of graft loss, death accounted for 55% of failures in the elderly in Aza therapy. Chronic rejection was the main cause of failure in all the other groups. In the older Aza population no kidney was lost because of acute rejection or rupture, while 10/33 were lost in the < 50 yrs Aza patients.

CONCLUSIONS

In view of these results, elderly patients appeare suitable for successful renal transplantation. Notably, graft survival rates, rejection rates and immunological causes of graft failure are superimposable in the two age groups. Anyway, it should be remarked that an higher rate of overall complications and 10 deaths occurred in older pts, even if infections, in our experience, are not the major cause of death. These results are in keeping with those of some other Authors (2,3,4,5,6) and giustify our policy of a cautious and less aggressive immunosuppression, adequate to the immunological characteristics of these patients.

REFERENCES
1) Segoloni G.P., Messina M., Colla L., Piccoli G.B., Triolo G., Vercellone A. Transpl. Proc., XX, n° 3, S3 1988, in press
2) Albrechtsen D., Fauchald P., Leivestad T., Talseth T., Flatmark A. Transpl. Proc. XX, 1:367-369, 1988
3) Fryd D.S., So S.K.S., Kruse L., Canafax D.M., Sutherland D.E.R., Simmons R.L., Najarian J.J. Transpl. Proc. XIX, 1:1530-1531, 1987
4) Lundgren G., Fehrman I., Gunnarsson R., Lindholm B., Tillegard A., Öst L., Groth C.G. Transpl. Proc. 14,3,601-604, 1982
5) Cardella C.J., Oreopoulos D.G., Uldall R., Honey J., Cook G., De Veber G.A. Transpl. Proc. XVIII, 1:151-152, 1986
6) Sommer B., David M.N., Mandelbaum M., Henry M.L., Ferguson M. In: Geriatric Nephrology. Martinus Nijhoff Publishers 1986, pp.157-168

KIDNEY TRANSPLANTATION AT AN ADVANCED AGE

I FEHRMAN, C BRATTSTRÖM, L ÖST

Dept of Renal Medicine and Transplant Surgery, Karolinska Institute, Huddinge Hospital, 141 86 Huddinge, Sweden

INTRODUCTION

Due to an ageing dialysis population and a wish from most patients to receive a transplant, we have expanded our age limits for kidney transplantation. This is a presentation of the results obtained in the very old recipients, namely those over 65 years of age.

MATERIAL AND METHODS

During the period 1980-1987, 38 such recipients, with a mean age of 68 ± 2.4 (SD) years, received a kidney transplant. 35/38 (91%) were on regular dialysis treatment before transplantation, 25/38 (66%) had received blood transfusions and 5/38 (13%) were PRA-positive (for definition see below). Between 1980-1985, exchange of kidney grafts within Scandinavia was based on HLA-DR matching criteria. After that kidneys were exchanged if HLA-A, B-matching could be obtained in a PRA-positive recipient. PRA-positive recipients were defined as those having lymphocytotoxic antibodies against >10% of panel T lymphocytes in a current (< 3 months) serum.

All patients were treated with Cyclosporine A (CyA) in combination with corticosteroids. 11 recipients received a higher initial CyA dose of 17-15 mg/kg/day (1, 2); 8 received a medium dose of CyA, initial dose 8 mg/kg/day (3) and 19 received a low dose CyA, initial dose 8 mg/kg/day (3). In the latter group Azathioprine was added at a dose of 1 mg/kg. Prednisolone was given at a low dose, starting at 100 mg daily and then quickly tapered to 20 mg daily after 10 days. The maintainance dose of 7.5 mg-10 mg daily was reached after 3 months.

Diagnosis of rejection was mostly confirmed with core biopsy. Rejection treatment consisted of 0.5 g Solumedrone on the first day and then 250 mg daily for the next 3 consecutive days. Anti-thymo-cyteglobuline was not given to these old recipients. Occasionally local radiation therapy with 150 RAD daily for 3 consecutive days was also given. Since 1986, Bactrim has been given as pneumocystis carinii prophylaxis after rejection treatment.

Since the beginning of 1987, CMV-serology of donors and recipients has been analysed. A CMV negative donor to a CMV negative recipient was one of the selection criteria for PRA-negative recipients.

Statistics

Actuarial survival curves were calculated using life-table methods. For comparison of groups student's t-test was used.

Results and discussion

Actuarial graft survival was 65% at one year which does not differ significantly from 83% found in recipients of primary cadaveric grafts aged 7-45 years (n=68). Graft survival was not correlated to HLA-matching. However, only 5/38 patients received grafts with maximum 0-1 HLA-AB and DR incompatibilities. Interestingly, 21/38 (55%) of the old patients experienced acute rejection episodes, which is the same frequency found in the much younger group (56%). Ten patients had more than one rejection episode and the rejections were not due to the fact that the prophylactic immunosuppression could not be maintained.

Five patients lost their grafts in irreversible rejections, two patients lost their grafts due to thrombosis.

Actuarial patient survival at one year was 71%, this is significantly lower than 100% found in the much younger age group (p<0.001). Lifethreatening infections occurred in 6 patients. All of these died in general CMV infections or CMV pneumonitis. 3 were primary and 3 were secondary CMV infections. Two patients died of infections while back on dialysis shortly after loosing their transplants in irreversible rejections. All patients who succumbed to infections had received rejection treatments. Patients with no rejection treatment had no severe lifethreating infections.

460

Concerning the long time survival, none of the grafts were lost in chronic rejection. Most patients lived a pretty normal life with a stable kidney function. The actuarial patient survival at three years was 61%. The later losses were due to cardiovascular diseases and malignancies.

In comparison to dialysis treatment, the greatest differences are seen in long term survival. Much poorer results are seen on dialysis treatment (own observations, 4).

In conclusion, we find it justified to perform kidney transplantation in old patients. However, rejection episodes occurred in 56% of the patients entailing a risk of life threatening infections. The most serious infection is CMV. Elderly patients seems to be more prone to severe CMV-infections than younger patients, 16% of the old patients died because of CMV-infections compared to 0% of the younger patients during the same period. 3 of the lethal CMV-infections in elderly were primary infections and 3 were secondary CMV-infections. To avoid primary CMV-infections we have started to match CMV seronegative kidneys with seronegative recipients. CMV-prophylaxis with immunoglobuline is given when CMV-matching is not possible. It may also be justifiable to give CMV-prophylaxis to seropositive elderly patients who receive antirejection therapy.

REFERENCES

1. Ringden, O., Öst, L., Klintmalm, G., Tillegård, A., Fehrman, I., Wilczek, H. and Groth, C.G. Transplant Proc 15:2507-2512, 1983.

2. Klintmalm, G., Brynger, H., Flatmark, A., Frödin, L., Husberg, B., Thorsby, E. and Groth, C.G. Transplant Proc 17:1026-1031, 1985.

3. Lundgren, G., Albrechtsen, D., Brynger, H., Flatmark, A., Frödin, L., Gäbel, H., Persson, H. and Groth, C.G. Transplant Proc 19:2074-2079, 1987.

4. Albrechtsen, D., Fauchald, P., Leivestad, T., Pfeffer, P., Talseth, T., Flatmark, A. Transplant Proc (in press).

CADAVERIC RENAL TRANSPLANTATION IN THE ELDERLY

M. SLAPAK, D. THOMPSON, N. DIGARD, B. GARDNER, F. GOODALL
Wessex Regional Transplant Unit, St. Mary's Hospital, Milton Road,
Portsmouth, Hampshire, England.

INTRODUCTION

Cadaveric renal transplantation is now the accepted optimal
therapy for end stage renal failure, since it provides, when successful, a quality of life considerably greater than that resulting from
either haemodialysis (HD) or continuous ambulatory peritoneal dialysis (CAPD). Patient survival is, in most units, greater than 90%
at 1 yr with concommitant graft survival for cadaveric donor transplantation at over 75%. Contributing to this increased success has
been the more judicious use of immunosuppressive (IS) agents, greater
clinical experience in the management of complications, better
quality donor kidneys and more precise histocompatibility. Recently
there has been a significant benefit from the use of a more effective
and more specific IS agent in the form of Cyclosporin A (CYA). In
addition, over the last three years combination IS therapy using
triple therapy (1) or quadruple therapy with polyclonal or monoclonal
antibodies has provided even better graft survival.

However, transplantation of patients in the over 60 age group is
still controversial. The risks of surgery, the shorter expected life
span, the scarcity of donor organs and the obviously greater risk of
complications from cardiac disease are the major reasons for reluctance. Frequently, however, the complications of the alternative
treatment, HD or CAPD are insufficiently appreciated, as is the grati-
fying true reversal of the symptoms of renal failure which may result
from a well functioning allograft. The main questions raised when
transplantation of the elderly is considered are :
Is the morbidity and morality of transplantation unacceptably high?

Does the age of the recipient affect the vigour of the immune
response?
In an attempt to answer these questions we record our experience in a
small group of elderly patients who received a cadaveric renal transplant.

MATERIALS AND METHODS
     27 patients aged between 60 and 73 yrs of age received a renal
transplant from a cadaveric donor. There were 15 male and 12 female.
4 patients were over 70 yrs. The majority of patients had been maintained on CAPD (21) for 0.5 to 3.0 yrs. 1 of the 6 patients who had
received HD had been on that form of treatment for 8 yrs. 6 of the
patients had significant ischaemic heart disease requiring specific
medication, of whom 2 had had, in addition, coronary artery bypass
surgery. There were 3 diabetics and 2 other patients with symptoms
of peripheral vascular disease due to atherosclerosis. The underlying renal pathology in this group was glomerulonephritis 18, pyelo-
nephritis 6, diabetic nephropathy 3. The mean age of the donors was
41.6 yrs, the range being 16 to 65 yrs. 23 or the 27 were from
heart-beating donors. There were 18 local kidneys, removed by the
Portsmouth non-snatch technique using an intra-aortic double balloon
catheter and $4°C$ Hyperosmolar Citrate as the preserving solution (2).
The warm ischaemic interval was always less than 4 minutes. The cold
ischaemic times of the 24 kidneys donated locally or within the U.K.
ranged from 10 to 39 hrs compared to a range of 48 to 72 hrs in the
kidneys which were transported from the U.S.A.

MATCHING
     All the patients were given ABO compatible kidneys. The mean
HLA match is indicated in Charts I and II, which also list some other
characteristics of the recipient and donor cohort. All recipients
had a negative donor specific cytotoxic crossmatch to T lymphocytes.
2 were positive against the B cells of the donor. Of the 27 recipients 6 had greater than 50% reactivity against a panel of 40 individuals. 1 patient received a second transplant.

CHART I PATIENT COHORT

Number	Mean Age	Age Range	M:F	H D	C A P D
27	64.1	60 - 73 (3 over 70)	15:12	6 (2 - 8 yrs)	21 (0.5 - 3 yrs)

Immunological Factors

Mean HLA A & B Match	Mean DR Match	% First Transplant	Panel Reactivity > 50%
2.8	0.7	96%	22%

CHART II DONOR COHORT

Number	Mean Age	Age Range	W I T	C I T	ILSF
27	33.00	16 - 65	< 4 min	26.4 hrs	55%

IMMUNOSUPPRESSIVE THERAPY

Three main forms of IS were used. 5 patients received conventional therapy using Azathioprine (AZA) 1.25 - 2.0 mg/kg body wt, depending on white cell and platelet count, together with Prednisolone (PRED) 14 - 15 mg daily. 16 patients received CYA beginning with the equivalent of an oral dose ranging from 12 - 16 mg/kg body wt, sometimes combined with 10 - 12 mg of PRED. CYA was then decreased over 90 days to an average dose of 5 - 7 mg/kg body wt. The blood IRA assay was used as a help in the diagnosis of nephrotoxicity. Generally levels between 300 and 600 ng/ml were aimed for. The third group of 6 patients received triple therapy (3) starting with CYA 12 mg/kg body wt, reducing to 3 mg/kg by the 30th day; AZA was given at 1 - 1.5 mg/kg and maintained according to white cell and platelet count; PRED was begun at 40 mg daily, reducing to

15 mg by the 30th day and was stopped in most instances by the 6th
month. In this group, kidneys in which immediate life supporting
function (ILSF) was not present were given antithymocyte globulin
(ATG) prophylactically at 3 mg/kg body wt for 6 days (3). In all
instances rejection was treated with Methyl Prednisolone intravenously 0.5 g for three consecutive days. If unresponsive to two
doses of this therapy, with a three day interval, the patient received ATG (Fresenius or Dutch) given after biopsy-proven vascular
rejection was found. Transplantation was performed using standard
techniques and the transplants were monitored using the usual clinical and biochemical criteria. In addition, US, radioactive DPTA
scanning and fine needle aspiration biopsies as well as Trucut
biopsies were used. None of the patients received OKT3.

RESULTS

Of 27 patients 21 (77%) are alive and 20 (74%) have functioning
grafts 6 weeks to 5 years after transplantation. 12 of these
patients have a life-supporting graft longer than 2 years post-
transplant. The actuarial 1 yr patient and graft survival was 81%
and ·78% respectively. Mean serum creatinine at 1 yr was 186 umol/l
$\pm$ 62. Of the 20 patients with a life supporting graft 16 were
judged to have a good or excellent quality of life.

There were 6 deaths. Sepsis was the underlying factor in 5. Two
had myocardial infarction, but in one it was a terminal event after
a septic course. One patient had acute diverticular disease. The
possible risk factors in these six patients who died compared to the
21 who survived are shown in Chart III

CHART III   ? Contributory Factors to Mortality in 6 Patients

Number	Outcome	ILSF	CYA ($\pm$ PRED)	HLA A,B	DR	MEAN DONOR AGE	CIT
6	Death	1	5	2.6	0.8	45.3	23
21	SurvivL	16	14	3.6	0.8	31.2	17

Chart IV shows the mortality and survival of 67 consecutive patients aged less than 60 yrs, transplanted in our Unit in 1987 and the actuarial 1 yr graft survival. The chart also includes, for comparison, the survival of 54 consecutive patients over age 60 yrs receiving HD or CAPD who have never been transplanted. The mortality is 28%.

CHART IV

Number	Mean Age	Age Range	Patient Survival	1 yr Actuarial Graft Survival
Transplanted				
67	41	18 - 59	92%	78%
HD and CAPD				
54	69	60 - 80	72%	-

DISCUSSION

Clearly a patient's age is only a very approximate guide to the higher risk of atherosclerosis and other factors which are the consequence of the aging process. In addition, the small number of patients described in this publication precludes any weighty conclusions. Nevertheless, the mortality rate is significantly higher than that of younger patients transplanted in our unit, whilst the graft survival rate is not significantly different. When comparisons are made with patients who have never been transplanted, there is no clear advantage for the transplant group, 77% 1 yr patient survival versus 72% (but this comparison may be misleading since fitter patients may be more numerous in the transplant group.

Between the 6 deaths and the 21 patients surviving (Chart III) there appears to be a suggestion that ILSF, present in only one of the patients who died) and poorer HLA A & B matching as well as a higher donor age, might be factors which contribute towards the increased mortality. Certainly the effect of prolonged cold ischaemia

in the presence of CYA acting to produce extended primary non-
function has been previously reported (4). The use of prophylactic
ATG whilst withholding CYA has been strongly suggested as an alternative method (3). A feature of our clinical experience has been
the extraordinary resilience and well being of some elderly patients.
Thus one of the patients (CC, Fig 1) aged 73, was discharged on the
11th day post-transplantation and has shown full rehabilitation on a
dose of 4.5 mg/kg body wt of CYA only. ILSF of graft was certainly
a feature in his particular case.

Figure 1.   Post-transplant Course of Patient CC

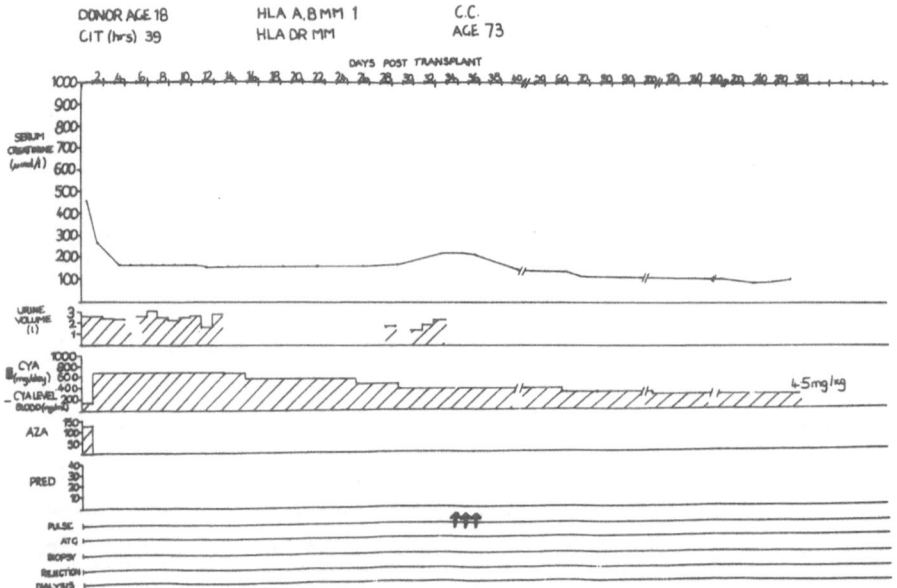

CONCLUSIONS

     On the basis of limited data we conclude that kidney transplanta-
tion in the elderly is fully justified. The mortality may be higher
than in younger groups unless stringent selection criteria for both
recipient and donor are exercised. Amongst these criteria we would
particularly emphasise factors leading to ILSF of the graft. The
individual patient's own wishes and the mortality on HD or CAPD
are factors which should be balanced.

REFERENCES

1. Slapak, M., Geoghegan, T., Digard, N., Ahmed, K., Sharman, V.L.,
   Crockett, R. Trans. Proc. XIX 2, 41-45, 1987
2. Digard, N., Geoghegan, T., Harris, K.R., and Slapak, M. Trans.
   Proc. XVI 1, 107-108, 1984.
3. Slapak, M., Thompson, F.C., Digard, N., Shell, T., Crockett, R.,
   Ahmed, K. Nephrol. Dial. Transplant. 3, 96-97, 1988.
4. Belitsky, P., MacDonald, A.S., Gajewski, J., Boudreau, J.,
   Bittesauermann, H., Cohen, A. Trans. proc. 19, 2096-2099, 1987.

RENAL TRANSPLANTATION IN ELDERLY RECIPIENTS.

J.M.MORALES, A.ANDRES, C.PRIETO, A.RODRIGUEZ, E.HERNANDEZ, T.ORTUÑO,
J.M.ALCAZAR, E.RODRIGUEZ PATERNINA, J.L.RODICIO.
Hospital 1º Octubre. Madrid. SPAIN.

Recently, several articles have been published by different centers
that show good results of renal transplantation (RT) in elderly patients (1,2). We present herein our experience in patients over 50
years old.

PATIENTS AND METHODS.

Between January 84-August 87 we have performed in our hospital 185
renal transplants (RTs). 40 cadaveric RTs (21.6%), 31 males and 9
females, were done in elderly recipients (ER): more than 50 years,
22 of them between 51-55 and the remaining 17 >55 years, X 56.2
years. Two patients received a second graft and one was hyperinmuni-
zed (HP). 31 received steroids (S) and cyclosporine (CsA) and 9 S
and Azathioprine (Aza). These protocols have been published previously (3). The results in the older group were compared to those
obtained in a group of 99 low risk RTs (non HP, younger that 50
years and receiving their first graft) performed during the same period and with similar follow-up: 1/84 - 3/88. 73 patients received S
and CsA and the remaining 26 received S and Aza. Graft an patient
survival times were calculated by the actuarial life table method
(Kaplan-Meyer curves wiht Mantel Test). In addition, the results of
ER were compared with a group of similar age in hemodialysis (HD).

RESULTS

	Patients >50 yr N=40			Low risk patients N=99			p
	6m	1yr	2yr	6m	1yr	2yr	NS
Patient actuarial survival %	95	93	89	96	95	90	NS
Graft actuarial survival %	79.5	77	67	85.5	83.5	76	NS
Acute tubular necrosis	26 (64.5%)			61 (61%)			NS
Acute rejection	17 (35%)			49 (50.5%)			NS
CsA nephrotoxicity	7/31 (22.5%)			30/73 /41%)			NS
Infections	30 (75%)			38 (38.3%)			<0.001
Sepsis	2 (5%)			4 (4.4%)			NS

In the Table we show the principal characteristics of both groups of patients. There were no significant differences between ER and low risk patients in the actuarial survival rates. Actuarial survival of HD patients group was at 12 and 24 mo, 89% and 80% respectively, without significant difference between the ER. The incidence of posttransplant acute tubular necrosis was similar and there was a tendency to show less frequent acute rejection and CsA neprotoxicity. During the follow-up in 30 ER (75%) we saw some episode of infection, mainly of urinary origin. Five of them were related to urological complications: urinary fistula or obstructive uropathy. Although infections were more frequent in ER, the incidence of sepsis was similar in both groups. Graft failure in ER was due to acute rejection in 3, chronic rejection in 2 and arterial thrombosis in 1. Five patients died, four of them with a functioning allograft (one, a diabetic patient). The causes of patient death were citomegalovirus in 2, pulmonary edema in 1, acute pancreatitis in 1 and the last one for unknown cause. It is important to emphasize that 16 ER (40%) did not suffer severe complications nor did they require readmittance to the hospital and 15 ER (37.5%) only needed one readmission.

DISCUSSION

As shown in the present analysis, a 2-year patient survival rate is 89% and near 70% of patients have a functioning graft. These results are not significantly inferior to those in a younger patient population, nor HP and with first transplant. Also, a slightly better survival rate in ER vs HD was seen. Therefore, we have demonstrated in our small group that RT in ER is a good therapy. Possibly, as other groups have demonstrated (2), CsA immunosupression may contribute to these results. On the other hand we would like to emphasize that in CsA ER more severe cardiovascular complications were not seen and the CsA nephrotoxicity incidence was similar in older and younger groups. Although, infections were more frequent in ER, mainly of urinary origin, the incidence of sepsis was similar: 5% ER vs 4.4% low risk patients. Remarkably, 40% of ER did not suffer severe complication nor did they require readmittance to the hospital during the follow-up.Therefore,the ER morbility was not very different than in low risk patients. Our results confirm previous findings that RT in patients over 50 years is a satisfactory therapy with a survival rate not different than that of a group of low risk RTs.

REFERENCES

1) TAUBE D, CAMERON JS, CHALLAH S. In: Renal function an disease in the elderly (Eds. Macias FJ and Cameron JS), Butler & Tanner Ltd, London, 1987, pp 529-537.
2) RINGDEN O, OST L, KLINTMALM G. et al. Transplant Proc. 14: 2507-2512, 1983.
3) MORALES JM, ANDRES A, PRIETO C. et al. Transplant Proc 19: 4005-4007, 1987.

RENAL TRANSPLANTATION WITH ELDERLY DONOR

C.PRIETO, J.M.MORALES, A.ANDRES, T.ORTUÑO, E.RODRIGUEZ PATERNINA, J.M.ALCAZAR, J.L.RODICIO.
Servicio Nefrologia. Hospital 1º Octubre. Madrid. SPAIN.

INTRODUCTION

For a long time, 50 yr was considered the age limit for cadaveric donor (1). We present herein our experience with renal transplantation (RT) using elderly donors.

PATIENTS AND METHODS

Between July 1982-December 1987 we have performed 258 (RT); 33 of them (12.7%), 31 males and 2 females, received a cadaveric graft from elderly donors (ED): aged more than 50 years. The average age was 56.6(50-68 yr) and 11 of them were>60 yr. The average age of recipients was 37.8 (17-60 yr) and in 6 of them it was their second graft. The treatment was steroids(S) and cyclosporine A(CsA) in 30 recipients and S and Azathioprine (Aza) in 3. These protocols have been published previously (2). The cumulative graft and patient survival of ED was compared to a group of 35 patients, 22 males and 13 females, that received a cadaveric graft from young donors (YD). The average age of YD was 25.2 (17-33 yr) and in 2 of them it was their second graft. The average age of recipients with YD graft was 41.2 (17-57 yr). The treatment was S and CsA in 25 and in the remaining

10 S and Aza. These protocols have been published previously (2). The average follow-up period was 25 mo (6-70).

RESULTS

In the table we show the principal features of both groups. The cumulative graft and patient survival rate was similar in patients with ED and in patients with YD. There was no difference in the incidence of posttrasplant acute tubular necrosis, acute rejection, arterial hypertension nor average of current serum creatinine levels. Remarkably, there was only one graft lost due to chronic rejection in the group of patients that received a transplant from a cadaveric donor >60 yr. Finally, the incidence of infections and the number of readmission to the hospital were not different in the group with the ED.

	Elderly donor(n=33) average age 56.6 (50-68 yr)	Young Donor(n=35) average age 25.2 (17-33 yr)	P
Average age receptor	37.8	41.2	NS
Second graft	6	2	NS
Acute tubular necrosis(ATN)	20(62%)	23(65%)	NS
No Readmittance	14(42.4%)	20(57%)	NS
Serum Creatinine (X mg%)	1.48	1.27	NS
Arterial hypertension	10(30%)	10(28%)	NS
Acute rejection	16(51.5%)	18(48.5)	NS
Graft survival	81.8%	85%	NS
Patient survival	95%	92%	NS

DISCUSSION.

Until now it has generally been throught that older donors would have more vascular lesions as consequence of aging. Theoricatelly, it could exacerbate postrasplant acute tubular necrosis and cause bad graft function. The scarcity of donor for organ transplantation togheter with the increase in patients on dialysis waiting for renal transplantation have been the principal reasons for changing the upper age limit of cadaveric donors. Our study demostrates three important features: First, the cumulative patient and graft survival rates were similar in patients with ED and in patients with YD. Second, there was no difference in the incidence of acute tubular necrosis, arterial hypertension nor level of renal function. Third the incidence of infections and the number of readmissions to the hospital were similar in both grups. These results do not indicate that renal graft function in CyA patients is dependent on donor age(3). In conclusion, in our experience RT with ED did not represent an important risk in the evolution of graft and recipient.

REFERENCES

1.- ACS/NIH Organ Transplant Registry. The 11th Report of the Human Renal Transpl.

2.- MORALES JM, ANDRES A, PRIETO C. et al. Transplant Proc. 19: 4005-4007, 1987.

3.- KML LENNISSEN, F.BOSMAN, GA KOTSTRA and JP VAN HOOF. In the second International Congress on Cyclosporine (Abstracts). Washington. Nov. 1987, pp 438.

Miscellany

CALCIUM ANTAGONISTS PREVENT LYMPHOCYTE ACTIVATION IN KIDNEY
ALLOGRAFT RECIPIENTS

S. LAMPERI, S. CAROZZI, M.G. NASINI

Nephrology Department, St. Martin's Hospital, Genoa, Italy

INTRODUCTION

It ha been shown that the inhibition of the proliferative
arm of the immune response induced by Cyclosporine-A,(Cy-A) a
calmodulin antagonist, in kidney allograft recipients(KAR) is
accompanied by a reduced T-lymphocyte(T-Ly)Ca++ concentration
(which is essential in cell proliferation and activation) and a
decreased in vitro release of Interleukin-2 (IL-2) and Interferon-
gamma (IFN-gamma) (1,2).
As the toxic effects of Cy-A are well known, in an attempt to
reduce the dosage of this drug, we determined the effect in vitro
of a calcium-antagonist, verapamil(V), on the immunosuppressive
activity of Cy-A in KAR, by evaluating T-ly Ca++concentration and
IL-2 and IFN-gamma release during phases of tolerance or acute rejection.

PATIENTS AND METHODS

Thirthy-five KAR were prospectively studied. Thirthy healthy
volunteers constituted the control group.
T-Ly Ca++ concentration was determined using a Quin-2 fluorescent
indicator (3). IL-2 and IFN-gamma release by T-Ly were assayed by
Gillis's (4) and radioimmunoassay techniques, respectively. Studies
were performed by incubating T-Ly with medium alone, and with medium
plus V in concentrations ranging from 5×10^{-7} to 5×10^{-5} M.

RESULTS

In the KAR treated with Cy-A alone, one week after transplantation, in the absence of acute rejection, T-Ly Ca++ was about half of that seen before grafting, or in the control group. However, in the 28 patients who showed acute rejection, T-Ly Ca++ was almost twice the steady-state levels. In vitro IL-2 and IFN-gamma production exhibited a similar behavior. When T-Ly from controls or from uremic patients in the pre-transplantation phase were incubated in vitro with V , a dose-dependent decrease in CA++ concentration and IFN-gamma and IL-2 production was seen. In the KAR, both in the steady-state and at the onset of acute-rejection, in vitro incubation of T-Ly with V induced marked decreases in Ca++ levels for all drug concentrations tested. When maximal doses of V were added to T-Ly from transplanted patients in the steady-state, Ca++, IL-2 and IFN-gamma levels were almost undetectable (Fig. 1).

DISCUSSION

Results show that in KAR treated with Cy-A, tolerance is associated with reduced T-Ly Ca++ levels, and IL-2 and IFN-gamma release, while during acute rejection episodes significantly increased levels occur. Our in vitro studies have demonstrated that V is able to decrease both Ca++ levels in the T-Ly, and the release of IL-2 and IFN-gamma in healthy subjects, in uremic patients before transplantation, and in KAR both in the steady-state and during acute rejection. From this we hypothesize that the in vitro potentiation of the Cy-A mediated immunosuppression induced by V may be due to a direct additive effect on cellular mechanisms that are in some way calcium-dependent (5).

Although further in vitro and in vivo studies are necessary to confirm these data, these results offer a potential therapeutic strategy to decrease the dose of Cy-A needed for effective immuno-suppression, thus lessening its dose-related side effects.

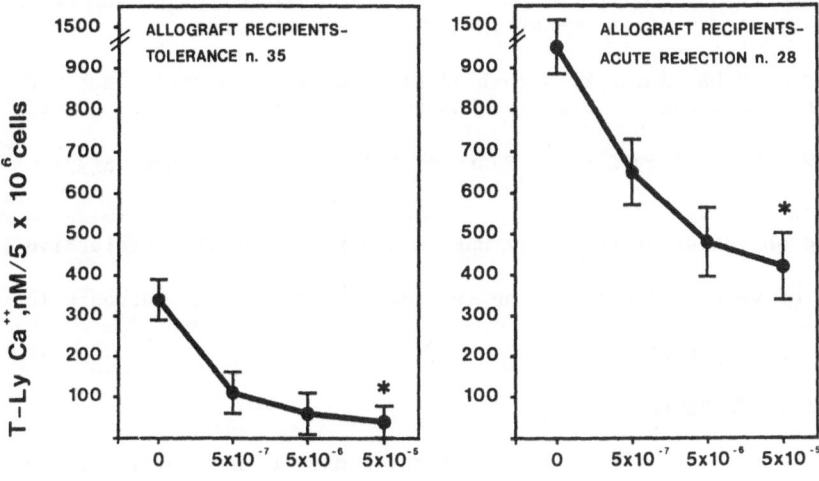

VERAPAMIL CONCENTRATION (M)

* SIGNIFICANTLY DIFFERENT FROM MEAN VALUE OBSERVED WHEN NO VERAPAMIL
WAS ADDED (P<0.05)

Fig. 1. Effects of in vitro incubation with V of T-Ly from KAR both in the steady state and the onset of acute rejection on the cellular concentration of Ca++.

REFERENCES

1.   Hesketh, T.R., Smith, G.A. ann Moore, J.P. J. Immunol. 258: 4876-4880,1983.

2.   Lamperi, S., Carozzi, S.and Nasini,M.G. Transpl. Proc. XIX: 1613-1617, 1987.

3.   Tsien, R.Y., Pozzan, T.and Rink, T.J. J. Cell. Biol. 94: 325-328, 1982.

4.   Gillis, S., Ferm, M.and Ou, M. J Immunol. 120: 2027-2030,1978.

5.   Gelfand, E.W., Cheung, R.K. and Mills G.B. J. Immunol.138: 1115-1120, 1987.

A PROSPECTIVE RANDOMIZED STUDY OF THE PORTECTIVE EFFECT OF VERAPAMIL ON THE ISCHAEMIC RENAL INJURY IN RENAL ALLOTRANSPLANTS.

Mohamed A. Sobh, Ahmed B. Shehab El-Din, Fatma E. Moustafa, Mohamed A. El-Far, Mowafake E. Hussein, Hossam M. Gad and Mohamed A. Ghoneim

Urology & Nephrology Center, Mansoura University, Mansoura, Egypt

The objective of this work was to study the possible protective effect of verapamil against the ischaemic acute tubular necrosis in kidney transplantation.

MATERIALS AND METHODS:

54 consecutive living related donor kidney transplantations were randomly distributed among two groups.Group I cases were given vera-pamil and group II cases served as control.Verpamil was given to the donor during muscle dissection prior to manipulating the renal pedicle, this was given as 5 mg slow I.v. within 10 min., other 5 mg verapamil was added to each 500 ml bottel of graft perfusate. Furthermore, anot-her dose of verapamil was given to the recepient during construction of the vascular anastomosis, this was repeated after 6 hours. Recipie-nts were assessed after kidney transplantation with special stress on:

1. Ischaemia time, diuresis after revascularization
2. Daily urine out put, serum creatinine and, urinary enzyme activity
3. The third post operative day was considered as the end of the study , at that time patients were subjected to Fine Needle Aspiration Biopsy (FNAB) and isotop renal scanning.

RESULTS

In this work, 28 received verapamil(groupI) and 24 served as control(groupII) Acute tubular necrosis was observed in 2 cases in the verapamil treated group (7.1 %) and in 8 cases in the control group

(33.3 %), the difference between the two groups was found to be sta-
tislicaly significant (P=0.049).Haemodialysis was needed in only two
cases,both were in the untreated group.The mean serum creatinine in
the verapamil treated group was 1.42±0.52mg/dl while in the untreated
group it was 2.30±2.26mg/dl, the difference was statisticaly significant (P = 0.027). The mean urine out put value at the third day was
10400±5663 c.c in the verapamil treated group while it was 8083±6649
c.c in the untreated group. The difference was statistically insignificant (P = 0.091). Regarding the urinary enzym NAG activity, there
was significant (P<0.05) difference in enzyme activity between the
two groups. Regarding the isotope scanning of the transplanted kidneys it was observed that there was no significant difference between
the two groups on evaluating the graft/Aorta ratio. Nevertheless,on
on estimating the perfusion index it was highly significant (P=0.014)
better in the verapamil treated group (P.I. = 19.79 ± 8.39%)than in
the non treated group (P.I. = 32.86 ± 16 %).

DISCUSSION

It was reported that treatment with verapamil will protect again-
est acute tubular necrosis in rats and dogs when renal ischaemia is
inflected with noradrenalin or by renal artery clamping (1,2).

In this, work treatment with verapamil resulted in significant protection of the renal transplants against the ischaemic tubular necrosis. The incidence of ATN was 7.1% in the verapamil treated group and
33.3 % in the control group. Further more, the serum creatinine was
significantly lower in the treated than in the control group and the
perfusion index was significantly better in the treated than in the
control group. Similar observations were reported using Diltiazem or
Nifidipine (3,4). Wagner et al (3) adding Diltiazem to Eurocollin's

solution at donor nephrectomy and giving it to the transplant recipients for 2 days post operative, observed a significant reduction in
the incidence of posttransplant ATN. Grekas et al (4) infused Euroco-
llins solution pluse Nifidipine into the left renal artery and placebo
into the right renal artery of dogs, ischaemia was inflected by renal
artery clamping. They observed functional but not morphologic protection against ATN by Nifedipine . In our study verapamil was given to
the donor so as to protect the kidney against ischaemia which may
occure due to renal artery spasm during dissecting the renal pedicle,
another dose was added to the graft perfusate to protect it during the
cold ischaemia, furthermore, two doses were given to the recipients to
protect the graft after reconstruction of the vascular anastomosis as
well as late after reflow. This late protection is important since it
has been reported that during the reflow phase, a further increase in
the cytosolic and mitochondrial calcium concentration leads to cellular and mitochondrial dysfunction and, consequently to progressive
organ damage(5), by perventing the calcium influx during reperfusion,
calcium antagonists could thus preserve renal function.

We have concluded that treatment with verapamil may protect
against the ischaemic ATN after kidney transplantation.

REFERENCES

1. Burke T.J., Arnold P.E., Gordon J.A., Bulger RE, Dobyan D.C.,
   Schrier R.W. J. Clin. Invest. 74 : 1830-1841. 1984

2. Loutzenhister R., Epstein M, Horton C. J. Cardiovasc. Pharmacol 9:
   Suppl. 1,70-75, 1987.

3. Wanger K, Albrecht S, Neumayer H. Am. J. Nephrol. 7:187-291, 1987.

4. Grekas D.M., Kalekou H.N., Christodoulou S., Tourkantions A.
   Nephrol Dial Transpl. 2 : 179-182, 1987.

5. Wilson D.R., Arnold P: Burke Th.J., Schrier R.W. J. Clin. Invest.
   74:1156-1164, 1984.

EFFECTS OF SYSTEMIC ADMINISTRATION OF THE PGE-1 ANALOGUE ALPROSTADIL IN THE EARLY PHASE OF RENAL TRANSPLANTATION.

G. Civati, B. Brando, C. Brunati, M.L. Broggi, G. Busnach, A. Sperandeo*, M. Seveso, E.E. Minetti, L. Minetti.
Dept. of Nephrology, Niguarda-Ca' Granda Hospital, Milano, and *Upjohn S.p.a, Caponago, Italy.

INTRODUCTION

The pathogenesis of acute post-transplant renal failure (ARF) is multifactorial, including the reduction of renal blood flow and the metabolic damage during cold and warm ischemia, causing intracellular depletion of cyclic AMP (cAMP). The advent of Cyclosporine (CSA) has added drug-related mechanisms which contribute to the sustaining of ARF, namely tubular toxicity, endothelial arterial damage and vasoconstriction (1). Rejection occurring during the early phase may further impair the ARF recovery. Prostaglandin (PG) of E series are known to stimulate the cAMP synthesis even with reduced oxygen supply, stabilize cell membrane and lysosome enzyme release, have a marked vasodilator effect, causing renal blood flow redistribution, inhibit platelet aggregation and also exert some immunosuppressive effect acting on T and B cells (2-5). The relationships between CSA and PG metabolism are however still controversial (6, 7), but some studies suggest a beneficial role of PGE on CSA-induced renal damage (8).

The PGE mechanisms of action and the demonstration of their protective effects on organ ischemia in some animal and human models (9, 10), together with the recent availability of stable PGE analogues for human use, have prompted us to study the effects of a PGE-1 derivative, Alprostadil (Prostin VR, Upjohn, Kalamazoo, Mich.) on ARF incidence and outcome and on early renal graft function in man.

PATIENTS AND METHODS

Twenty-three renal transplant patients received 500µg Alprostadil i.v. daily over 12 hours, starting from graft vessels anastomosis, for 4 days (PGE group). Other 23 randomly selected patients served as controls (NPG group). All patients received CSA and Methylprednisolone. Orthoclone OKT 3 antibody was given in case of refractory rejection (for details, see G. Civati et al, this issue). The i.v. protocol included fluids, 400 mg Furosemide and 100 ml 20% Mannitol every 6 hours, to maintain an urinary output of at least 300 ml/h. Diuretics were reduced in case of abundant diuresis. ARF was defined by dialysis requirement.

RESULTS

The following table summarizes our results. Functional data refer to immediately functioning kidneys.

	PGE	NPG	
Age (Years)	41±11	37.6±12	
ARF Incidence	5/23	4/23	P ns
Urine Output (l) Day 1	12.3 ± 6.5	9.8 ± 4.8	P ns
Urine Output (l) Day 2	9.6 ± 4.6	10.6 ± 4	P ns
Urine Output (l) Day 3	8.9 ± 3.8	7.3 ± 3.5	P ns
Furosemide Dose (g) Day 1	0.91 ± 0.65	1.55 ± 0.2	P <0.005
Furosemide Dose (g) Day 2	0.70 ± 0.56	1.42 ± 0.28	P <0.001
Furosemide Dose (g) Day 3	0.56 ± 0.51	1.23 ± 0.42	P <0.001
Mannitol Dose (g) Day 1	57 ± 36	80 ± 0	P <0.05
Mannitol Dose (g) Day 2	18 ± 33	57 ± 36	P <0.005
Mannitol Dose (g) Day 3	0	33 ± 39	P <0.000
Arterial Perfusion Index (U)	205 ± 93	236 ± 139	P ns
CSA BTL (1st Determin.)	289 ± 152	384 ± 177	P ns
Rejections within Day 30	16/23	9/23	P ns
Days to PCreat <2 mg/dl	16.4 ± 16.7	36.5 ± 32.5	P <0.05
PCreat at Day 30 (mg/dl)	1.7 ± 0.7	2.1 ± 0.8	P ns

DISCUSSION

Our results indicate that PGE and NPG patients had a similar ARF incidence (expected rate 22% in our Unit). Therefore, Alprostadil seems not to influence the occurrence of ARF in the recipient once a severe warm ischemic damage has been induced in donor kidneys during coma and surgical procedures. Renal transplant ischemia, however, may be present in the grafted organ in milder form and may account for delayed functional recovery. Alprostadil seems to be effective in such instances, as demonstrated by the significantly lower diuretic requirement, by the shorter time required to reach a PCreat < 2 mg/dl, and maybe by the slightly lower PCreat level at 1 month. Alprostadil does not seem to affect CSA requirement. All patients were given similar daily and cumulative CSA doses, and mean CSA BTL were also similar in both groups. No apparent beneficial effect was observed on rejection incidence. The PGE group had a slightly higher rejection rate during the first month, which should be verified with a larger patient series. No interferences were observed between Alprostadil and Orthoclone OKT3 in the four patients in which it was required.

This study is in progress to evaluate the long-term effects of Alprostadil on graft outcome. A cohoperative study should be designed, in order to evaluate the prophylactic effect on ARF incidence of Alprostadil administration also in the cadaver donors from all organ procurement Centers during coma and organ removal procedures.

REFERENCES
1) Ryffel B, Mihatsch MJ: Transplant Proc 19: 1635, 1987.
2) Horton R, Zipser R, Fichman M: Med Clin N America 65: 891, 1981.
3) Kaufman RP, Kobzik L, Shephro D et al: Ann Surg 205: 195, 1987.
4) Kelly CJ, Zurier RB, Krakauer KA et al: J Clin Invest 79: 782, 1987.
5) Simkin NJ, Jelinek DF, Lipsky PE: J Immunol 138: 1074, 1987.
6) Coffman TM, Carr DR, Yarger WE et al: Transplantation 43: 282, 1987.
7) Jorkasky D, Audet P, Williams S: Transplant Proc 19: 1742, 1987.
8) Ryffel B, Donatsch P, Hiestand P et al: Clin Nephrol 25(S1): 95, 1986.
9) Harjula ALJ, Starkey TD et al: Ann Chir Gynaecol 76: 56, 1987.
10) Koyama I, Neya K, Ueda K et al: Transplant Proc 19: 3542, 1987.

INTERLEUKIN-2 (IL2) PRODUCTION BY PERIPHERAL BLOOD LYMPHOCYTES (PBLS)
IN THE DIAGNOSIS OF RENAL ALLOGRAFT REJECTION (R) IN CYCLOSPORIN
(CsA) TREATED PATIENTS

S. H. BALLAL

Division of Nephrology, Veterans Administration Medical Center and
St. Louis University School of Medicine, St. Louis, Missouri USA

In CsA treated renal allograft recipients R episodes can be
confused with CsA nephrotoxicity. Since rejection causes activation
of T lymphocytes and increase in IL2 production whereas CsA acts to
decrease IL2 production, we evaluated the diagnostic value to serial
IL2 levels produced by lectin stimulated PBLS (Human Immunology 17,
297, 1986) in 15 patients with biopsy proven R [9 acute (AR), 6
chronic (CR)]. In addition, in these patients IL2 levels were
correlated with trough whole blood CsA levels (measured by RIA in
ng/ml, when CsA levels were normal (< 600 ng/ml) and toxic (> 1000
ng/ml). Demographics: Age 21 to 57 years (mean 35 years), 9 males
and 6 females, 10 were cadaver and 5 living related transplants.
IL2 levels increased from 0.26 ± 0.20 to 1.03 ± 0.73 units (u) with R
($p = 0.001$). In AR IL2 increased from 0.20 ± 0.17 to 1.11 ± 0.90 u
($p = 0.01$). In CR IL2 increased from 0.33 ± 0.22 to 0.90 ± 0.40 u
($p = 0.002$). Baseline CsA level was 560 ± 290 and did not change
with R (476 ± 182). IL2 levels at baseline and during R were not
significantly different between the AR and CR groups (0.20 ± 0.17 vs
0.33 ± 0.22 and 1.11 ± 0.90 vs 0.90 ± 0.40 respectively). At normal
(451 ± 168) CsA levels, the IL2 level was 0.22 ± 0.14 u and decreased
to 0.14 ± 0.08 u ($p = 0.05$) with toxic (1271 ± 189) CsA levels.

In conclusion, IL2 levels increased significantly both in AR and
CR but decreased with toxic CsA levels. A rise in IL2 level in the
face of worsening renal function strongly suggests R as compared to
CsA toxicity.

CHANGES OF ANTI-THROMBIN III (AT III), PROTEIN C (PC), AND PROTEIN S (PS) IN RENAL TRANSPLANTATION

K.N. Lai*, J. Yin+, P. Li*, P. Yuen+. Departments of Medicine* and Paediatrics+, The Chinese University of Hong Kong, HONG KONG.

INTRODUCTION

Patients undergoing regular hemodialysis are subjected to a special risk of thrombotic complications related to low plasma AT III and PC during dialysis (1,2). A recent study showed that cyclosporin A [CyA] – treated transplanted patients had a number of hemostatic changes which favor thrombosis (3). Enhanced platelet aggregation with CyA therapy has been suggested to result in the increased thrombotic phenomenon (4). Our present work studied the changes of plasma PC, PS, and AT III in renal transplantation.

METHODS

Five uremic patients on regular hemodialysis receiving living related renal allografts were studied. They were treated with Prednisolone [30 mg/day] and CyA [10 mg/kg/day] during the first two weeks of transplantation. Blood samples were collected before transplantation [pre-dialysis], and regularly at day 2, 7, 30, 100 after renal transplantation.

Plasma samples were collected into anticoagulant mixture and stored at -70°C until assay. Protein S and Protein C related antigens were measured by the sandwich technique of enzyme immunoassay using assay kits [Diagnostica Stago, Asnieres, France]. The anti-thrombin III was measured by amidolytic assay using assay kits [Diagnostica Stago]. The values were expressed as percentage of reference plasma. Urine samples from 2 patients collected before and 2-4 days after renal transplantation were studied for the concentrations of these coagulation inhibitors. Blood samples from 3 patients with nephritis and normal renal function receiving

CyA were obtained during their first 2 weeks of treatment to assess the effect of CyA on PS, PC, and AT III.

RESULTS

All 5 allografts functioned immediately after transplantation. All patients developed significant diuresis [4-10 litres/day] lasting 6-14 days. The mean serum creatinine fell from 870+124 umol/l to 136+34 umol/l within the first two weeks after transplantation. The mean daily urine output increased from 230+63 ml/day during dialysis to 6500+2550 ml/day at one week after transplantation.

Anti-thrombin III in Renal Transplantation

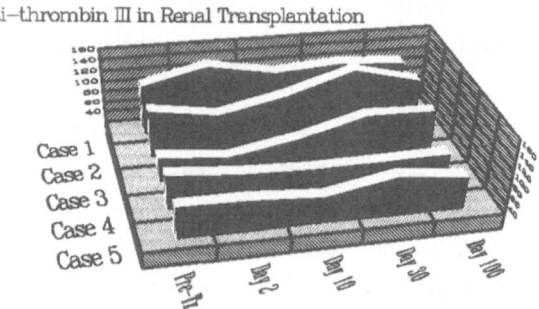

Figure 1.
Changes of AT III in renal transplantation.

Protein C in Renal Transplantation

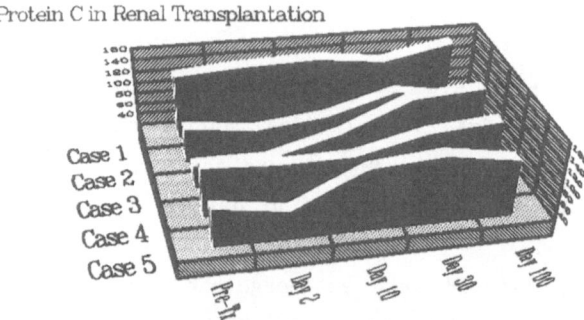

Figure 2.
Changes of Protein C in renal transplantation.

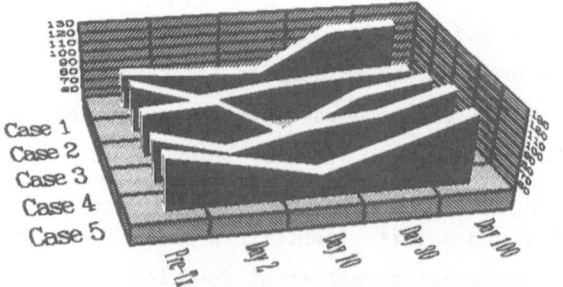

Figure 3.
Changes of Protein S in renal transplantation.

Protein S in Renal Transplantation

The mean pre-transplantation PS, PC, and AT III were similar to the control although the number of patients was too small for proper statistical assessment. A transient fall of plasma PS and PC was observed during the first week after transplantation. Similar fall of AT III was observed in 4 of the 5 patients. A progressive rise of plasma PS, PC, and AT III was observed at 4th and 14th weeks after transplantation with values 19%, 40%, and 13% respectively higher than the values measured during the period of maintenance dialysis therapy. The urinary concentrations of PS, PC, and AT III were similar before and after transplantation but their daily losses were manifold higher due to marked diuresis. No obvious changes in PS, PC, and AT III were observed in the three patients after two weeks of CyA therapy.

DISCUSSION

In our study we have observed an initial reduction of plasma PS, PC, and AT III during the first week after renal transplantation with good functioning allografts. Despite the small number of patients studied, a consistent overall pattern is definitely demonstrated in these patients. The fall in the plasma inhibitors of coagulation is believed to be due to urinary loss related to massive diuresis following acute tubular necrosis in the allograft. The loss could be up to 50 times the normal urinary loss prior to transplantation. CyA was less likely to be responsible for reduced plasma PS, PC, and AT III as similar changes of plasma coagulation inhibitors were not observed in nephritic patients receiving CyA. Furthermore, a progressive rise of these plasma proteins was evident when acute tubular necrosis subsided while the patients continued to receive CyA for anti-rejection therapy. In conclusion, our study suggests PS, PC, and AT III increased with functioning renal allograft but a potential risk of increased thromboembolism could occur during early post-transplantation period due to massive urinary loss of such plasma coagulation inhibitors.

REFERENCES
1. Brandt, P., Jespersen, J., Sorensen L. Nephron 1981; 28: 1-3.
2. Alegre, A.. et al. Nephron 1987; 46: 386-387.
3. Vanrenterghem, Y. et al. Lancet 1985; 1: 999-1002.
4. Grace, A. et al. Kidney Int 1987; 32: 889-895.

KAPOSI'S SARCOMA AFTER KIDNEY TRANSPLANTATION, AN ETIOLOGIC STUDY AND SUCCESSFUL TREATMENT.

M. SOBH, F. Moustafa, A. Shehab El Din, H. Abd El Ghafar, M. Abd El. Razic, H. Mowafi, G. El Wehidi, M. Ghoniem.

Urology And Nephrology Center, Mansoura University, Egypt.

MATERIALS AND METHODS

Kidney transplant recipients under follow up were examined and those with suspecious lesions for Kaposi's Sarcoma(K.S) were subjected to:

1. <u>Histopathologic Examination</u> 2. <u>Clinical Assessment</u> 3. <u>Virologic work-up</u> (HBs Ag, Epestien Barr virus, CMV and HIV).

4. <u>Evaluation of patients immune competence</u> :

a- Skin reactivity to Dinitro Chloro Benzene (DNCB). b- Antibody Dependent Cell mediated Cytotoxicity (ADCC). c- Natural Killer cell (NK). d) Lymphocyte proliferation in response to mitogens. e- T-cell Subsets : OKT_3, OKT_4 & OKT_8.

5. <u>Determination of the patients HLA - DR typing</u>.

6. <u>Therapeutic approaches</u> :

a) Modification of the immune suppressive regimen : This was done either by immediate arrest of azathioprine and/or ciclosporin as well as rapid withdrawal of the prednisolone in rapidly progressive life endangering cases. In cases with mild to moderate lesions, only variable degrees of reduction of immuno suppressive drugs was performed. b) Cytotoxic drugs : Vincristine was given in life endangering cases. c) Superficial irradiation: When there was no satisfactory response to simple reduction of immuno suppressive drugs. g) Intralesional injection of bleomycin sulphate:For residual lesions.

RESULTS

Out of 250 patients with renal allografts ,Seven cases were found

to be suffering from K.S.(2.8%). Time of discovery of the tumour
following kidney transplantation varied from 3 to 15 months. Prior to
discovery of the tumour four patients were under triple immuno
suppression, two were given ciclosporin plus prednisolone and one was
treated by prednizolone and azathioprine. All had been subjected to at
least one histologically proven rejection episode and all except one
patient had perfect graft function.

Two types of presentations with K.S. were observed in our cases :
1. Oropharyngeal K.S.:(two cases)Developed rapidly with lesions
related to the gum, floor of the mouth and the soft palate cervical
lymphadenopathy. 2.Cutaneous K.S.(five cases)these were multicentric
reddish blue,indurated nodules or plaques confined to the lower limbs.

Hislopathologic Evaluation :

It revealed ill defined areas in the dermis formed of multiple
thin walled capillaries lined by plump endothelial cells and in between these capillaries exist fusiform cells running in different
directions, the degree of mitosis among these fusiform cells was not
so marked.

Virologic, genetic and immunologic evaluations :

These cases were negative for HBsAg, CMV, EbV and HlV.

HLA typing of six patients showed presence of $HLA-A_1 \& DR_5$ in four
patients (The A_1 in the general Egyptian population being 20% and
DR_5 is 6.1%) ($P < 0.05$). Skin testing using DNCB showed that those
who later on developed K.S. were all non responders. T lymphocyte
subsets analysis showed reduced T_4/T_8 (0.9-1.2) Furthermore, there was
always significant reduction in the NK and the ADCC activities while
the response to mitogen was variable.

Response to treatment :

In the first two cases with aggressive oropharyngial K.S., the tumour showed rapid complete regression within 3-4 months. In cases with cutaneous K.S., there was partial ($\pm$ 30%) reduction in the tumour in two cases. These two patients were subjected to superficial irradiation which was followed by complete resolution of the tumour in one case, while the other showed some residual lesions. The remaining three cases, showed regression of the tumour 3-6 months after simple reduction of the immuno supperssive drugs with some residual lesions in one of them. The residual lesions were treated by intralesional bleomycin therapy.

DISCUSSION AND CONCLUSION

Penn I, 1981 (1) reported an over all incidence of K.S. of 0.06-0.4 % for whole kidney transplant recipients. In our series we discovered seven cases ammong 250 Egyptian kidney transplant recipients under follow up, making an incidence of 2.8% which is very high.

We have concluded that K.S. is more common among Egyptian kidney transplant recipients, racial and genetic predisposing factors are probably working, lack of immune survillance is an important factor in the pathogenesis of the disease, regression of the tumour can be achieved without sacrifying the graft even in the severe oropharyngeal cases.

REFERENCES

1. Penn I. : Transplant Proc., 11 : 1047-1051, 1979.

RENAL ARTERIAL STENOSIS IN RENAL TRANSPLANTATION:
A MATHEMATICAL PATHOGENETIC HYPOTHESIS AND ITS POSSIBLE
CLINICAL IMPLICATIONS

Colì L., Pallotti G.*, Pettazzoni P.*,Gaviani G.*,
Buscaroli A., Stefoni S., Campieri C., Bonomini V.

Institute of Nephrology and *Department of Physics,
University of Bologna

The pathogenesis of the renal artery stenosis in renal
transplantation is not yet completely clear. A possible
role may be played by the impaired progression of the
sphigmic wave and of the blood pulse at the point of the
vascular anastomosis, caused by an anastomosis between two
artery segments with different straining characteristics
(1).

The factors influencing the artery straining are mainly
the microvascular lesions following surgery, the
immunological reactions, the aging structural involvement
and the degenerative processes (atherosclerosis)(2,3). In
particular the biological aging produces a progressive
lack in the resilience and straining properties of the
arterial wall and consequently an alteration of the
elastic response to the sphigmic wave and the blood pulse.
In kidney grafting, the age gap between donor and
recipient is often considerable, and so the vascular
anastomosis is characterized by different straining
properties of the two artery segments (4).

This study regards a mathematical elaboration of a
pathogenetic hypothesis: the straining properties of an
artery wall are mathematically expressed by the impedance
(Z) formula:

$$z(v) = \sqrt{r^2 + \left(m\,\omega - K/\omega\right)^2}$$

where m is the fluid mass, K is the elastic constant, and r expresses the damping properties of the system (v is the frequency and ω the period of the pulsation).

The different biomechanical impedance between donor (Z_1) and recipient (Z_2) arteries, generates a discontinuity on the artery wall, and only a part of the incident blood energy intensity can be transmitted across the anastomosis, whereas the remainder of energy intensity is reflected by the system. The amount of blood energy reflected by the system depends on the difference in mechanical impedance ($Z_1 - Z_2$) between the two arterial walls:

$$I_t = I_o \frac{4\,Z_1\,Z_2}{(Z_1 + Z_2)^2}$$

$$I_r = I_o \frac{(Z_1 - Z_2)^2}{(Z_1 + Z_2)^2}$$

where I_o, I_t, I_r are respectively the incident, the transmitted and the reflected intensity. If the difference ($Z_1 - Z_2$) is negligible nearly all the energy crosses the suture; if it is not negligible, the energy transmitted is smaller than the reflected. In this case the blood flow loses its laminar characteristics and generates turbulent fluxes, which may cause vascular complications (5).

To support with clinical data this pathogenetic hypothesis, considering that the main factor influencing the vascular difference impedance between recipient and donor is patient's age, we made a retrospective study on 132 Renal transplants, performed in the Department of Nephrology of the University of Bologna, in the period from 1982 to 1985.

The patients were divided into 2 groups: the first group

included 61 patients with donor/recipient age difference ≥ 15 years; the second group included 71 patients with donor/recipient age difference < 15 years. In the first group 6 cases of artery stenosis, corresponding to 9,8 % appeared; no cases in the second group; the difference was statistically significant (p<0.025).

We can conclude: 1) The mathematical model described, shows that factors favouring artery stenosis (turbulent fluxes) can be caused by the great difference between the impedance in the two anastomotic segments. 2) The clinical data confirm that the impedance difference is strictly correlated with the donor/recipient age.gap 3) It would be advisable to avoid, when even possible, a great age gap between donor and recipient at the moment of the choice of the graft recipients.

Supported in part by grant 60% MPI

REFERENCES:
1. Bonomini,V. Fifth International Conference on Mechanics in Medicine and Biology, Bologna, July 1-5 1986 ; pp.387-389
2. Doyle, T.J., McGregor, W.R., Fox, P.S., Maddison, R.E., Rogers, R.E., Kaufmann, H.M. Surgery 77: 53, 1975
3. Ricotta, J.J., Shaff, H.V., Williams, G.M., Rolley, R.J., Whelyon, P.K., Harrington, D.M. Surgery 84: 595, 1978
4. Grossman, R.A., Defoe, D.C., Schoenfeld, R.B. Transplantation; 34:339-343, 1982
5. Perrucca E. in:Fisica generale e sperimentale, Volume I, pp.135-145; Torino 1949

"RENAL FUNCTIONAL RESERVE" IN RENAL TRANSPLANT PATIENTS
ON CYCLOSPORINE THERAPY.

Papa A., Fuiano G., Lotito M.A., Rampino T., Campolo G.,
Pacchiano G., Imperatore P., Memoli B., Libetta C.,
Reggio R., Milone D., Andreucci V.E.

Dept. of Nephrology, 2nd Faculty of Medicine, Napoli
(Italy).

The increase in glomerular filtration rate (GFR) due
to afferent and efferent arterioles vasodilation induced
by protein-load or aminoacids and/or dopamine is termed
"Renal Functional Reserve" (RFR). The simultaneous
infusion of aminoacids and dopamine has been showed to
be additive in their effects on GFR (1).

RFR has been demonstred in healthy subjects and in
patients with different renal diseases, but only with
initial degrees (GFR > 50 ml/min) of renal
insufficiency. Aim of this study was to estabilish if
any RFR exists in transplanted patients on Cyclosporine
A therapy.

PATIENTS AND METHODS.
The study was carried out on seven renal transplanted
patients, who had received the graft 4-30 months prior
to the study. All patients were on immunosuppressive
therapy with prednisone (10-17.5 mg/day) and
cyclosporine (3.5-7.8 mg/Kg/day); three received also
azathioprine (50-150 mg/day). Renal function (as
assessed by creatinine clearance twice a month) was
steady in all. Mean age was 34.1 years (range: 23-64).
Experimental design: briefly, in all patients a moderate
water diuresis was induced by mouth and

maintained by 5% glucose infusion. Inulin and PAH were also infused. After 60 minutes of stabilization, 3 control clearances were performed. At this point, an infusion of aminoacids (4 ml/min of a 7.5% solution) and dopamine (2 µg/Kg/min) was started. After an additional 1 hour period of stabilization three experimental 30-minutes clearances were performed.

RESULTS.

Renal plasma flow, as assessed by PAH clearance, increased moderately in 4 patients and markedly in 3. GFR also increased parallely to RPF. Mean percent increase of RPF was 16.1 ± 15.4 SD (p < 0.05 vs basal); GFR increased by 22.4 ± 24 %. (p < 0.05 vs basal). Individual data of GFR and RPF are plotted in Fig 1 and 2.

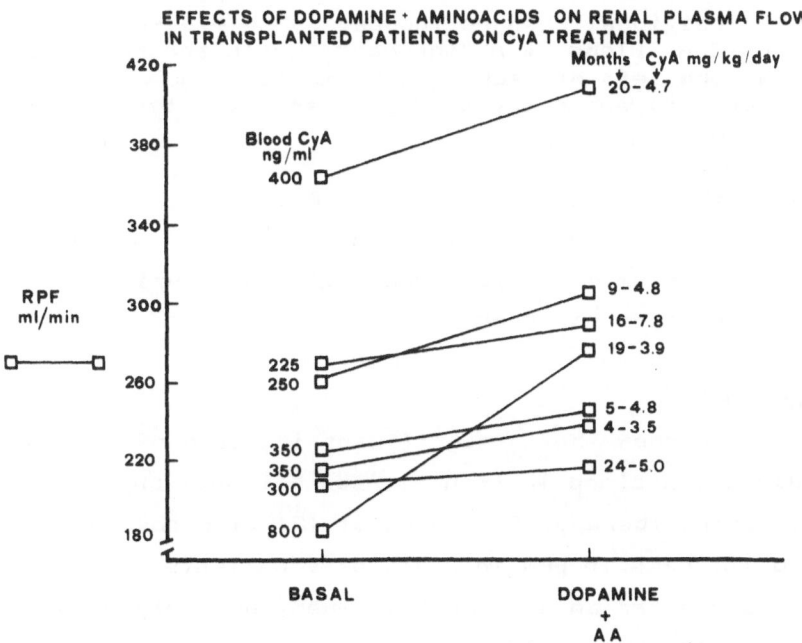

EFFECTS OF DOPAMINE + AMINOACIDS ON RENAL PLASMA FLOW
IN TRANSPLANTED PATIENTS ON CyA TREATMENT

Fig1. Individual changes induced by AA + D infusion on RPF. Blood Cy A "through" levels are reported on the left of each line; time to tranplant (months) and daily Cy dosage are reported on the right.

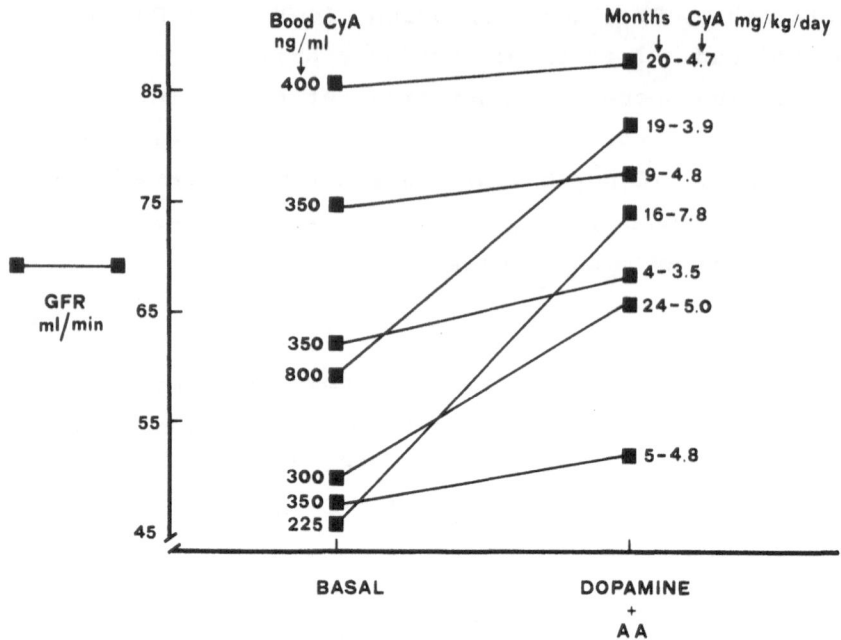

Fig. 2. Individual changes induced by AA + D infusion
on GFR. Blood Cy A "through" levels are reported
on the left of each line; time to tranplant
(months) and daily Cy dosage are reported on the
right.

Due to the similar increase of GFR and RPF,
filtration fraction did not change after AA + D. No
change of sodium excretion (UNa x V) and of urinary
sodium excretion occurred.

CONCLUSIONS

Our data show that a significant increase of RPF and
GFR can be obtained in transplanted patients on
Cyclosporine therapy. Dhaene et al (2) also observed a
marked increase in GFR in 3 out of 7 patients studied
before and after an oral protein load, but only 3 were
on Cy and the basal GFR was greater than in our
patients.

Mean basal GFR of our patients was 61 ml/min (range

48-86): therefore our patient had a mild to moderate
renal insufficiency: with similar values of GFR, no or
poor improvement of renal function was reported by
other authors (1)(3) . Consequentely, other factors could
influence the significant rise of the GFR observed in
our patients. Since Cy A is well known to cause renal
vasconstrictive effects it is reasonable to ascribe the
observed increase of GFR to the reversion of such
effects induced by AA and D. Moreover, since an
increment of RPF and GFR was observed unrespectively of
the time to transplant, the negative effects of Cy on
renal function appear to be still present and
reversible also after long time from the transplant.

REFERENCES

1.ter Wee,P.M., Rosman,J.B., van der Geest ,S., Sluiter
  W.J., Donker ,A.J.M. Kidney Int. 29: 870-874, 1986.
2.Dhaene,M., Sabot,JP. Philippart ,Y., Doutrelepont ,J.
  M., Vanherweghem, J.L., Toussaint, C.,. Nephron, 44:
  157-158, 1986.
3.ter Wee,P.M., Smit ,A.J., Rosman, J.B., Sluiter,
  W.J., Donker, A.J.M. Am J. Nephrol. 6: 42-46, 1986.

V. CYCLOSPORINE

Drug Interaction

S A N D I M M U N®/ AN APPRAISAL OF DRUG INTERACTIONS

I.T.R. COCKBURN, P. KRUPP
Drug Monitoring Centre, Sandoz Ltd., 4002 Basle, Switzerland

INTRODUCTION

During the last five years many papers have been published summarising the more significant drug interactions observed with the use of Sandimmun (Cs) in animals and man (1-9). The Drug Monitoring Centre (DMC) of Sandoz Basle has monitored all information concerning this topic. Sources of data are the medical literature, the on-going post-marketing surveillance (PMS) study and spontaneous reports. Although the exact mechanisms for many interactions reported for Cs are still not understood, at least some can be explained either by alterations in absorption, metabolism or elimination or from deviation of expected pharmacological effects. The clinical outcome may vary from a minor disturbance requiring dose adjustment to more major consequences including nephrotoxicity or graft rejection. This paper summarises the results from this compilation.

PHARMACOKINETICS

Cs is a highly lipid soluble cyclic polypeptide consisting of 11 aminoacids. It is formulated either in ethanol and polyoxyethylated castor oil for the intravenous composition or in ethanol, polyoxyethylated glycerides and olive or maize oil for the oral solution or capsules. Following oral administration peak blood concentrations are achieved within 1-6 hours; the absolute bioavailability has an inter-individual variability of 20-50% at steady state (10,11). Cs is largely distributed outside the blood volume, in the plasma approximately 90% is bound to proteins, mostly lipoproteins, and in the blood 41-58% is contained within erythrocytes (7,12). Experiences from animal and clinical work have led to the conclusion that Cs is largely metabolised by the hepatic monooxygenase system including cytochrome P-450. The main route of elimination is biliary secretion, with only 6% of the oral dose excreted in the urine (10), and it appears that the parent compound does not undergo enterohepatic recycling (13).

CONSEQUENCES OF DRUG INTERACTIONS

The frequency of reports concerning interactions with Cs is continuously increasing. Those interactions in which a clear underlying mechanism has been demonstrated or confirmed by subsequent reports are classified as "substantiated" and labelled in the product literature. All other interactions are classified as "suspected". Any further information concerning these latter interactions are individually considered and reclassification is implemented where appropriate.

As Cs is mostly metabolised by the hepatic monooxygenase system, in particular cytochrome P-450, inducers or suppressors of cytochrome P-450 will be expected to correspondingly reduce or increase Cs concentration. It has been reported that P-450 inducers (a) may reduce the concentration/dose ratio of Cs, (b) reduced Cs concentration may become evident after approximately 48 hours and (c) Cs concentration will normalise after discontinuation of a P-450 inducer after a period of 2-3 weeks (14).

Conversely, those agents known to inhibit hepatic metabolism or Cs, usually by competitive effects on microsomal enzymes including cytochrome P-450, will be expected to increase Cs concentration by a reduction of metabolism.

In considering the likely clinical implication of interactions with Cs, drugs are further sub-categorised according to their primary effects:

(1) Increase of Cs concentration

(2) Decrease of Cs concentration

(3) Additive nephrotoxicity

(4) Miscellaneous

Substantiated drug interactions

Table 1 summarises those interactions that have become, in the course of time, substantiated by the weight of clinical experience or corroboratory evidence.

Drugs increasing the concentration of Cs. The **calcium channel antagonists** **nicardipine** (17-17), **verapamil** (18) and **diltiazem** (19-22) have been shown to increase Cs concentration by interfering with hepatic metabolism. Diltiazem has an apparent direct inhibitory effect on cytochrome P-450 (21). However, this increased Cs concentration could be demonstrated by radioimmunoassay (RIA) but not by high pressure liquid chromatography (HPLC) suggestive of different effects on the parent compound and its metabolites (22).

Corticosteroid preparations including **prednisolone** and **methyl-prednisolone** are often used conjointly with Cs. Cs has been shown to potentiate prednisolone therapy by reducing clearance (23), or conversely during high-dose steroidal therapy the clearance of Cs may be increased, whereby it was recommended that HPLC should be used instead of RIA because of the accompanying rapid clearance of Cs metabolites (24). One centre, however, has reported that, at least for a short period after transplantation, patients have a normal metabolism of prednisolone when receiving Cs (25).

There is clear evidence from dechallenge and rechallenge of a single well documented spontaneous report that **doxycycline** increases the Cs concentration during concomitant administration.

The increase in Cs concentration, occasionally to dangerous levels, has been frequently reported after the concomitant administration of **ketoconazole** (26-32). Although most authors have suggested that this is a result of cytochrome P-450 induction, one group has noted changes in the distribution of Cs by competitive competition for cell binding sites (32). However, it has been noted that it is safe to combine Cs with ketoconazole as long as there is an appropriate reduction in Cs dosage (33). An interesting finding was the observation of increased immunosuppression in mice (as measured by a delayed hypersensitivity response) receiving Cs and ketoconazole (34).

Several papers have described an increased concentration of Cs during the concomitant administration of macrolide antibiotics including **erythromycin** (35-47) and **josamycin** (48). Originally it was felt that this may have been the end-result of either an interference with hepatic metabolism (35,37, 39,42) or a direct inhibition of cytochrome P-450 (45). Recently it has been noted that erythromycin also increases the area under the curve (AUC) in the pharmacokinetic profile (41,43,46,47). This evidence of an increase in absorption or alteration in the apparent volume of distribution (44) is currently unexplained, but it has been proposed that the undesirable increase in Cs concentration may be avoided by reducing the dosage of Cs in those patients who must by necessity receive erythromycin (47).

Androgenic steroids including **levonorgestrel** (49,50), **danazol** or **norethisterone** (51) and **methyltestosterone** (52) have all been shown to increase Cs concentration. As oral contraceptive steroids are weak inhibitors of hepatic microsomal enzymes, this may be a possible mechanism of action. Those interactions reported with levonorgestrel were also shown to have an accompanying increase in hepatic enzymes (49,50).

Drugs reducing the concentration of Cs. One of the best known inducers of cytochrome P-450 are the **barbiturates** and their **derivatives.** It is not surprising, therefore, that there have been publications referring to the same, including **phenobarbitone** (53,54). Another anticonvulsant, **valproic acid**, has also been shown to reduce Cs concentration (55).

Although it had been shown that **phenytoin** may reduce Cs concentration (56), presumably by an increased metabolism of Cs cytochrome P-450 (14), it now appears that phenytoin may decrease Cs concentration not by enzyme induction but by decreasing absorption and thereby bioavailability (57). No explanation has been offered for this finding.

Similarly decreased concentration of Cs has been observed with **carbamazepine,** another known cytochrome P-450 inhibitor (58).

In three individual well documented spontaneous reports, **metamizole**, an active component of the antipyretic agent Novalgin, has been shown in each case to decrease the concentration of Cs during concomitant administration.

In one publication it has been shown that **nafcillin** can decrease the Cs concentration in renal transplant recipients (59). As this semi-synthetic penicillin is primarily eliminated by hepatic inactivation, the suggested mechanism has been that of an enhanced Cs hepatic clearance due to cytochrome P-450 enzyme induction. Nafcillin has also been shown to enhance warfarin elimination through hepatic microsomal enzyme induction (60).

The antituberculous drug **rifampicin** is known to induce hepatic microsomal enzymes. There have been reports of rifampicin causing reduction in Cs concentration (61-65) with further evidence of decreased bioavailability (64) or an increased rate of elimination of Cs (65).

Several papers have described a significant decrease in Cs concentration during concomitant intravenous administration of **sulphadimine** with or without **trimethoprim** (66-68).

Drugs causing additive nephrotoxicity. Those agents known either to have direct nephrotoxic effects or synergistically interact with Cs at the level of the nephron, thereby increasing the potential of nephrotoxicity, should be used with extreme caution in patients receiving Cs.

There have been warnings concerning the use of **aminoglycosides** in Cs-treated patients (69), and there has been evidence of severe nephrotoxicity when Cs is given concomitantly with **gentamycin** (70). Cs-treated patients who received **amphotericin B** were also noted to develop increased nephrotoxicity (71).

The antimitotic agent **melphalan** has been shown to have an additive nephrotoxic effect with Cs, with an elevation of serum creatinine (72).

A marked but reversible deterioration in renal function has been reported in CS-treated patients receiving **trimethoprim** either singly or in combination with **sulphamethoxazole (co-trimoxazole)** (73-75).

Miscellaneous interactions. It is well established that both Cs and **nifedipine** can cause gingival hyperplasia. It is therefore not surprising that an increased incidence of gingival hyperplasia has been observed when the two drugs are given together (76,77). It is still unclear whether this is an additive or synergistic effect.

Suspected drug interactions

Table 2 summarises those interactions which have not yet been validated.

Drugs increasing the concentration of Cs. It has been noted in a single publication that patients given a heavy intake of **alcohol** developed an increased concentration of Cs (77). Those patients with a light to moderate intake of alcohol had no disturbance of their Cs concentration.

In one poorly documented spontaneous report an apparent increase in Cs concentration was observed during the concomitant administration of **acetazolamide**. No further information was available to substantiate this claim.

A single poorly documented spontaneous report concerning **coumarin** and later a paper referring to **warfarin** (78) have both described an increased Cs concentration, and in the latter case a decrease in efficacy of warfarin, during administration of these agents to Cs recipients.

In another poorly documented spontaneous report it was suggested that **dioctyl sodium sulfosuccinate** had caused an apparent increase in Cs concentration. Further information was unavailable.

Several unpublished spontaneous reports have suggested that Cs clearance is decreased by the concomitant use of the H2-antagonist **cimetidine** and that as a consequence the Cs concentration may be expected to show an increase. There has been another spontaneous report suggesting that **ranitidine**, another H2-antagonist, increased the risk of nephrotoxicity in Cs-treated renal transplant recipients. Conflicting results have been published. It was described that cimetidine does not alter the pharmacokinetics of Cs (79) and that ranitidine can be used without risk in the treatment and prevention of peptic ulcer in renal transplant patients immunosuppressed with Cs (80). Deleterious effects on blood concentration of Cs and creatinine have been reported for some renal and cardiac transplant recipients receiving concomitantly Cs and an H2-antagonist (81).

Although the beta-lactam antibiotic **imipenem** given in conjuction with **cilastatin** has also been described as increasing Cs concentration by inhibiting hepatic metabolism (82), a partial degree of nephroprotectivity from this combination has also been reported (83).

Less understood, however, is the increased concentration of Cs which was noted with changes in absorption and distribution for **itraconazole** (84). It has been suggested that the metabolites of itraconazole may interfere with Cs metabolism (85), but in another paper there is an apparent lack of interaction between itraconazole and Cs (86).

It has been reported that **metoclopramide** can increase the bioavailability of Cs and thereby increase Cs concentration by altering gastric transit time (87).

According to a single well documented spontaneous report the quinolone derivative **norfloxacin** increases Cs concentration. This drug has been shown previously to inhibit cytochrome P-450 metabolism of theophyllin, and therefore this competitive inhibition may be the mechanism of action for this reported interaction. **Pristinamycin**, a depsipeptide antibiotic with a structural similarity to macrolides (88), has been shown to increase Cs concentration by a presumed inhibition of hepatic metabolism. **Ticarcillin**, a penicillin derivative, was noted to cause an increase in Cs concentration, confirmed by dechallenge and rechallenge, in a single spontaneous report.

Two other spontaneous reports described increased Cs concentrations during concomitant administration of either **pentazocine** or **tamoxifen**. No further information is available to substantiate these interactions.

Drugs reducing the concentration of Cs. Some anticonvulsants including **mesuximide** and **primidone** have been reported spontaneously as decreasing Cs concentration, presumably by induction of cytochrome P-450.

The beta-antagonist **metoprolol** has been shown in a group of patients with end-stage renal failure to reduce the median plasma Cs concentration without altering the overall profile of the plasma Cs curve (89).

In a single poorly documented spontaneous report an apparent reduction in the concentration of Cs with subsequent normalisation after the introduction and discontinuation of **omeprazole** in a Cs recipient was described.

The somatostatin analogue **Sandostatin** is a potent inhibitor of pancreatic exocrine function. The resultant inhibition or delay of fat absorption arising from the use of such analogues probably explains the reduced Cs concentration which has been observed in renal and pancreatic transplant recipients (90,91).

The uricosuric agent **sulfinpyrazone**, a phenylbutazone analogue, was reported to have caused a threefold increase of Cs blood concentration after its discontinuation in a Cs recipient (92). It was proposed that this agent may have interfered with Cs assays. No other similar reports have been received.

Drugs causing additive nephrotoxicity. An additive nephrotoxic effect has been reported both with **acyclovir** (93) and **ganciclovir** (94).

An enhancement of **adriamycin**-induced proteinuria in rats receiving Cs has been reported (95).

In two spontaneous reports **captopril** was described as causing an increased serum creatinine concentration in two patients on Cs therapy.

In several spontaneous, poorly documented reports There have been suggestions that an elevation of serum creatinine may be expected in Cs recipients during the concomitant administration of the cephalosporines **ceftazidine** or **latamoxef**. However, in a single publication it has been published that ceftazidine does not affect the serum creatinine in Cs recipients (96).

Although it is established that **digoxin** can interact with many other drugs, there has been only one publication of increased digoxin toxicity accompanied by acute renal failure in cardiac transplant recipients receiving digoxin and Cs concomitantly (97). The authors proposed that these changes were due to alterations in the apparent volume of distribution of digoxin.

The anti-arrhythmic agent **disopyramide** has been noted to cause an increase in serum creatinine concentration (98). Whether this was due to haemodynamic changes of renal vascular flow compounding Cs nephrotoxicity is yet to be established.

It can be understood that patients whose kidneys are already under stress either from Cs toxicity or other aetiology may suffer additive effects from diuretics. Although diuretics are frequently used in transplanted patients receiving Cs, there have only been two papers referring to deterioration in renal function while receiving either **metolazone** (99) or **furosemide** (100).

It is postulated that prostaglandin depletion plays a role in the development of acute nephrotoxicity from Cs. Therefore **non-steroidal anti-inflammatory drugs** (NSAID), which deplete prostaglandins by cyclooxygenase inhibition, will enhance Cs toxicity, and this hypothesis has been supported by animal studies with either

indomethacin (101) or **diclofenac** (102).

Miscellaneous interactions. The precise immmunological action of Cs is still not fully understood. In the case of **verapamil** it is interesting to note that there is a potentiation of the immuno-suppressive action of Cs (103, 104), which results from inhibition of the protein kinase C-mediated events in lymphocyte activation (105). The reported synergistic effects of increased immunosuppression after combining Cs with certain agents including **etoposide** (101,106) and **mizoribine** (107) will need further investigation. The synergistic effect of **etoposide** has been shown to be similar to that observed with calcium antagonists (verapamil) or with **anti-anticalmodulin agents** (106). A synergism between **1,25-dihydroxyvitamin D3** (vitamin D3) and Cs with regard to thymidine incorporation of IL-2 production has been demonstrated, but this effect requires validation for its clinical implication (108).

Although a precautionary warning concerning a potential "antabuse" or facial flushing effect with the ethanol excipient of the i.v. formulation of Cs has been published (98), no other reports, either spontaneous or from the medical literature, have been received to substantiate this claim.

In a recent publication it has been suggested that the incidence of myopathy among recipients of **lovastatin** may be increased in cardiac transplant recipients receiving Cs (109). Although this interaction has not been formally studied, it would appear appropriate to monitor creatinine phosphokinase in patients receiving both drugs.

A previously unreported potentiation of the action of a neuromuscular blocking agent, **atracuronium**, possibly due to an interaction with the solvent of Cs, Cremophor EL, has been described in some experiments in cats (110). No mechanism is available to explain this effect, and no such effects have been reported in man.

CONCLUSION

Whereas initially most interactions were thought to be due to an interference with the metabolism of Sandimmun, other mechanisms of action have recently been proposed, including effects on absorption, distribution, renal function and immunomodulation. However, it is clear that any drug that induces or inhibits cytochrome P-450 or has deleterious effects on renal function will either interfere with Cs elimination or have additive effects on Cs nephrotoxicity.

Those drugs considered as "substantiated" in their potential to interact with Cs are labelled in the product literature. The process of the addition of new drugs to those known to interact with Cs is a continuous one, necessitating persistent review of all potential sources of data. Although "suspected" interactions are not currently included in the product literature, they are discussed in this review as they may become clinically relevant in the future.

When prescribing drugs known or potentially liable to interact with Cs the clinician should be aware of the possible consequences:

(1) The bioavailability of Cs may be altered and therefore regular monitoring of Cs concentration, particularly during the introduction or withdrawal of the drug, is required.

(2) When prescribing drugs with a known nephrotoxic potential there is a risk of an additive effect with Cs. During periods of concomitant administration parameters of renal function, for example serum creatinine, should be closely monitored.

(3) Certain drugs may potentiate the immunosuppressive effect of Cs, resulting in the development of risks inherent to over-immuno-suppression. The dosage of Cs during this period should be carefully adjusted to minimise this risk.

TABLE 1

SANDIMMUN: SUBSTANTIATED DRUG INTERACTIONS / CONSEQUENCES

Drugs Increasing the Concentration of Cs	Drugs Reducing the Concentration of Cs	Drugs Causing Additive Nephrotoxicity	Miscellaneous (Described Effect)
Calcium channel antagonists (incl. diltiazem, nicardipine, verapamil)	Barbiturates & derivatives (incl. phenytoin and phenobarbitone)	Aminoglycosides (incl. gentamycin and tobramycin)	Nifedipine (gingival hyperplasia)
Corticosteroids (incl. prednisolone and methylprednisolone)	Carbamazepine	Amphotericin B	
	Metamizole	Melphalan	
Doxycycline	Nafcillin	Trimethoprim (incl. co-trimoxazole)	
Ketoconazole	Rifampicin		
Macrolide antibiotics (incl. erythromycin and josamycin)	Sulphadimidine with trimethoprim (i.v.)		
Oral contraceptives/ Androgenic steroids (incl. danazol, levo- norgestrel, northisterone)			

TABLE 2

SANDIMMUN: SUSPECTED DRUG INTERACTIONS / CONSEQUENCES

Drugs Increasing the Concentration of Cs	Drugs Reducing the Concentration of Cs	Drugs Causing Additive Nephrotoxicity	Miscellaneous (Described Effect)
Alcohol (heavy intake)	Anticonvulsants, others (incl. mesuximide, primidone)	Acyclovir (incl. ganciclovir)	1,25 Dihydroxyvitamin D3 (immunomodulation)
Acetazolamide	Metoprolol	Adriamycin	
Coumarin anticoagulants (incl. dicoumarin, warfarin)	Omeprazole	Captopril	Atracuronium (potentiation of neuromuscular blocking)
Dioctyl sodium sulfosuccinate	Somatostatin analogues	Cephalosporins (incl. ceftazidine and latamoxef)	
H2-antagonists (incl. cimetidine and ranitidine)	Sulfinpyrazone	Digoxin	Chlorpropamide/disulfiram/ metronidazole (antabuse-effect)
Imipenem/cilastatin		Disopyramide	
Itraconazole		Furosemide	
Metoclopramide		Metolazone	Etoposide (immunomodulation)
Norfloxacin		NSAID's (incl. diclofenac and indomethacin)	
Pentazocine			Lovastatin (myopathy)
Pristinamycin			
Tamoxifen			Mizoribine (immunomodulation)
Ticarcillin			
			Verapamil (immunomodulation)

REFERENCES
1. AJ Wood, G Maurer, W Niederberger et al.Transplant Proc 1982; 14:659
2. LE Kerr. Clin Pharm 1984; 3:346
3. PA Keown, CR Stiller, M Stawecki et al. In: "Cyclosporin in Autoimmune Diseases", 1st International Symposium, Basle (CH), 18-20 March 1985
    Editor: R. Schindler. Publ: Springer-Verlag, Berlin, Heidelberg, New York, Tokyo 1985; 39-42
4. Anonymous Editorial. Pharmacy International, February 1986; 31-32
5. PH Whiting, MD Burke, AW Thomson. Transplant Proc 1986; 18(suppl 5): 56-70
6. ITR Cockburn. Transplant Proc 1986; 18(suppl 5):50-55
7. J Grevel. In: "Ciclosporin in Renal Transplantation", International Workshop on Ciclosporin in Renal Transplantation, Milan (I), 25-26 October 1985. Editor: C Ponticell, A De Vecchi. Publ: Karger, Basel, München, Paris, London, New York, New Delhi, Singapore, Tokyo, Sidney 1986; 23-30
8. A Orfila, L Lloveras, M Mir et al. Kidney Int 1987; 32:610
9. NK Wadhwa, TJ Schroeder, AJ Pesce et al. Ther Drug Monit 1987; 9:399-406
10. T Beveridge, A Gratwohl, F Michot et al. Curr Ther Res 1981; 30:5
11. G Burckhart, T Starzl, L Williams et al. Transplant Proc 1985; 17:1172
12. J Grevel, E Nuesch, E Abisch et al. Europ J clin Pharmacol 1986; 31:211-216
13. R Venkataramanan, R Ptachinski, G Burckhart et al. J Clin Pharmacol 1984; 24:528
14. PA Keown, A Laupacis, G Carruthers et al. Transplantation 1984; 38:304-5
15. B Bourbigot, J Guiserix, J Airiau et al. Lancet 1986; i:1447
16. M Kessler, E Renoult, B Jonon et al. Therapie 1987; 42:273-5
17. M Cantarovich, C Hiesse, F Lockiec et al. Clin Nephrol 1987; 28:190-3
18. A Lindholm, S Henricsson. Lancet 1987; i:1262-3
19. HH Neumayer, K Wagner. Lancet 1986; ii:523
20. JM Grino, I Sabate,, AM Castelao et al. Lancet 1986; i:1387
21. JM Pochet, Y Pirson. Lancet 1986; i:979
22. U Kunzendorf, G Walz, HH Neumayer et al. Klin Wschr 1987; 65:1101-3
23. L Ost. Transplantation 1987; 44:533-5
24. RJ Ptachinski, R Venkataramanan, GJ Burckhart. Transplant Proc 1987; 19(1):1728-9
25. FJ Frey, A Schnetzer, FF Horber et al. Transplantation 1987; 43:494-8
26. TK Daneshmend. Lancet 1982; ii:1217
27. H Dieperink, J Moller. Lancet 1982; ii:1217
28. RM Ferguson, DER Sutherland, RL Simmons et al. Lancet 1982; ii:882-3
29. C Cunningham, MD Burke, PH Whiting et al. Lancet 1982; i:1464
30. DJG White, NR Blatchford, G Cauwenbergh. Transplantation 1984; 37(2): 214-5
31. JH Shepard, RL Simmons, JS Najarian. Clin Pharm 1986; 5:468

32. JM Smith. Clin Sci 1983; 64:678-9
33. TJ Schroeder, DB Melvin, CW Clardy et al. J Heart Transplant 1987; 6:84-9
34. JE Anderson, RE Morris, TF Blaschke. Clin Res 1987; 35:115A
35. RJ Ptachinski, BJ Carpenter, GJ Burckhart et al. New Engl J Med 1985; 313:1416-7
36. M Hourmant, JF Le Bigot, L Vernillet et al. Transplant Proc 1985; 17: 2723-7
37. JRP Godin, IS Sketris, P Belitsky. Drug Intelligence and Clin Pharm 1986; 20:504-5
38. RC Venuto, BM Murray, L Edwards et al. Kidney Int 1986; 29:438
39. DE Kohan. New Engl J Med 1986; 314:448
40. R Martell, D Heinrichs, CR Stiller et al. Ann intern Med 1986; 104: 660-1
41. TA Gonwa, DD Nghiem, JA Schulak et al. Transplantation 1986; 41:797-9
42. M Kessler, J Louis, E Renoult et al. Europ J clin Pharmacol 1986; 30: 633-4
43. DJ Freeman, R Martell, SG Carruthers et al. Clin Pharmacol Ther 1986; 39:193
44. FY Aoki, R Yatscoff, J Jeffery et al. Clin Pharmacol Ther 1987; 41:221
45. JD Harnett, PS Parfrey, MD Paul et al. Transplantation 1987; 43(2): 316-8
46. NK Wadhwa, TJ Schroeder, EO O'Flaherty. Ther Drug Monit 1987; 9:123-5
47. P Vereerstraeten, P Thiry, P Kinnaert et al. Transplantation 1987; 44:155-6
48. C Kreft-Jais, EM Billaud, C Gaudry et al. Europ J Clin Pharmacol 1987; 32:327-328
49. G Leimenstoll, P Jessen, P Zabel et al. Deutsch Medizin Wschr 1984; 109:1989-90
50. G Deray, P Le Hoang, P Cacoub et al. Lancet 1987; i:158-9
51. WB Ross, D Roberts, PJA Griffin. Lancet 1986; i:330
52. BB Moller, B Ekelund. New Engl J Med 1985; 313:1416
53. H Carstensen, N Jacobsen, H Dierpink. Brit J clin Pharmacol 1986; 21:550-1
54. Anonymous. Pharm Int 1986; 7(II):269-70
55. G. Hillebrand, LA Castro, W Van Scheidt et al. Transplantation 1987; 43:915-6
56. PA Keown, CA Stiller, AL Laupacis et al. Transplant Proc 1982; 14: 659-61
57. M Rowland, SK Gupta. Brit J clin Pharmacol 1987; 24:329-34
58. P Lele, P Peterson, S Yang et al. Kidney Int 1985; 27:344
59. SA Veremis, MS Maddus, R Pollak et al. Transplantation 1987; 43:913-5
60. GD Qureshi, TP Reinders, GJ Somori et al. Ann Intern Med 1984; 100:527
61. E Langhoff, S Madsen. Lancet 1983; ii:1031
62. NJ Daniels, JS Dover, RK Schacter. Lancet 1984; ii:639
63. P Howard, TJ Bixler, B Gill. Drug Intell Clin Pharm 1985; 19:763-4
64. G Offermann, F Keller, M Molzahn. Amer J Nephrol 1985; 5:385-7
65. MJD Cassidy, R van Zyl-Smit, MD Pascoe et al. Nephron 1985;

41:207-8
66. J Wallwork, CGA McGregor, FC Wells et al. Lancet 1983; i:366-7
67. DK Jones, M Hakim, J Wallwork. Brit med J 1986; 292:728-9
68. PF D'Arcy. Pharm Int 1986; 7:138
69. JM Hows, S Palmer, S Want et al. Lancet 1981; ii:145-6
70. A Termeer, AJ Hoitsma, RAP Koene. Transplantation 1986; 42:220-1
71. MS Kennedy, HJ Deeg, M Siegel et al. Transplantation 1983: 35(3):211-5
72. GR Morgenstern, R Powles, B Robinson et al. Lancet 1982; ii:1342
73. JF Thompson, DHK Chalmers, AGW Hunnisett et al. Transplantation 1983; 36(2):204-6
74. G Nyberg, H Gäbel, P Althoff et al. Lancet 1984; i: 394-5
75. O Ringden, P Myrenfors, G Klintmalm et al. Lancet 1984; i:1016-7
76. AA Shaftie, LL Widdup, MA Abate et al. Drug Intell Clin Pharm 1986; 20(7):602-5
77. MD Paul, PS Parfrey, M Smart et al. Amer J Kidney Dis 1987; 10(2): 133-5
78. DS Snyder. Ann intern Med 1988; 108:311
79. D Freeman, A Laupacis, P Keown et al. Ann R Coll Physicians Surg Can 1984; 17(4):301
80. J Zazgornik, J Schindler, F Gremmel et al. Kidney Int 1985; 28:401
81. M Jarowenko, CT Van Buren, WC Kramer et al. Transplantation 1986; 42:311-2
82. J Zazgornik, W Schein, K Heimberger et al. Clin Nephrol 1986; 26:265-6
83. B Sido, C Hammer, W Mraz et al. Transplant Proc 1987; 19(1):1755-8
84. MA Shaw, M Gumbleton, PJ Nichols. Lancet 1987; ii:637
85. D Trenk, W Brett, E Jahnchem et al. Lancet 1987; ii:1335-6
86. I Novakova, P Donelly, T de Witte et al. Lancet 1987; ii:920-1
87. NK Wadhwa, TJ Schroeder, EO O'Flaherty et al. Transplantation 1987; 43:211-3
88. R Garraffo, B Monnier, P Lapalus et al. Med Sci Res 1987; 15:461
89. MK Chan. In: "Proceedings", 2nd Asian Cyclosporin Workshop, Hong Kong 12-13 April 1986. Editor: BD Kahan. Publ: Excerpta Medica, Amsterdam, Hong Kong, Princeton, Sydney, Tokyo 1986; 38-40
90. L Rosenberg, DC Dafoe, R Schwartz et al. Transplantation 1987; 43: 764-6
91. T Van den Akker, R Benner, J Radl. Transplantation 1987; 44:724-5
92. JB Dossetor, T Kovithavongs, M Salkie et al. Ann Roy Coll Physicians Surg Can 1984; 17:363
93. Anonymous Editorial. Ann Intern Med 1983; 99:851-4
94. A Erice, MC Jordan, BA Chace et al. J Amer med Ass 1987; 257:3082-7
95. BM Murray, MS Paller. Kidney Int 1986; 29:434
96. BE de Pauw, T de Witte, RM Janssen et al. Krankenhausarzt 1984;57: 854-8
97. P Dorian, C Cardella, M Strauss et al. Transplant Proc 1987; 19(1): 1825-7
98. G Nanni, SC Magalini, F Serino et al. Transplantation 1988; 45:257
99. P Christensen, M Leski. Brit med J 1987; 294:578
100. PH Whiting, C Cunningham, AW Thompson. Biochem Pharmacol 1984;

33:1075
101. O Kloke, R Osieka. Klin Wschr 1985; 63:1081-2
102. G Deray, P Le Hoang, B Aupetit et al. Clin Nephrol 1987; 27:213-4
103. MA McMillen, RJ Tesi, WB Baumgarten et al. Transplantation 1986; 40: 444-6
104. RJ Tesi, J Hong, KMH Butt et al. Transplant Proc 1987; 19(1):1382-4
105. MA McMillen, WK Baumgarten, HC Schaefer et al. Transplantation 1987; 44:395-401
106. R Osieka, S Seeber, R Pannenbäcker et al. Cancer Chemother Pharmacol 1986; 18(3):198-202
107. S Suzuki, T Hijoka, I Sakakibara et al. Transplantation 1987; 43 (5):743-4
108. D Fas. M Shimizu, B Vayuvegula et al. J Allergy Clin Immunl 1988; 81(1):199
109. P Hansten. Drug Interact News Letter 1984; 4:29
110. JA Tobert. New Eng J Med 1988; 318:47-48

DRUG INTERACTION BETWEEN CYCLOSPORIN A AND MACROLIDES ANTIBIOTICS : STUDY IN VITRO AND IN VIVO.

P. BERTAULT-PERES*, Y. BERLAND**, L. VERNILLET***, P. BRES*, A. DURAND*, M. OLMER**.

*Laboratoire de pharmacocinétique de la Faculté de Pharmacie.**Service de Néphrologie, Hôpital de la Conception 13005 MARSEILLE ***Laboratoires Sandoz FRANCE

Cytochrome P450 from liver microsomes is the generic name used to design a family of monooxygenase hemoprotein involved in the metabolism of an impressive number of endogenous and exogenous compounds. Cyclosporin A (CYA) metabolism in rabbit and humans is cytochrome P450 dependent, as we demonstrated from the Lm3C isozyme [1-2]. Thus we developed a model using human liver microsomes to establish and quantify drug interactions between CYA and several other drugs. Six macrolides antibiotics (TAO, Josamycin, Midecamycin, Erythromycin, Roxithromycin and Spiramycin) were assayed with this human model. At varying concentrations from 10 to 1000 μMol of macrolide, inhibition of CYA metabolism ranges from 19 to 90 % save for Spiramycin which exhibits no interaction. We tried to correlate these data in kidney transplant recipients.

PATIENTS

Six kidney graft recipients, one woman and five men ; mean age, 32 years (range, 18 to 50) were studied. They had received a cadaveric transplant since 17 months (range 5 to 34) and were treated by an average dose of 5.8 mg/kg/day (range 3.6-9.1) of CYA and 10-15 mg/day of prednisolone. The CYA dose was individually adjusted to maintain plasma trough levels between 80 to 180 ng/ml (plasma separated from red blood cells at 37°C ; RIA polyclonal Sandoz).

METHODS

6 million units of Spiramycin were administered daily to the patients during 15 days (JO to J+14). Plasma kinetic of CYA was realised on J-1, J+1 and J+14 and consisted of 12 blood samples distributed over 24 hours. Serum creatinine, bilirubin, ASAT and ALAT were determined on J-1 and J+14.

RESULTS

Results of the in vitro study are summarized on figure 1. For a given concentration of 1000 μM, all tested Macrolides except Spiramycin inhibit cyclosporin-oxydase activity in hepatic microsomes. Spiramycin shows only a moderate inhibition (%). At a concentration of 10 μM spiramycin has no inhibition potential whereas other macrolides still have a moderate inhibitory role. Table 1 depicts the absence of a significant change of serum creatinine, bilirubin, ASAT and ALAT during Spiramycin administration to the 6 transplant recipients treated by CYA. The pharmacokinetic profile of CYA is not altered by the administration of Spiramycin as shown on figure 2. One patient expressed paresthesias during concomittant intake of CYA and Spiramycin.

Table 1 BIOCHEMICAL DATA AT J-1 (A) AND J+14 (B) DURING SPIRAMYCIN ADMINISTRATION (Mean values ± S.D) N = 6

S.CREATININE (μmol/l)		S.BILIRUBIN (μmol/l)		ASAT (I.U.)		ALAT (I.U.)	
A	B	A	B	A	B	A	B
113	118	23	17	16	18	17	17
± 26	± 21	± 14	± 11	± 5	± 9	± 7	± 11

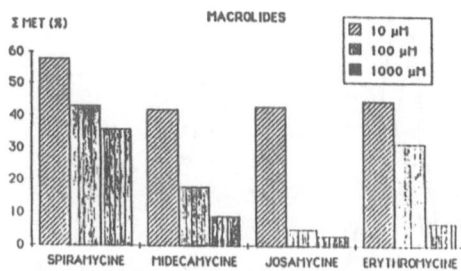

FIGURE 1:Sum of CyA metabolites
with increasing macrolide concen
trations.

DISCUSSION

Metabolic interactions occur between CYA and Erythromycin (3). We have developed a simple and reproducible model establishing metabolic interferences with CYA. The use of human hepatic microsomes help avoid extrapolation of results as observed with animal models. This model has allowed to select a macrolide Spiramycin, which does not interact with CYA metabolism. Pharmacokinetic study carried out in the 6 kidney-graft recipients confirm the results obtained in vitro. No change has been observed in renal and hepatic functions.

Spiramycin thus appears to be the only Macrolide devoid of metabolic interaction with CYA.

1 - BERTAULT-PERES P, BONFILS C, FABRE G, JUST S, CANO J.P., MAUREL P. Drug metabolism and disposition. 15, 391-398, 1987.

2 - SATO R and OMURA T.
"Cytochrome P 450" (Kondaska Tokyo, ed) Academic Press, New York, 1978.

3 - HOURMANT M, LE BIGOT J.F, VERNILLET L, SAGNIEZ G, REMI J.P, SOULILLOU J.P. Transplant Proceed. 17, 2723-2727,1985.

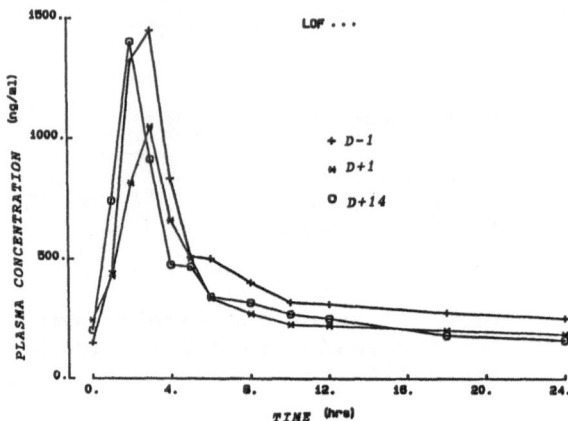

FIGURE 2: An exemple of CyA plasma kinetic curve during the study.(D-1 without spiramycine(s̄p),D+1 and D+14 with sp treatment)

INTERACTION OF CALCIUM ANTAGONISTS AND CICLOSPORINE A

H.-H. NEUMAYER, J. BROCKMÖLLER*, G. HEINEMEYER*, U. KUNZENDORF, I. ROOTS*, K. WAGNER

Departments of Internal Medicine and Nephrology and Clinical Pharmacology*, Klinikum Steglitz, Freie Universität Berlin, Federal Republic of Germany

INTRODUCTION

Our group has previously demonstrated that the combined treatment of donor and recipient with the calcium antagonist (CA) diltiazem (Dil) reduced the incidence of delayed graft function in cadaveric kidney transplants, although significantly elevated ciclosporine A (CsA) whole-blood trough levels were observed (1). This first observation of an interaction of Dil and CsA induced us to investigate in a retrospective study the influence of initiation or discontinuation of Dil and nifedipine (Nif) on CsA therapy. In a second prospective clinical trial, the effect of Dil on kidney graft function and CsA pharmacokinetics was investigated in patients with stable graft function to elucidate possible mechanisms of this interaction.

METHODS

In a retrospective investigation of nonhospitalized patients, at least three months after kidney transplantation, CsA whole-blood trough levels, doses and clearances were recorded before the start of either Dil (n=23) or Nif (n=24) and after achieving CsA blood levels comparable to those before the initiation of CA. The same parameters were determined after withdrawal of Dil or Nif and after stable CsA blood levels had been achieved without further dose adjustment. Patients (n=20) receiving no CA were used for reference.

After informed consent and according to the guidelines of the declaration of Helsinki, 22 nonhospitalized patients without previous CA therapy and with stable graft function (at least 6 months after cadaveric kidney transplantation, plasma creatinine levels

< 150 µMol/l and no changes exceeding ± 10% during the last 3 months, no rejection episodes during this period) were included in this prospective study. An initial pharmacokinetic profile of the oral CsA maintenance dose was obtained together with measurements of glomerular filtration rate (GFR) and renal blood flow (RBF), using single-shot techniques with inulin and PAH (2). Dil was then initiated at an oral dose of 2x60 mg/d. After 1 and 4 weeks, phar-macokinetic investigations and measurement of renal function were repeated. Over the subsequent 3 weeks, CsA dose was tapered down to achieve CsA whole-blood trough levels comparable to those before Dil therapy. These levels were determined by RIA using polyvalent and monovalent unspecific antibodies according to the method of Donatsch (3). In addition, CsA blood levels and concentrations of the metabolites M1, M17, M18, and M21 were measured by HPLC accord-ing to the method of Christians et al. (4). Data are given as mean ± SEM. Statistical significance was accepted at the 5% level (Student's t-test).

RESULTS
Initiation of calcium antagonists (Tab. I).

CA therapy was initiated 349 ± 63 days (Dil) and 164 ± 27 days (Nif) after renal transplantation. Application of CA was indicated in all patients by mild or moderate arterial hypertension. CsA pa-rameters were recorded before and after 214 ± 40 (Dil) or 169 ± 42 (Nif) days of continuous intake. The same parameters were recorded in the control group 311 ± 41 days after renal transplantation and after an additional period of 185 ± 4 days. None of the groups showed significant changes in plasma concentrations of creatinine or liver enzymes (GOT, GPT, AP). During the observation periods, CsA dose was reduced by $16\pm2\%$ in controls ($p\leq0.001$), by $21\pm4\%$ in patients on Nif ($p\leq0.01$) and by $43\pm5\%$ in the Dil-treated group ($p\leq0.0001$). CsA whole-blood levels (RIA) remained stable in the Dil group ($+5\pm3\%$), but fell in the Nif group ($-15\pm6\%$) and controls ($-7\%\pm4\%$). These findings were reflected by changes in CsA clearances: $-50\pm9\%$ in the Dil patients ($p\leq0.05$), $-11\pm3\%$ in the Nif group (ns) and $-17\pm4\%$ in controls ($p\leq0.001$).

Discontinuation of calcium antagonists (Tab. I).

Dil (n=20) was applied for 206±39 days and Nif (n=13) for 272±50 days. The indications for discontinuation were retrospectively not established in most cases. Parameters of CsA therapy were recorded 103±16 (Dil) or 146±28 (Nif) days after termination of calcium blocker therapy (Tab. II). CsA dose was raised by +14±3% after discontinuation of Dil, but significantly reduced by -17±4% after withdrawal of Nif (p≤0.05). An analogous dose reduction of -16±2% was observed in the control group (p≤0.001). In contrast to a significant reduction of CsA whole-blood trough levels in the Dil-treated patients by -37±6% (p≤0.001), only minor changes occurred after abandonment of Nif (+2±5%, ns) and in controls (-7±4%, ns). This was confirmed by the alterations calculated for CsA clearances in all 3 groups: Dil: +77±11% (p≤0.05), Nif: -37±4% (p≤0.0001), controls: -17±4% (p≤0.001). During the observation period, 6 rejection episodes occurred in the Dil group compared to only 3 in the Nif group. Corrected for an equivalent period of 100 days, 0.29 rejection episodes per patient occurred in the Dil group compared to 0.15 episodes in the Nif group (p≤0.05).

Table 1. Influence of Calciumantagonists (CA) on Ciclosporin-A-Therapy (CsA)

		Diltiazem	Nifedipin	Control
Initiation of CA				
Patients	(n)	23	24	20
CsA parameters before initiation of CA				
dose	(mg/kg/d)	4.47 ± 0.3	5.62 ± 0.4	4.57 ± 0.3
blood level	(ng/mL)	404 ± 50	472 ± 41	375 ± 32
clearance	(mL/min/kg)	8.6 ± 0.6	9.1 ± 0.8	9.8 ± 1.2
CsA parameters under therapy with CA				
dose	(mg/kg/d)	2.55 ± 0.2*	4.4 ± 0.2†	3.85 ± 0.3‡
blood level	(ng/mL)	425 ± 29	403 ± 25	350 ± 27
clearance	(mL/min/kg)	4.3 ± 0.3§	8.1 ± 0.5	8.1 ± 0.7‡
Discontinuation of CA				
Patients	(n)	20	13	20
CsA parameters before discontinuation of CA				
dose	(mg/kg/d)	3.47 ± 0.4	5.21 ± 0.5	4.57 ± 0.3
blood level	(ng/mL)	493 ± 50	399 ± 43	375 ± 32
clearance	(mL/min/kg)	5.2 ± 0.5	11.1 ± 2.2	9.8 ± 1.2
CsA parameters after discontinuation of CA				
dose	(mg/kg/d)	3.96 ± 0.4	4.27 ± 0.4§	3.85 ± 0.3
blood level	(ng/mL)	319 ± 26‡	405 ± 35	350 ± 27
clearance	(mL/min/kg)	9.2 ± 0.8§	8.1 ± 1.2*	8.1 ± 0.7*

Note: Results are mean, SEM. P values reflect comparison to initial values.
§P < .05, †P < .01, ‡P < .001, *P < .0001,

<u>Influence of Dil on CsA pharmacokinetics and kidney function (Fig. 1).</u>

After 1 week of Dil application (2x60 mg/d), CsA blood trough levels (RIA) had raised from 348±18 ng/ml to 595±35 ng/ml (p≤0.0001). HPLC determination showed an increase from 118±8 to 173±12 ng/ml (p≤0.001). Mean trough levels of M17 increased from 184±13 to 335±25 ng/ml (p≤0.0001), whereas the concentrations of M1 (70±9 vs 82±8 ng/ml), M18, and M21 were found unchanged (Fig. 1). There was a clear trend towards an increase in the maximal concentration (C_{max}) from 1,638±200 to 2,035±304 ng/ml with Dil, but no change in the invasion rate (K_{inv}) or elimination rate (K_{elim}). After 1 week of Dil application, a slight but significant reduction in RBF, parallel to the increase in CsA blood levels, from 324±17 ml/min to 295±16 ml/min (91±4%, p≤0.05) was seen. There was also a tendency towards a moderate decrease in GFR (57±5 vs 64±6 ml/min, ns). After 4 weeks of Dil, the intial CsA dose was reduced by 29±3% from 3.62±0.2 mg/kg/d to 2.61±0.2 mg/kg/d (p≤0.0001), but CsA blood levels were significantly higher than at the starting point (435±32 vs 348±16, p≤0.05). It was calculated that a dose reduction by 40% (2.02±0.2 mg/kg/min) would bring about the initial CsA levels. At the end of the investigation, neither GFR, RBF nor plasma creatinine (128±4 μmol/l) leves differed from the initial values.

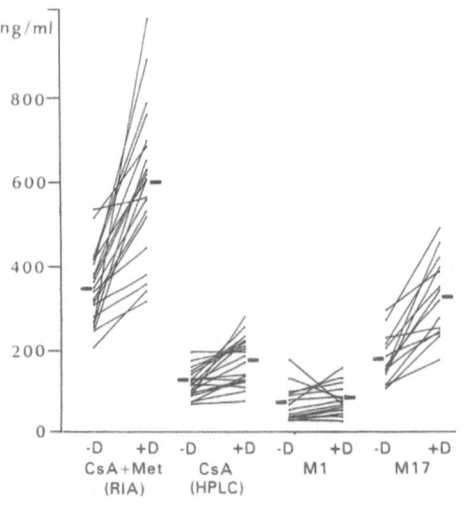

Whole blood trough levels of CsA, M1, and M17 before (-D) and during (+D) diltiazem application

Mean values are indicated by bars

DISCUSSION

In contrast to our findings with Nif, the results of the retrospective investigation revealed a striking effect of Dil, a CA
of the benzothiazeoine-type, on CsA pharmacokinetics. After initiation of Dil, a dramatic drop of CsA clearance by $50\pm9\%$ occurred,
which led to a reduction of the CsA dose by $43\pm5\%$. This reduction
was twice as high as in controls and might at least reduce the
costs of aftercare in organ transplantation. It must, however, be
mentioned that the reversibility of this interaction may lead to an
untoward situation after discontinuation of Dil. Since CsA clearance increased by $77\pm11\%$ and CsA was only augmented by $14\pm3\%$ in our
patients, a clinically relevant decrease in CsA blood levels occurred. After withdrawal, the incidence of rejection episodes was
twice as high as in the Nif group. It is therefore mandatory to
intensify CsA blood level control in organ recipients who receive
CA like nicardipine (5), verapamil (6) or Dil, especially when
those drugs are discontinued. The increase in CsA blood levels
after Dil measured by mono- and polyclonal RIA kits and HPLC might
in part be due to alterations in the metabolite composition, since
HPLC showed a marked increase in M17, whereas M1, M18, and M21 remained unchanged. The main mechanism of this drug interaction seems
to be an inhibition of hepatic CsA metabolism by Dil. This is confirmed by our in vitro studies with human liver microsomes, which
showed a dose-dependent non-competitive inhibition of CsA metabolism by Dil. In parallel with the observed alterations in plasma
concentrations, formation of M1 was more strongly inhibited than
that of M17. A major step of metabolite formation is hydroxylation
in position 9 (M1), which is also the main secondary metabolisation
step for further degradation of M17 to M8 or M26 via M18.

In summary, the present data as well as previously determined
CsA levels in our study on the prevention of delayed graft function
by Dil (7,8) clearly demonstrate that the elevated CsA blood levels
are caused, at least in part, by accumulation of CsA metabolites.
This might be of great clinical relevance, since the inhibitory
potency of M17 on interleukin-2 formation is comparable with native
CsA (9), while its nephrotoxicy seems to be lower (10). This would
also explain the results of our previous clinical trial, where we

demonstrated a reduced incidence of rejection episodes under concomitant therapy with Dil and CsA, although CsA blood levels were kept in the same range by a drastic dose reduction (1). This would only be possible, if Dil led to an accumulation of metabolites with lower nephrotoxicity but equivalent immunosuppressive activity.

REFERENCES
1. Neumayer, H.H. and Wagner, K. J. Cardiovasc. Pharmacol 10: 170-177, 1987.
2. Hall, J.E., Guyton, A.C., Farr, B.M. Am. J. Physiol 232: 72-76, 1977.
3. Donatsch, P., Abisch, E., Homberger, M. et al. J. Immunoassay 2: 19, 1981.
4. Christians, U., Zimmer, K.-O., Wonigeit, K. and Sewing, K.-Fr. J Chromatogr. 413: 121-129, 1987.
5. Bourqbigot, B., Giuserix, J., Airiau, J. et al. Lancet 2: 1447, 1987.
6. Lindholm, A., Hericsson, S. Lancet 2: 1262, 1987
7. Kunzendorf, U., Walz, G., Neumayer, H.H. et al. Klin. Wochenschr. 65: 1101-1103, 1987.
8. Walz, G., Kunzendorf, U., Keller, F., Neumayer, H.H., Offermann, G. Clin. Transplantation 2: 21-25, 1988.
9. Freed, B.M., Rosano, T.G., Lempert, N. Transplantation 43: 123 - 127, 1987
10. Ryffel, B., Hiestand, P., Foxwell, B. et al. Transplant. Proc. 18: 41-45, 1986.

CYCLOSPORIN A - H2 RECEPTOR ANTAGONISTS DRUG INTERACTION IN THE SPRAGUE-DAWLEY RAT.*

R. GIACOMELLI, V. FILINGERI°, G. FAMULARO, A. CALOGERO'', F. STORTONI°, S. NARDI°, R. ROSATI°, A. IACONA^, S. SACCHETTI, V. CERVELLI°, R. VERNA'', G. TONIETTI, and C.U. CASCIANI°

Clinica Medica and ''Patologia Clinica, University of L'Aquila; °Clinica Chirurgica, University of Rome 'Tor Vergata'; ^Ist. Tipizz. Tessutale CNR, L'Aquila; Italy.

INTRODUCTION

The H2 receptor antagonists (H2ra) such as cimetidine (C), ranitidine (R), and famotidine (F) seem to be effective in the
prevention and treatment of stress ulcer in transplant recipients
receiving cyclosporin A (CyA). A major problem in the management
of these patients is to define the possible influence of H2ra on
CyA metabolism and the possible synergistic nephro- and hepatotoxicity of these drugs, when co-administered (1). The aim of this
research was to study the possible interaction between CyA, on one
hand, and C, R, and F, on the other hand by evaluating the serum
creatinine (SC), the serum alanine aminotransferase (ALT), the
serum aspartate aminotransferase (AST) levels in experimental rats,
in order to determine whether H2ra may be used with CyA without
risk. Histological observations of the liver and kidneys of all rats
studied were performed at the end of the experimental period.

MATERIALS AND METHODS

80 young male Sprague-Dawley rats, averaging 250 g in weight,
were entered into the study. Table 1 shows the drugs administered
to each group. After 5 days of treatment, blood was sampled from the
animals of groups 5, 6 , 7, 8 and whole blood CyA levels were measured
by radioimmunoassay; after 10 days all animals were sacrificied,
their blood was collected to assay SC, ALT, AST and serum CyA levels

TABLE 1

DRUGS ADMINISTERED FOR EACH STUDIED GROUP

GROUP 1: Controls	GROUP 5: CyA 5 mg/Kg/daily i.p.
GROUP 2: C 10 mg/Kg/daily i.p.	GROUP 6: CyA 5 mg/Kg/daily i.p. + C 10 mg/Kg/daily i.p.
GROUP 3: R 5 mg/Kg/daily i.p.	GROUP 7: CyA 5 mg/Kg/daily i.p. + R 5 mg/Kg/daily i.p.
GROUP 4: F 2 mg/Kg/daily i.p.	GROUP 8: CyA 5 mg/Kg/daily i.p. + F 2 mg/Kg/daily i.p.

TABLE 2

SC, AST, ALT, AND CyA LEVELS IN STUDIED GROUPS

	SC mg/100ml	AST U/L	ALT U/L	CYA(5d) ng/ml	CYA(10d) ng/ml
GROUP 1:	0.7+0.2	73+15.4	36+10.8		
GROUP 2:	0.7+0.1	79+18.7	50+14.3		
GROUP 3:	0.6+0.1	78+19.3	45+17.6		
GROUP 4:	0.7+0.2	84+22.7	51+19.2		
GROUP 5:	0.8+0.1	65+15.4	48+15.7	2271+280.6	1543+552.6
GROUP 6:	0.6+0.2	220+130.5 [a]	111+41.2 [a]	2220+544.6	2448+250.6 [a]
GROUP 7:	0.8+0.2	92+ 35.8	55+14.6	2298+455.3	2420+410.8 [b]
GROUP 8:	0.6+0.2	80+ 19.3	41+12.5	2174+450.3	1587+521.6

a: P< 0.01; b: P< 0.05

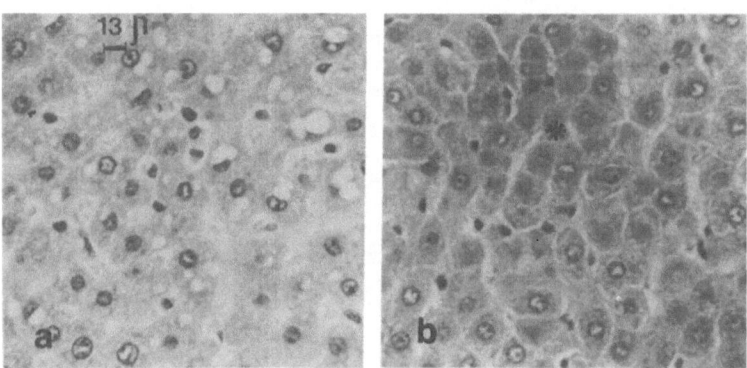

Fig. 1. The micrograph shows: a) micro- and macro-vesicular steatosis without balloning cells and flogistic infiltrates; b) eosinophilic degeneration of some hepatocytes (*).

at the end of the experimental period. Furthermore, their liver and kidneys were removed, immediately fixed in Bouin fluid and processed for light microscopy. Statistical analyses were performed by the

Student's T test.

RESULTS

Our results are shown in Table 2 and Fig. 1. After 10 days
serum CyA levels were increased only in the animals of group 6 and
group 7. SC levels were normal in all groups, and ALT and AST levels
were increased only in the animals of group 6 . Steatosis in the liver of the rats of group 6 and 7 was observed. The liver of some
rats of group 7 showed limited areas of eosinophilic degeneration.
No histologic alterations were observed in the kidneys. Controls
were all negative.

DISCUSSION

The main finding of our study is that animals co-treated with low
dosage of CyA and C or R, show an increase of serum CyA levels,
histological liver changes and, as far as animals receiving CyA + C
are concerned, a deterioration of liver functional parameters:

These data suggest an inhibition of CyA hepatic metabolism by
the Citochromes P-450 induced by C and R (2). The high serum CyA
levels seem to play a major role in the appearance of histological
changes. Unlike C and R, F seems to not interfere with Cytochromes
P-450 (3). The normal biochemical and histological patterns of
kidneys studied seem to indicate a higher resistance of this
organ to damage induced by CyA treatment (4).

REFERENCES

1. Cockburn, I. Transplan. Proc. XVIII: 50-55, 1986.
2. McCarthy, D.M. Ann. Int. Med. 99: 551-553, 1983.
3. Humphries, T.J. Scand. J. Gastroenter. (suppl) 134: 55-60,
   1987.
4. Scolari, F., Sandrini, S., Savoldi, S., Cristinelli, L., Prati,
   E., Brunori, G., Sacchi, G., Tardanico, R., Cancrini, G.C., and
   Maiorca, R. Transplant. Proc. XIX: 1745-1748, 1987.

*THIS WORK WAS SUPPORTED IN PART BY CNR GRANT No. 86.00598.44.

CYCLOSPORIN A (CSA) DRUG INTERACTIONS.

A.M.CASTELAO, I.SABATE, J.M.GRIÑO, S.GILVERNET, E.ANDRES, R.SABATER, J.ALSINA.
Nephrology Department. Hospital Universitario de Bellvitge. Barcelona, Spain.

INTRODUCTION.

Because CsA is subject to extensive hepatic metabolism (1), the possibility of pharmacokinetic drug interaction can be anticipated if drugs which enhance or inhibit its metabolism are co-administered (2-4). In addition to this, there is the possibility of interaction if other drugs given with CsA are nephrotoxic, since they may enhance the toxicity of CsA (5).

An important number of interactions nave been described, being the aim of this study to show the observed inter actions in our transplanted patients.

MATERIAL AND METHOD.

Two hundred patients who received a kidney transplant in our hospital between March 1984 and March 1988 were treated with a CsA-Prednisone or a CsA-PNS-Antilymphocyte globuline protocol.

We studied the influence of certain drugs on CsA blood levels (polyclonal RIA in whole blood, n= 300- 800 ng/ml), in 42 patients (24 men, 18 female, mean age 37 yr) who presented variations in the CsA levels because of the treat - ment with some different drugs.

RESULTS.

We observed a rise in the CsA levels in 38 patients because of the treatment with erythomycin in 12 cases, ketoconazole in one, diltiazem in seventeen, verapamil in one, cimetidine in one or a decrease when we stopped cimetidine in three cases, ranitidine in two or nifedipine in one case. All the patients received a steady dose of CsA for a minimun of four days before starting the treatment.

The influence of erythromycin on CsA levels presented individual variability of interaction (Table 1).

Two patients required diltiazem and one patient verapamil because of angor pectoris. In these cases we performed a CsA clearance study, calculated as the area under the curve (AUC) with and without the questioned drug.

CsA clearance with diltiazem was 1,18 ml/min/kg and without diltiazem 3,8 ml/min/kg. The rise in CsA level was significant (before treatment 290 ng/ml, after 1100 ng/ml but not the increase in plasma creatinine (before treatment 180 umol/l, after 158 umol/l).

CsA clearance with verapamil was 1,2 ml/min/kg and without verapamil 2,03 ml/min/kg. The rise in CsA level was significant (before treatment 460 ng/ml, after 920 ng/ml) but not the increase in plasma creatinine (before 743 umol /l, after 530 umol/l).

In the patients treated with H2 receptor antagonists the increase in CsA dose needed to maintain normal CsA levels was $1,1 \pm 0,8$ mg/kg/day.

We observed a decrease in CsA blood levels or persistently low levels in four patients receiving phenytoin or phenobarbitone. The mean CsA level decrease was 209 ± 197 ng/ml and plasma creatinine diminished 123 ± 56 umol/l.The four patients required an increase of $1,55 \pm 0,6$ mg/kg/day to maintain normal CsA blood levels.

Table 1. Influence of Erythromycin on CsA blood levels.

	Before	After	p
CsA levels(ng/ml)	608 ± 352	1080 ± 504	0,002
CsA dose (mg/kg/d)	$8,3 \pm 3,2$	$3,5 \pm 1,7$	0,001
Pl. creatinine (umol/l)	451 ± 318	490 ± 302	0,05

Table 2. Influence of Diltiazem on CsA blood levels.

	Before	After	p
CsA levels (ng/ml)	342 ± 166	796 ± 480	0,001
CsA dose (mg/kg/d)	$9,2 \pm 4,9$	$6,6 \pm 3,8$	0,001
Pl. creatinine (umol/l)	262 ± 161	230 ± 123	n s

DISCUSSION.

CsA is a potent immunosuppressive drug metabolized in the liver by the cytochrome P-450 enzyme system. Drugs that may enhance or inhibit this system could interact with CsA when they are co-administered. Many of the interactions are well kmown, but some others are presently under discussion.

In addition to this, the nephrotoxicity of other new agents, like acyclovir (6) could be enhanced by CsA.

In conclusion: 1) Care should be taken when co-adminis tering drugs that could enhance CsA levels because of the danger of nephrotoxicity, and with others that decrease CsA levels, raising the risk of rejection. 2) The interaction presents very marked individual variability. 3) Diltiazem and verapamil could minimizeCsA nephrotoxicity by decrea-sing the CsA dose, but very careful monitoring of CsA level must be taken into account, specially if we measure CsA levels by means of the new specific monoclonalRIA.

So we agree with other authors   that research on the CsA metabolites may reveal important information on drug interactions.

REFERENCES.

1. Maurer,G., Loosli,H.R., Schreiner,E. and Keller,B. Drug Metab. Disp. 24: 120-126, 1984.
2. Gumbleton,M., Brown,J.E., Hawksworth,G. and Whiting,P.H Transplantation 40:454-455, 1985.
3. Griñó,J.M., Sabater,I., Castelao,A.M., Guardia,M. and Serón,D. Ann. Intern. Med. 105:467-468, 1986.
4. Griñó,J.M., Sabater,I., Castelao,A.M. and Alsina,J. Lancet 1: 1387, 1986.
5. Bennet,W. Clin. Nephrol.25:126-129, 1986.
6. Jhonson,P.C., Kumor,K., Welsh,M.S., Woo,J. and Kahan,B. D. Transplantation 44: 329-331, 1987.

CYCLOSPORINE A + GLYBENCLAMIDE. EFFECT ON GLUCOSE METABOLISM: PRELIMINARY RESULTS

A. GALIONE, V. HOPPS*, F. VACCARO, F. BIONDI*

Department of Organ Transplantation, University of Palermo, Italy
* Institute of Pharmacology and Pharmacognosy, University of Palermo, Italy

INTRODUCTION

Cyclosporine A (CsA) is an immunosuppressive drug which determines, at high dosage, glucose intolerance (1). Different drugs present a pharmacological interaction with CsA increasing or reducing its blood level (2). To investigate the role of Glybenclamide (HB419), a sulphonilureic oral antidiabetic drug of large use, on CsA glucose metabolic effect, we have administered CsA + HB419 in rats. The aim of our work is to evaluate if HB419 influences CsA blood levels and if it improves glucose tolerance.

MATERIALS AND METHODS

Sixty Wistar male rats, weighing 240 ± 20 g, were divided into 10 experimental groups marked by letters. "A" group was tube fed with acacia gum (a.g.) 5% and olive oil (10 ml/kg). "B, C and D" groups were tube fed as the "A" group for the first ten days and then they were treated with 1, 2 and 3 doses of CsA (100 mg/kg) dissolved in olive oil, respectively. "E, F and G" groups were treated with HB419 (Euglucon, Boehringer R.) (0.2 mg/kg) daily suspended in a.g. for 11, 12 and 13 days, respectively. "H, I and L" groups were treated with HB419 (0.2 mg/kg) for the first ten days and then they were treated with 1, 2 and 3 doses of HB419 (0.2 mg/kg) + CsA (100 mg/kg), respectively. After drug administration animals were fasted for 24 hours and then killed to take blood samples to test CsA, Glucose, Insulin and Glucagon. At 12th day "B, E and H" groups were killed; at 14th day "C, F and I" groups were killed and at 19th day "A, D, G and L" groups were killed. Statistical comparison of results was performed by variance analysis and the difference among control treated animals were measured by Dunnett's method.

RESULTS

CsA blood levels are presented in table I. Twenty-four hours after the I dose of

	Group B mean ± SE	Group H mean ± SE	Group C mean ± SE	Group I mean ± SE	Group D mean ± SE	Group L mean ± SE
24 hs after I dose	2833,3 55,8	2800,0 51,6	–	–	–	–
	p: ns					
24 hs after III dose	–	–	2066,0 49,4	2144,0 84,0	–	–
			p: ns			
6 hs after III dose	–	–	–	–	594,0 87,0	350,0 51,0
					p < 0,05	

Table I — CsA Blood Levels (ng/ml)

CsA, there is no significant difference between CsA and CsA + HB419 treated groups. Twenty-four hours after the III dose CsA decreases unaccountably. No significant difference is present. Six days after the III dose CsA blood levels decrease and there is a significant difference (P < 0.05) between the two groups. Table II shows that CsA is

Groups	Treatment	BLOOD		
		Glucose mg % mean ± SE	Insulin μU · ml $^{-1}$ mean ± SE	Glucagon pg · ml $^{-1}$ mean ± SE
A	Control	82.34 1.08	2.52 0.33	28.07 0.50
B	24 hs after I dose of CsA	92.66 1.24 P > 0.05	3.74 0.51 P < 0.01	25.17 0.90 P > 0.05
C	24 hs after III dose of CsA	112.34 4.48 P < 0.01	2.38 0.35 P > 0.05	20 85 1.44 P < 0.01
D	6 days after III dose of CsA	90.00 2.06 P > 0.05	1.46 0.10 P < 0.05	24.95 0.80 P > 0.05
E	24 hs after XI dose of HB419	97.00 2.12 P > 0.05	0.87 0.12 P < 0.01	34.88 5.00 P > 0.05
F	24 hs after XIII dose of HB419	111.0 13.3 P < 0.01	1.08 0.14 P < 0.01	29.55 2.89 P > 0.05
G	6 days after XIII dose of HB419	118.0 0.66 P < 0.01	0.73 0.05 P < 0.01	35.70 2.51 P < 0.05
H	24 hs after XI dose of HB419 + 24 hs after I dose of CsA	111.66 7.04 P < 0.01 P_1 > 0.05	1.01 0.11 P < 0.01 P_1 < 0.01	20.13 1.72 P < 0.05 P_1 > 0.05
I	24 hs after XIII dose of HB419 + 24 hs after III dose of CsA	105.34 6.48 P < 0.01 P_2 > 0.05	1.30 0.11 P < 0.01 P_2 < 0.01	24 95 3.27 P > 0 05 P_2 > 0.05
L	6 days after XIII dose of HB419 + 6 days after III dose of CsA	152.0 4.50 P < 0.01 P_3 < 0.01	0.82 0.16 P < 0.01 P_3 > 0.05	35.82 2.79 P < 0.05 P_3 < 0.01

Table II — Glucose, Insulin and Glucagon (mean ± SE) in experimental groups of rats

P = P versus control - P_1 = P versus group B - P_2 = P versus group C - P_3 = P versus group D
HB419 = Glybenclamide - CsA = Cyclosporine A

able to determine a light hyperglicemia only after the III dose (group C). HB419 increases serum glucose levels in group "F and G". In group "H and L" serum glucose is enhanced if data are compared to control. Insulin blood levels increase in "B" group and decrease in "D, E, F and G" groups significantly. "H, I and L" groups show a significantes decreased levels too. About glucagon CsA reduces its serum levels in "C" group and HB419 in "G" group. In HB419 + CsA treated groups CsA has a predominatly effect after the I dose and HB419 six days after the XIII dose.

DISCUSSION
    As frequently observed from the leterature CsA exerts different actions in different conditions. Hahn (3) reports the toxic effects of CsA on the endocrine pancreas of Wistar

rats; however in BB rats Laupacis (4) has shown that CsA prevents the onset of IDDM. Recently (5) CsA has also been tested as a therapeutic alternative for immunosuppressive therapy in Insulin Dependent Diabetes Mellitus (IDDM). Impaired glucose tolerance with CsA has also been reported in animals (3) and in man (1). The toxic effects of CsA on endocrine pancreas of Wistar rats increase after an high administration of this drug. In rats high doses of CsA produce severe morphological and functional alteration of the pancreatic β Cells. The degranulation and hydropic degeneration of the β Cells (6) correspond to the decrease of pancreatic insulin content, insulin plasma levels and to hyperglicaemia of the animals. In our study to improve glucose tolerance we have used HB419 + CsA. The aim of our study was to test if HB419, when administered with CsA, improves glucose tolerance. Our results show a significant increase of glucose and glucagon only six days after the III dose of CsA + HB419 if data are compared to controls; whereas in the group of animals data show a significant decrease of insulin.

The results reported in this study are consistent with the possibility that a long HB419 pre-treatment (10 days) could leed to severe degranulation of islet β cells. This could trend cellular metabolism towards neoglycogenesis. In a former study of ours, accordingly with this hipothesis, we have reported hypopiruvicemia and high hepatic glicogen concentration. We can conclude, at least, in this sperimental condition, that HB419-CsA association could worsen CsA glucose intollerance.

REFERENCES
1. Gunnarsson R., Klintmalm G., Lundgren G., Wilczek H., Ostman J., Groth C.G The Lancet vol. 1, n. 8324, 1983.
2. Hopps V., Galione A., Biondi F., Vetri P., Sorrentino M.C., Leone F. In: Atti XXVIII Congr. Soc. Ital. Nefrol. (Eds. Acta Medica), p. 507-510 1987.
3. Hahn H.J., Laube F., Lucke S., Kloting I., Kohnert K.D. and Warzock R. Transplantation vol. 41, n. 1, 1986.
4. Laupacis A., Gardell C., Dupre J., Stiller C.R., Keown P., Wallace A.C., Thibert P. The Lancet vol. 1, n. 8315, 1983.
5. Stiller C.R., Dupre J., Gent M., Jenner M.R., Keown P.A., Laupacis A., Martell R., Rodger N.W., Graffnried B.V. Wolfe B.M.J. Science 223: 1362-67, 1984
6. Nielsen J.H., Mandrup-Poulsen T. and Nerup J. Diabetes, vol. 35, 1049-1052 1986.

Side Effects

ACUTE CYCLOSPORINE A NEPHROTOXICITY

V.E. ANDREUCCI, G. CONTE, M. SABBATINI, G. FUIANO, P. STANZIALE, L. DE NICOLA, V. SEPE, M. BALLETTA

Department of Nephrology, Second Faculty of Medicine, University of Naples, Naples, Italy

ACUTE EFFECTS OF CYCLOSPORINE A (CyA) ON THE KIDNEY

Experimental studies in rats have demonstrated that CyA causes tubular necrosis only when given at very high dosage. At a dosage of 20 mg/kg b.w./day proximal tubular changes are subtle and can be detected only by electron microscopy after a week of treatment (1). Some authors have suggested a direct toxic effect of the drug on proximal tubular cells. But the lack of early histopathologic lesions during CyA therapy (2), the increase of fractional proximal tubular reabsorption after acute or short-term administration of the drug (3-6) and the reversibility of renal dysfunction upon discontinuation of CyA (7,8) have supported the hypothesis that acute renal function impairment by CyA is due to reversible changes in renal hemodynamics, a form of "prerenal" failure.

The renal hemodynamics under the effect of CyA has been recently studied in rats. Acute or short-term administration of CyA caused a fall in PAH clearance and inulin clearance (CIn), and a decrease of the ratio lithium clearance (CLi) to CIn, indicative of proximal tubular overreabsorption, (3,4,9,10) and a rise in renal vascular resistance (10). All these changes are consistent with a renal vasoconstriction as a primary effect of CyA on the kidney.

Renal micropuncture studies were performed in Munich-Wistar rats in our laboratory to define the hemodynamic changes induced acutely by CyA at a single nephron level. The acute i.v. infusion of CyA (20 mg/kg b.w.) caused a decrease of afferent and efferent arteriole blood flow, whole kidney GFR and GFR in single nephron (SNGFR) and glomerular ultrafiltration coefficient (Kf), and an increase in afferent and efferent arteriole resistance. No changes occurred in glomerular, tubular and effective filtration pressures. All these data were reflecting a marked glomerular vasoconstriction in both pre- and post-glomerular vessels and in glomerular capillaries, as suggested by the fall in Kf (6). Similar results were obtained by others (11). Glomerular arteriolar vasoconstriction by CyA has been observed also by scanning electron microscopy (12). When dopamine was infused with CyA in rats at dopaminergic dosage, all the above changes were reversed (13).

We have also performed clearance studies in normal humans on CyA effects on renal hemodynamics (5,14). When CyA was given orally, at a dosage of 12 mg/kg b.w., to 8 healthy volunteers during maximal water diuresis, a decrease of PAH clearance, CIn, urine output, fractional excretion of sodium and free-water clearance was observed. The addition of dopamine (2 microg/kg b.w./min i.v.) reversed these changes. Other authors have observed a similar positive effect of dopamine but only on RBF (15).

ROLE OF THE RENIN-ANGIOTENSIN SYSTEM

After seven days of CyA treatment hyperplasia of the juxtaglomerular apparatus has been demonstrated in ruts and rabbits that was dose-dependent (16) and is consistent with the demonstrated stimulatory effect of CyA on renin-angiotensin system (17). CyA, in fact, has been shown to increase renin production in rat kidney slices (18) and plasma renin activity (PRA) has been found raised after a single i.v. infusion and after 3-7 days (10,17,19) or even 20-28 days of CyA treatment (19,20).

In a recent study the acute CyA-induced changes in RBF and GFR were shown to be blunted by captopril, with complete normalization of renal vascular resistance (11). In another study, bolus injection of captopril caused a fall in blood pressure suggesting that the beneficial effect of the drug was due to an autoregolatory response to captopril-induced hypotension; when BP was maintained constant, RBF and GFR were improved, but not normalized by captopril injection (21). Identical results have been obtained with saralasin (21). These studies suggest an important, but not exclusive, role of angiotensin II (AII) in CyA-induced renal dysfunction.

Is AII involved because of the activation of tubuloglomerular feedback (TGF) system? Studies in rats by micropuncture technique have demonstrated an increased NaCl concentration in fluid from the thick ascending limb (TAL) of Henle's loop both after a single i.v. dose of CyA and after oral administration over 10 days; this has suggested that an impairment of salt reabsorption in TAL may increase NaCl concentration at the macula densa level thereby causing activation of TGF, with the consequent decrease of GFR (22). Henle's loop microperfusion studies in rats pretreated with CyA, however, gave no indication of impairment in Henle's loop electrolyte transport (23). Even the distal delivery of tubular fluid was not found to be elevated in CyA-treated rats; actually it was decreased because of the reduction in SNGFR (21). Finally the interruption of tubular flow to the macula densa in single nephrons of CyA-treated rats did not restore the SNGFR reduced by CyA, thereby excluding the possibility that the reduction in SNGFR was a response to a CyA-induced fall in proximal tubular reabsorption (with a consequent increase in distal delivery) and was TGF mediated (21).

ROLE OF SYMPATHETIC NERVOUS SYSTEM

It has been demonstrated that renal denervation prevents and α-adrenergic blocking agents reverse the impairment of RBF and the increase of renal vascular resistance caused by CyA in rats (10,24). These data suggest that renal vasoconstriction by CyA is mediated by an increase of either renal sympathetic nerve activity or circulating levels of catecholamines.

ROLE OF THROMBOXANE (TX) AND VASODILATING PROSTAGLANDINS (PGs)

After the first demonstration of increased urinary excretion of TX by rats treated with CyA over 14 days (25), conflicting results have been reported. Thus, rats treated for 3-7 days with CyA exhibited no change in renal slice release of TX, as well as of PGE_2 and 6-cheto-$PGF_{1\alpha}$ (prostacyclin metabolite), despite the fall in GFR and the increase in PRA (17). But the oral administration of the drug for up to 3 months caused a progressive increase in urinary excretion of TXB_2, which was already significant after one month of therapy and was inversely correlated with GFR; the intraperitoneal administration of a selective TX inhibitor, UK-38,485, resulted in a decrease in urinary excretion of TXB_2 with increase (but not normalization) of GFR (26). In a more recent study rats treated over 14 days with CyA had very high TX concentration in renal cortical tissue which was associated with a fall of GFR; when the conventional vehicle (olive oil) used for solubilization of CyA was replaced by fish oil, rich in eicosapentaenoic acid (an inhibitor of renal cortical eicosanoids, including TX), a reduction of CyA-induced renal functional impairment was observed, in association with a depressed renal cortical level of TX (27). These differences in the behaviour of TX in experimental studies may be related to difference in duration of CyA treatment: acute or short-term administration of CyA does not, while long-term administration of the drug does increase TX synthesis by the kidney.

Some authors have found either a decrease (28) or no change (20) of PGE_2 and no change of PGI_2 production by isolated glomeruli of normal rats treated for 20 days with CyA (20,28). No increase of urinary PGs was observed during oral doses of CyA for a period up to 3 months (26). But after a single i.v. infusion or daily administration over 7 days of CyA, others have reported an increase of urinary excretion of 6-cheto-$PGF_{1\alpha}$ (10). When meclofenamate was given to rats prior to the i.v. infusion of CyA a fall in RBF was observed, suggesting that PGs production have a protective effect against CyA-induced renal vasoconstriction (10).

An attempt to prevent CyA nephrotoxicity by using a PG has been performed in rats. The concomitant administration of CyA and 16,16-dimethyl PGE_2 ($dmPGE_2$) (a synthetic PG) resulted in a significant improvement in animal survival, creatinine clearance and renal histology when compared to rats treated with CyA alone (29). But a recent study in rats has shown that $dmPGE_2$ reduces the intestinal absorption of CyA and abolishes the immunosuppressive effect of the drug (30).

Since acute CyA administration in Brattleboro rats produced a less marked impairment of renal function than in normal rats, it has been postulated that the presence of ADH (which is known to decrease Kf) is somehow necessary for a full nephrotoxic action of CyA (11).

CYCLOSPORINE A AND RENAL ISCHEMIA

Studies in laboratory animals have demonstrated the interaction between CyA and renal ischemia (31-33). Thus, the effects of CyA (10 to 25 mg/kg b.w./day for

14-28 days) alone or associated with 30 to 60 min
ischemia (clamping of renal artery) were evaluated in
rats after unilateral nephrectomy was performed to mimic
the condition of the single transplanted kidney; under
such circumstances the drug exhibited adverse effects on
the initiation or progression of compensatory hypertrophy
and the repair of the ischemic insult (34,35).

The intraperitoneal administration in rats of 50
mg/kg b.w./day of CyA over 12-14 days after left kidney
denervation and 30 min renal artery clamping caused a
marked reduction of both RBF and GFR which was associated
with renal production and urinary excretion of both TXB_2
and PGI_2; increased was also PGE_2 production, but not
its urinary excretion (32).

It has been observed that renal damage by ischemic
injury was particularly exacerbated by CyA when the drug
was given after rather than before the ischemic insult
(33).

A recent study (36) has utilized NMR-spectroscopy and
electron microscopy to figure out, respectively,
functional and morphological effects of ischemia (30 min
renal artery clamping) on renal mitochondria and on
renal high-energy phosphate metabolism in rats treated
with CyA (15 mg/kg b.w./day for 20 days). Ischemia
caused a rapid functional impairment of mitochondria,
with a marked drop (to less than 10%) of ATP level; more
than 50% of the original ATP, however, was resynthesized
within 10 minutes after the onset of recirculation with
no difference between control and CyA-treated animals.
At the electron microscopy, however, control animals
maintained the morphological integrity of renal tissue,
while CyA-treated rats exhibited both degenerative
changes (swelling, myelin figures, fragmentation in
tubular inclusion bodies) as well as proliferation of
mitochondria, with increase of the number of cristae and
presence of megamitochondria. These results have

suggested that under the studied experimental conditions the morphological damage of mitochondria was compensated by mitochondria proliferation so that NMR spectrum was preserved even in CyA-treated rats. It is possible, however, that with higher doses of CyA and/or prolonged treatment the mitochondrial damage reaches such an extent that cannot be compensated, so that the functional impairment becomes detectable by NMR (36).

The mentioned studies appear to support the harmful effect of CyA nephrotoxicity on a freshly transplanted cadaver kidney that has undergone a prolonged ischemia and renews emphasis on the need of minimizing ischemic renal damage (37).

REFERENCES

1. Pfaller W, Kotanko P, Bazzanella A:
Morphological and biochemical observations in rat nephron epithelia following cyclosporine A treatment.
Clin Nephrol, 25 (Suppl 1): S105-S110, 1986.

2. D'Ardenne AJ, Dunnill MS, Thompson JF, McWhinnie D, Wood RFM, Morris PJ:
Cyclosporin and renal graft histology.
J Clin Pathol, 39: 145-151, 1986.

3. Dieperink H, Leyssac PP, Starklint H, Kemp E:
Nephrotoxicity of cyclosporin A. A lithium clearance and micropuncture study in rats.
Eur J Clin Invest, 16: 69-77, 1986.

4. Dieperink H, Leyssac PP, Starklint H, Jorgensen KA, Kemp E:
Antagonist capacities of nifedipine, captopril, phenoxybenzamine, prostacyclin and indomethacin on cyclosporin A induced impairment of rat renal function.
Eur J Clin Invest, 16: 540-548, 1986.

5. Conte G, Sabbatini M, Napodano P, De Nicola L, Gigliotti G, Fuiano G, Testa A, Russo D, Esposito C, Libetta C, Dal Canton A, Andreucci VE:
Dopamine counteracts the acute renal effects of cyclosporine in normal subjects.
Transplant Proc, 1988 (in press).

6. Sabbatini M, Esposito C, Uccello F, De Nicola L, Alba MM,
Conte G, Dal Canton A, Andreucci VE:
Acute effects of cyclosporine A on glomerular dynamics.
Micropuncture study in the rat.
Transplant Proc,   1988 (in press).

7. Chapman JR, Griffiths D, Harding NGL, Morris PJ:
Reversibility of cyclosporin nephrotoxicity after three months
treatment.
Lancet, 1: 128-129, 1985.

8. Palestine AG, Austin HA III, Nussenblatt RB:
Renal tubular function in cyclosporine-treated patients.
Am J Med, 81: 419-424, 1986.

9. Whiting PH, Simpson JG:
Lithium clearance measurements as an indication of cyclosporine A
nephrotoxicity.
Clin Sci, 74: 173-178, 1988.

10. Murray BM, Paller MS, Ferris TF:
Effect of cyclosporine administration on renal hemodynamics in
conscious rats.
Kidney Int, 28: 767-774, 1985.

11. Barros EJG, Boim MA, Ajzen H, Ramos OL, Schor N:
Glomerular hemodynamics and hormonal participation on cyclosporine
nephrotoxicity.
Kidney Int, 32: 19-25, 1987.

12. English J, Evan A, Houghton DC, Bennett WM:
Cyclosporine-induced acute renal dysfunction in the rat.
Transplantation, 44: 135-141, 1987.

13. Sabbatini M, Esposito C, De Nicola L, Uccello F, Altomonte M,
Romano G, Veniero P, Dal Canton A, Andreucci VE:
Dopamine reverses acute cyclosporine A nephrotoxicity.
Micropuncture study in the rat.
Proc. 2nd Int Sorrento Meeting on "Current Therapy in Nephrology",
Sorrento May 22-25, 1988, (Eds. VE Andreucci and A. Dal Canton),
Kluwer Academic Publ, Boston,   1988.

14. Conte G, Sabbatini M, De Nicola L, Gigliotti G, Fuiano G,
Testa A, Sepe V, Imperatore P, Dal Canton A, Andreucci VE:
Reversibility of acute cyclosporine renal impairment by
dopamine in healthy subjects.
Proc. 2nd Int. Sorrento Meeting on "Current Therapy in Nephrology",
Sorrento, May 22-25, 1988, (Eds. VE Andreucci and A. Dal Canton),
Kluwer Academic Publ, Boston,   1988.

15. Kho TL, Teule J, Leunissen KML, Heidendal GAK, Lijnen PJ,
Amery AK, van Hooff JP:
Nephrotoxic effect of cyclosporine-A can be reversed by dopamine.
Transplant Proc, 19: 1749-1753, 1987.

16. Verpooten GA, Wybo I, Pattyn VM, Hendrix PG, Giuliano RA, Nouwen EJ, Roels F, De Broe ME:
Cyclosporine nephrotoxicity: comparative cytochemical study of rat kidney and human allograft biopsies.
Clin Nephrol, 25 (Suppl 1): S18-S22, 1986.

17. Duggin GG, Baxter C, Hall BM, Horvath JS, Tiller DJ:
Influence of cyclosporine A on intrarenal control of GFR.
Clin Nephrol, 25 (Suppl 1): S43-S45, 1986.

18. Baxter CR, Duggin GG, Hall BM, Horvath JS, Tiller DJ:
Stimulation of renin release from rat renal cortical slices by cyclosporin A.
Res Commun Chem Pathol Pharmacol, 43: 417-423, 1984.

19. Siegl H, Ryffel B, Petric R, Shoemaker P, Muller A, Donatsch P, Mihatsch M:
Cyclosporine, the renin-angiotensin-aldosterone system and renal adverse reactions.
Transplant Proc, 15: 2719-2726, 1983.

20. Perico N, Benigni A, Bosco E, Rossini M, Orisio S, Ghilardi F, Piccinelli A, Remuzzi G:
Acute cyclosporine A nephrotoxicity in rats: wich role for renin-angiotensin system and glomerular prostaglandins?
Clin Nephrol, 25 (Suppl 1): S83-S88, 1986.

21. Kaskel FJ, Devarajan P, Arbeit LA, Partin JS, Moore LC:
Cyclosporine nephrotoxicity: sodium excretion, autoregulation, and angiotensin II.
Am J Physiol, 252: F733-F742, 1987.

22. Gnutzmann KH, Hering K, Gutsche H-U:
Effect of cyclosporine on the diluting capacity of the rat kidney.
Clin Nephrol, 25 (Suppl 1): S51-S56, 1986.

23. Muller-Suur R, Davis SD:
Effect of cyclosporine A on renal electrolyte transport: whole kidney and Henle loop study.
Clin Nephrol, 25 (Suppl 1): S57-S61, 1986.

24. Murray BM, Paller MS:
Beneficial effects of renal denervation and prazosin on GFR and renal blood flow after cyclosporine in rats.
Clin Nephrol, 25 (Suppl 1): S37-S39, 1986.

25. Kawaguchi A, Goldman MH, Shapiro R, Foegh ML, Ramwell PW, Lower RR:
Increase in urinary thromboxane B2 in rats caused by cyclosporine.
Transplantation, 40: 214-216, 1985.

26. Perico N, Benigni A, Zoja C, Delaini F, Remuzzi G:
Functional significance of exaggerated renal thromboxane A2 synthesis
induced by cyclosporin A.
Am J Physiol, 251: F581-F587, 1986.

27. Elzinga L, Kelley VE, Houghton DC, Bennett WM:
Modification of experimental nephrotoxicity with fish oil as the
vehicle for cyclosporine.
Transplantation, 43: 271-273, 1987.

28. Stahl RAK, Kudelka S:
Chronic cyclosporine A treatment reduces prostaglandin E2
formation in isolated glomeruli and papilla of rat kidney.
Clin Nephrol, 25 (Suppl 1): S78-S82, 1986.

29. Makowka L, Lopatin W, Gilas T, Falk J, Phillips MJ, Falk R:
Prevention of cyclosporine (CyA) nephrotoxicity by synthetic
prostaglandins.
Clin Nephrol, 25 (Suppl 1): S89-S94, 1986.

30. Ryffel B, Donatsch P, Hiestand P, Mihatsch MJ:
PGE2 reduces nephrotoxicity and immunosuppression of cyclosporine
in rats.
Clin Nephrol, 25 (Suppl 1): S95-S99, 1986.

31. Kanzai G, Stowe N, Steinmuller D, Ho-Hsieh H, Novick A:
Effect of cyclosporine upon the function of ischemically damaged
kidneys in the rats.
Transplantation, 41: 782-785, 1986.

32. Coffman TM, Carr DR, Yarger WE, Klotman PE:
Evidence that renal prostaglandin and thromboxane production is
stimulated in chronic cyclosporine nephrotoxicity.
Transplantation, 43: 282-285, 1987.

33. Bia MJ, Tyler KA:
Effect of cyclosporine on renal ischemic injury.
Transplantation, 43: 800-804, 1987.

34. Jablonski P, Harrison C, Howden B, Rae D, Tavanlis G, Marshall
Vc, Tange JD:
Cyclosporine and the ischemic rat kidney.
Transplantation, 41: 147-151, 1986.

35. Provoost AP, Kaptein L, Van Aken M:
Nephrotoxicity of cyclosporine A in rats with a diminished renal
function.
Clin Nephrol, 25 (Suppl 1): S162-S167, 1986.

36. Ellermann J, David H, Marx I, Grunder W, Pfeifer H, Scholz D,
Jung K:
31P-NMR spectroscopy and ultrastructural studies on nephrotoxicity
of cyclosporine A.
Exp Pathol, 32: 73-79, 1987.

RENAL PATHOLOGY AFTER LOW DOSE CYCLOSPORINE (CyA) IN PATIENTS WITH
PRIMARY SJOGREN´S SYNDROME

K.C.SIAMOPOULOS, A.A.DROSOS, H.M.MOUTSOPOULOS, M.J.MIHATSCH*
Departments of Medicine, Medical School, University of Ioannina,
Ioannina, Greece and Pathology* , University of Basel, Switzerland.

INTRODUCTION

Sjogren´s syndrome (Ss) is a lymphocyte-mediated exocrinopathy
with systemic manifestations (1). Today there is no therapeutic modality to control this lymphoproliferative disorder. A double-blind
study was undertaken to assess the efficacy of CyA in 20 patients
with primary Ss (pSs) and the results of this study were recently
reported (2). In this report, we present the clinical and laboratory
renal findings with emphasis to the histopathological renal lesions
in 8 pSs patients treated with a small dose of CyA for a short period
of time.

MATERIALS AND METHODS

All 8 patients were female, aged 38-73 years and satisfied the
clinical criteria for the diagnosis of pSs (1). The diagnosis was
confirmed in all patients by salivary biopsy findings compatible with
Ss. None of them had clinical or serological abnormalities characteristic of other autoimmune diseases. Renal function and blood pressure levels were within normal range. The patients were randomly allocated either to CyA (5 mg/kg/day) or to placebo for a 6 months period. After this period, the trial was continued as an open study and
all the patients were continued or started on CyA at the same dose
for an additional period of 6 months. After 7 months of treatment,
the patients underwent a percutaneous kidney biopsy. Informed consent
was obtained from all of them. Kidney tissues were examined "blindly"
using standard methods. The morphologic lesions were semiquantitavely
evaluated using a relative score of 0-4+ .

RESULTS

None of the patients showed serious side-effects during the study. After the histopathological examination of the renal tissues, the code of the study was broken. Three patients received placebo (6 months) and additional 1 month treatment with CyA (Group A), while the remaining 5 received CyA for 7 months (Group B). Hypertension was not recorded during the follow-up and renal function remained stable in both groups. No differences were also recorded in the urine analysis at the initial and the latest follow-up examination, although there was a notable reduction of proteinuria (from 3.5 to 1.3 g/24 h) in a patient of Group B, in whom membranous glomerulopathy was diagnosed. Non-specific mesangial matrix increase was found in 4 other patients associated with IgM or IgM and C_3 deposits. Arteriolar changes of the type of hyaline arteriolosclerosis were evident in 3 patients. Protein deposits in the arteriolar wall were identified as IgM or C_3. Typical CyA-associated arteriolopathy (3) was not found. Tubular atrophy and interstitial lesions of slight degree were seen in 3 patients. Tubular vacuoles and/or inclusion bodies were found by light and/or electron microscopy in 2 patients of Group A and in 4 of Group B. Typical giant mitochondria and isometric vacuolation were not found. Enlarged mitochondria, however, were present in 5 patients and inclusion bodies were identified as lysosomes by electron microscopy in 2 patients.

DISCUSSION

Although impressive results have been reported in small series of patients, the number of controlled trials with CyA in a variety of autoimmune diseases is limited (2,4). Moreover, its use has been complicated by the development of nephrotoxicity in more than 50% of patients (5) depending on the duration of treatment (5,6). In contrast to these studies, the renal function in our patients remained stable during the follow-up period. This could be attributed to the small doses of CyA as well as to the fact that there was no concomitant medication. In accordance with the clinical findings, the histopathologic evaluation did not show definite signs of acute or chronic toxicity (3). Six patients showed minor tubular lesions. Renal tubular lesions associated with CyA treatment are non-specific and may also be found in a wide variety of diseases and even in essentially normal kidneys (3). It cannot be ruled out however, that CyA may have contributed to the development of mitochondrial changes and/or vacuolation. The morphologic lesions of CyA chronic nephrotoxicity are of two different types: CyA-associated arteriolopathy and interstitial fibrosis with tubular atrophy. Typical CyA-associated arteriolopathy was not found. The interpretation of the interstitial changes (fibrosis and inflammation) is difficult. Both lesions have been described in transplanted and non-transplanted kidneys after long term CyA treatment. Interstitial inflammation and fibrosis with tubular atrophy, however, are very common histopathological findings in patients with Ss (1). Since no CyA-associated arteriolopathy was found in our patients and no episodes of acute neprhotoxicity were recorded, we believe that the interstitial lesions observed are probably not due to CyA treatment. In conclusion, neither definite clinical nor morphological signs of nephrotoxicity were found in these patients given CyA alone at small doses and for a limited period of time. However, the well documented nephrotoxic potential of the drug as well as the histopathological lesions observed, should be considered with scepticism.

REFERENCES
1. Moutsopoulos, H.M., Chused, T.M., Mann, D.L., Klippel, J.H., Fauci, A.S., Frank, M.M., Lawley, T.J., and Hamburger, M.I. Ann Int Med 92 (2): 212-216, 1980.
2. Drosos, A.A., Costopoulos, J., Papadimitriou, C., Moutsopoulos, H.M. Ann Rheum Dis 45: 732-735, 1986.
3. Mihatsch, M.J., Thiel, G., Basler, V., Ryffel, B., Landmann, J., Overbeck, J.von., Zollinger, H.U. Transplant Proc XVII (4) Suppl.1: 101-116, 1985.
4. The Lancet i: 909-911, 1985.
5. Palestine, A.G., Austin III, H.A., Balow, J.E., Antonovych, T.T., Sabnis, S.G., Preuss, H.G., Nussenblatt, R.B. N Engl J Med 314 (20): 1293-1298, 1986.
6. Von Graffenried, B., Harrison, W.B. In: Cyclosporin in Autoimmune Diseases (Ed. Schnider, R.), Springer, Berlin, Heidelberg, New York, Tokyo, 1985, pp. 59-73.

THE INFLUENCE OF CYCLOSPORIN ON CYTOMEGALOVIRUS-RELATED KIDNEY GRAFT SURVIVAL

EDWIN S SPENCER, OLE FJELDBORG & H KERZEL ANDERSEN

Renal Transplantation Unit and Department of Virology, University Hospital, Aarhus Denmark.

In 1981, we reported that one-year actuarial kidney graft survival was much better in recipients with no evidence of cytomegalovirus (CMV) infection than in recipients with primary CMV infection (1). At that time standard post-transplant therapy consisted of prednisone and azathioprine. Four-and-a-half-years ago azathioprine was replaced with cyclosporin. The present paper concerns graft survival in relation to CMV in these patients.

PATIENTS

From November 1983 to November 1987, 293 patients received kidney grafts at our center in Aarhus, Denmark. Among these 4 had been given a living donor kidney, and in 16 insufficient sera were available to ensure a 6-month period of observation from the day of transplantation. Thus 273 patients were included in the present study.

IMMUNOSUPPRESSION

Cyclosporin was started at transplantation and continued for the first week at 10 mg/kg/day unless signs of toxicity necessitated reduction in dosage. Prednisone was also given to all patients starting with 500 mg on day 1. On the second and third days 75 mg was given. From the fourth day 50 mg prednisone was given for 3 days, thereafter 40 mg for 3 days, 30 mg for 3 days and from approximately the third post-transplant week prednisone was slowly tapered from 20 mg/day to 5 mg/day at 9 months. Rejection crises were treated with intravenous methyl-prednisolone 1/2 to 1 g daily for 3 to 5 days.

Prior to November 1983, azathioprine 1-3 mg/kg/day
was used together with prednisone in dosages about 50%
higher than those given after November 1983. The therapy
of rejection crises has not changed during the last 15
years, 1/2 to 1 mg methyl-prednisolone being given
intravenously for 3 to 5 days.

SEROLOGIC METHODS

Blood specimens obtained at the time of transplantation and thereafter at 2 week intervals until the 3rd
post-transplant month together with samples after
6 and 12 months were tested for CMV antibodies of the IgM
and IgG class as reported previously (2).

RESULTS

Of the 273 patients, 199 had a positive CMV
complement-fixing (CF) titer at transplantation and thus
serologic evidence of previous CMV infection. The mean
age in this group was 44 years and 55% were men. Among
the 74 patients CMV sero-negative at the time of
transplantation, 46 or 62% later developed a positive CMV
CF titer and were considered to have had a primary
infection. Twenty-eight had no evidence of either past
or present infection. Mean ages in these two groups were
33 and 35 years, and 67 and 63 percent were men (table
1).

Table 1. Number in parenthesis give azathioprine treated.

	Number	Mean age	% men	graft surv. % 1 year
CMV positive	199 (71)	44 (43)	55 (54)	65 (54)
Primary infec	46 (34)	37 (33)	67 (71)	55*(32)#
No infection	28 (18)	37 (35)	63 (67)	70*(68)#

* non significant, # p = 0.01 (Fishers exact test).

As can be seen there was a tendency in both groups

for better graft survival in patients with no evidence of CMV infection compared with patients with primary infection, but only in the azathioprine-treated patients was this difference significant. Overall graft survival was also better after introduction of cyclosporin.

DISCUSSION

The introduction of cyclosporin in November 1983 not only increased general 1-year graft survival in our kidney transplant recipients, but also eliminated the negative effect of primary CMV infection on graft survival. Cyclosporin must modify some immunological effect of the CMV infection so that it no longer affects graft survival, since the incidence and severity of CMV infections in our patients has not changed after introduction of cyclosporin (2).

Other herpesvirus infections have been shown not to influence graft survival (3).

In an attempt to find a histo-pathological correlate to active CMV infection, we studied a series of graft biopsies taken from patients with and without CMV infection, but we could not find any association between active CMV infection and the glomerular lesion reported by Richardson et al. (4,5).

REFERENCES
1.   Spencer, E.S., Fjeldborg, O. and Andersen, H.K. Scand. J. Urol. Nephrol. Suppl. 64.128-131, 1981.
2.   Arnfred,J., Nielsen, C.M., Spencer, E.S. and Andersen, H.K., Scand. J. Infect. Dis. 19: 297-302, 1987.
3.   Spencer, E.S., Fjeldborg, O. and Mordhorst, C-H. Dan. Med. Bull. (in press).
4.   Jepsen, F.L. and Spencer, E.S. (in preparation)
5.   Richardson, W.P., Colvin, R.B., Cheeseman, S.H. et al. N. Engl. J. Med. 305: 57-63, 1981.

This work was supported by Aarhus Universitets Forskningsfond, grant no 1986-7131.

KAPOSI'S SARCOMA IN KIDNEY GRAFT RECIPIENTS TREATED WITH LOW DOSES OF CYCLOSPORINE.

G. Civati, B. Brando, G. Busnach, M.L. Broggi, C. Brunati, G.P. Casadei[*], M. Seveso, E.E. Minetti, L. Minetti.
Dep.ts of Nephrology and [*]Pathology, Niguarda-Ca'Granda Hospital, Milano.

INTRODUCTION

Kaposi's sarcoma (KS) is a neoplastic disease of endothelial cells, which accounts for some 3% of organ transplantation malignancies, and it is also common in HIV infection. KS incidence seems increased with Cyclosporine (CSA) therapy, as compared with conventional immunosuppression (1, 2). In our unit, 4 out of 150 CSA-treated recipients developed KS, while no other malignancies have been recorded. This occurred despite a low-dose CSA regimen (3), as compared with the absence of neoplasia in other 150 patients receiving conventional treatment. The clinical features of our KS cases were reviewed.

METHODS AND PATIENTS

Immunosuppressive therapy included CSA 10 mg/Kg orally on day 0, followed by 8 mg/Kg orally in two daily doses, then adjusted to keep blood trough levels (BTL) between 200 and 400 ng/ml. Methylprednisolone (MP) was tapered from 500 mg i.v. on day 0 to 40 mg i.v. on day 4, followed by 16 mg orally until day 180, then reduced to 8 mg/day. Rejections were treated with 5 500 mg i.v. MP pulses; steroid resistant rejections were treated with a 10 day course of 5 mg i.v. of Orthoclone OKT 3 monoclonal antibody (MAb). The clinical features of the four patients are summarized here.

Patient A. A 28-year-old man was grafted in Dec. 1985. In June 1986 fever, leukopenia and perineal nodes developed, with a biopsy diagnosis of KS. Therapy was withdrawn, excepted for 6 mg of MP This patient was retrospectively found to have anti-HIV-1 antibodies before transplantation, due to multiple blood transfusions. KS then spread throughout the skin and a suspected nodule in the liver was found. Two 7-day courses of 10 M Units of i.v. human recombinant alpha-2b interferon were undertaken, followed by long-term 1 M Units twice weekly subcutaneously. Skin lesions are currently stable.

Patient B. A 39-year-old woman was grafted in Oct. 1986. She had two rejection episodes, the second of which required OKT 3 MAb and recovered. In Mar. 1987 a KS nodule appeared on her forearm arterovenous fistula, soon followed by multiple lesions on her extremities. No visceral involvement up to now. CSA was withdrawn, 8 mg of MP were maintained, with improvement of KS lesions, which are to date stable and flattened.

Patient C. A 26-year-old woman was grafted in Feb. 1986, with an uneventful course. She required larger CSA doses. In Nov. 1986 anemia, amenorrhea, serum C-reactive protein, fever, oral candidiasis and a KS lesion on upper gum developed. On the next few days, multiple nodules appeared on her face, neck and back, with rapid clinical worsening and death for acute respiratory failure. Autopsy disclosed widespread visceral KS, with massive lung, spleen, lymph node, g.i. tract, adrenals and native kidneys involvement. The grafted kidney was entirely free of lesions.

Patient D. A 50-year-old man was grafted in Jun. 1986 from his HLA-identical sister, with a normal course. In Apr. 1987 a single KS nodule appeared at the forearm fistula. The lesion was removed, CSA and steroids were reduced and no other lesions have so far appeared.

In all patients the HLA-B 18 allele was present, while variable HLA-DR patterns were observed. The other immunological features were unremarkable. Only in pat. A leukopenia, inverted CD4/CD8 ratio, elevated polyclonal serum IgG were present. All patients were negative for HBs Ag and had detectable IgG for HSV and EBV. The CSA cumulative doses were as expected in all cases.

DISCUSSION

All patients were born in southern Italy. In Mediterranean countries, a genetic predisposition to the classic slowly progressive KS is known (4). It has been reported that HLA-DR 5 allele is associated with an increased risk of KS, while HLA-DR 3 seems to confer resistance to the disease (4, 5). The HLA-B 18 allele has a 15 - 20% frequency in Mediterranean area. We were unable to find reports about the association between KS and HLA-B 18, and our series is too small to calculate relative risk. It is interesting to stress the absence of KS lesions in the kidney of pat. C, which came from a B 18- DR3+ donor.

CSA and steroids influence the immune response against organisms and, maybe, malignancies. However, KS is known to occur in subjects not receiving immunosuppression. The exact immunologic mechanism involved in KS is to date unknown. Some studies describe the CMV tropism for endothelial cells, which may promote uncontrolled angiogenesis (6, 7). In summary, an unusual incidence of KS was observed in our series of transplanted patients receiving low dose CSA. In case of KS, the reduction or the withdrawal of CSA is recommendable and human alpha-2b interferon may be useful in generalized forms. CSA may have a facilitating role on KS occurrence in genetically predisposed patients.

REFERENCES

1) Little PJ, Farthing CF, Al Khader A, et al: Postgrad Med J 59: 325, 1983.
2) Al Suleiman M, Haleen A, Al Khader A: Transplant Proc 19: 2243, 1987.
3) Penn I: Transplant Proc 19: 2211, 1987.
4) Contu L et al:In Cerimele D (ed): Kaposi's sarcoma.Spectrum, Ph.1985,29.
5) Scorza Smeraldi R, Fabio G, Lazzarin A, et al: Lancet 2: 1187, 1987.
6) Levine AS: In Friedman-Kien AE, Laubenstein LJ (eds): The epidemic of Kaposi' sarcoma and opportunistic infections. Masson, N. Y. 1984, p 7.

A CELLULAR MECHANISM FOR CYCLOSPORINE A-INDUCED NEPHROTOXICITY

H.MEYER-LEHNERT*, R.W.SCHRIER+

*Med. Univ.-Poliklinik Bonn, West Germany, +Univ. of Colorado Sch. Med., Denver, CO, USA

INTRODUCTION

The immunosuppressive agent cyclosporine A (CyA) has been successfully used in organ transplantation and in the treatment of autoimmune diseases. A problem in CyA-therapy, however, is its nephrotoxicity (1) which is associated with a marked fall of glomerular filtration rate.

An important determinant of glomerular filtration is the glomerular filtration area. Experimental evidence suggests that filtration area is regulated at least partially by the contractile state of glomerular mesangial cells (2,3). Thus, we examined the hypothesis that CyA augments vasopressor-induced Ca^{2+} mobilization in glomerular mesangial cells; it may thus enhance mesangial cell contraction, a mechanism that may contribute to CyA-nephrotoxicity.

MATERIALS AND METHODS

CyA was obtained from Sandoz (Basel, Switzerland). The vehicle cremophore (Sigma, St.Louis, MO) was used in each control group in equivalent volumes.

Isolation of glomeruli and mesangial cell cultures were performed as described previously (3). Mesangial cells in primary cultures grew to confluence within 21-28 days. Further subculturing was performed at 7 to 10 days intervals using 0.25 % trypsin and 0.01 % EDTA.

$^{45}Ca^{2+}$ Efflux

After aspiration of culture medium and rinsing with phosphate buffered saline (PSS), cell monolayers were loaded with 8 µCi $^{45}Ca^{2+}$ in 1 ml of PSS at 37°C for 3 hrs and then washed with PSS. Efflux was determined by liquid szintillation counting at 1, 2, 3, and 4 min and at 30 sec intervals thereafter (3).

$^{45}Ca^{2+}$ Uptake

Cells were incubated for 5 min with 2 μCi of $^{45}Ca^{2+}$ in 1 ml of PSS in the presence and absence of any effector. $^{45}Ca^{2+}$ uptake was terminated by rinsing the culture dish five times at 4°C with Ca^{2+}-free PSS containing 2 mM EDTA. Intracellular radioactivity was extracted with sodium dodecyl sulfate (SDS)-containing alkaline solution (3).

RESULTS

AVP ($10^{-8}M$) increased $^{45}Ca^{2+}$ efflux within 30 sec after addition of the hormone (1322±83 vs 2674±146 cpm/mg prot, control vs AVP, p<.001). This stimulatory effect of AVP was significantly enhanced (p<.01) after preincubation with CyA (5 μg/ml)(1403±72 vs 3425±225 cpm/mg prot, p<.001), i.e. the peak efflux rates were significantly higher in the presence than in the absence of CyA. In contrast, CyA alone had no effect on spontaneous $^{45}Ca^{2+}$ efflux and was also ineffective when added simultaneously with AVP. CyA also enhanced the Ca^{2+}-mobilizing effect of AVP in Ca^{2+}-free medium. While, under these conditions, AVP induced an increase of 1048±122 cpm/mg/30sec, this differential increment was 2092±184 cpm/mg prot/30sec (p<.01) in the presence of CyA (5 μg/ml).

CyA significantly stimulated $^{45}Ca^{2+}$ uptake after 5 min (7924±414 vs 11928±760 cpm/mg prot, p<.05). This effect was in the same range as the rate of uptake stimulated by 10^{-8} M AVP . The combined effect of CyA plus AVP was somewhat higher than that of either CyA or AVP alone (12880±580 vs 11298±760 vs 11120±490 cpm/mg prot, AVP+CyA vs CYA and AVP, respectively), but this difference did not reach statistical significance.

DISCUSSION

The present study was designed to elucidate potential effects of CyA on glomerular filtration function at the cellular level. The results suggest that CyA stimulates Ca^{2+} uptake in glomerular mesangial cells and may thus increase the content of AVP-sensitive intracellular Ca^{2+} pools. Furthermore, we could demonstrate that AVP-induced Ca^{2+} mobilization as assessed by estimation of

$^{45}Ca^{2+}$ efflux is enhanced in the presence of CyA.

In order to demonstrate an effect of CyA on AVP-stimulated Ca^{2+} mobilization, cells had to be preincubated with CyA; the augmentory effect of CyA on AVP-induced $^{45}Ca^{2+}$ efflux was not only observed in Ca^{2+}-containing but also in Ca^{2+}-free medium. These observations indicated that if there was any direct effect of CyA on extracellular Ca^{2+}, it was likely to occur during the preincubation period prior to the addition of AVP and that it was not associated with a rapid Ca^{2+} influx in the presence of the vasopressor hormone. This assumption was supported by the results of the influx studies. CyA stimulated cellular Ca^{2+} uptake within 5 min, thereby presumably increasing cellular Ca^{2+} content prior to the exposure to AVP. These results are consistent with the effects of CyA reported for hepatocytes (4).

The potential augmentory effect of CyA on AVP-induced Ca^{2+} mobilization in mesangial cells is supported by studies from our laboratory that demonstrate an enhancement of AVP-stimulated intra-cellular free Ca^{2+} levels and AVP-induced contraction in mesangial cells (5).

Enhancement of mesangial cell contraction, however, is only one aspect of CyA-nephrotoxicity. Other factors like increased renal vascular resistance have also been implicated (6). In this regard it is of note that data from this laboratory indicate a similar effect of CyA on Ca^{2+} fluxes in vascular smooth muscle cells (7). Clearly, further studies will be needed for elucidation of the complex mechanisms in CyA-nephrotoxicity.

REFERENCES

1. Barger, A.C., Herd, J.A. N.Engl.J.Med. 284:482-490, 1971
2. Kreisberg,J.I., Venkatachalam, M., Troyer,D. Am.J.Physiol. 249: F457-F463, 1985
3. Takeda, K., Meyer-Lehnert, H., Kim, J.K, Schrier, R.W. Am.J. Physiol. 254:F254-F266, 1988
4. Nicchitta, C.W., Kamoun, M., Williamson, J.R. J.Biol.Chem. 260: 13613-13618, 1985
5. Meyer-Lehnert, H., Schrier, R.W., Kidney Int. in press
6. Centis, J.J., Dubovsky, E., Whelchel, J.D., Luke, R.G., Diethelm, A.G., Johns, P. Lancet 1986
7. Meyer-Lehnert, H., Schrier, R.W., Kidney Int. 31:464(Abs.), 1987

DOPAMINE (D) REVERSES ACUTE CYCLOSPORINE A (CyA) NEPHROTOXICITY. MICROPUNCTURE STUDY IN THE RAT.

M Sabbatini, C Esposito, L De Nicola, F Uccello, M Altomonte, G Romano, P Veniero, A Dal Canton*, VE Andreucci.

Dept. of Nephrology, University of Naples and *University of Reggio Calabria at Catanzaro.

We have recently shown, by renal micropuncture, that acute CyA-induced nephrotoxicity is entirely due to modifications in glomerular dynamics (1). Several vasodilating drugs have recently been tested in the attempt to prevent or reverse the acute renal dysfunction due to CyA, but, despite some beneficial effects, none of them was able to restore GFR to normal values. This study was carried out to evaluate whether D could counteract the hemodynamic modifications induced by CyA. D, in fact, has a renal vasodilating action if administered at low doses, which stimulate only dopaminergic receptors.

METHODS

Twenty-seven female Münich-Wistar rats were prepared for renal micropuncture as described elsewhere (2).The rats were divided into 3 groups: Group N (n=9), normal rats receiving saline as placebo; Group CyA (n=10), rats treated with CyA (20 mg/kg iv); Group CyA+D (n=8), rats treated with CyA as above and then with vasodilating doses of D (1.2-2.0 ug/100 g/min iv). As this dosage is variable in the rat, we have tested several concentrations of the drug, starting from a hypertensivant dosage and then decreasing it by steps until BP was similar as in the control period; such dosage was considered "dopaminergic", i.e. not associated to stimulation of adrenoceptors. In all rats we measured: total GFR, single-nephron GFR (SNGFR), afferent and efferent arteriole resistances (Ra and Re, respectively), glomerular plasma flow (GPF), hydrostatic pressures in glomerular capillaries (P_G) and in tubules (P_T), and ultrafiltration coefficient (Kf). Data are expressed as means ± SEM.

RESULTS

Body weight, BP and Hct were similar in all groups. GFR was significantly decreased by CyA; D infusion reversed such change, restoring GFR to normal values. Similarly, SNGFR was reduced after CyA but was normalized during D infusion. The fall of SNGFR was due to a striking reduction of GPF in Group CyA; again, during D infusion, GPF returned to normal values. These data are summarized in Table 1. Both Ra and Re were significantly increased after CyA (+65% and +107%, respectively) in Group CyA , and were normalized in Group CyA+D. P_G was increased in Group CyA, while P_T was higher in Group CyA+D; this resulted in a decreased glomerular capillary pressure gradient in Group CyA+D ($p < 0.05$ vs CyA) and, therefore, in a lower effective filtration pressure since oncotic pressures were similar in the three groups. Kf was greatly decreased by CyA, but during D infusion, was markedly increased even vs Group N (+18%, $p < 0.05$). CyA blood levels were similar in Group CyA and CyA+D, averaging 7421±1356 ng/ml. The average dosage of D was 1.67 ug/100 g/min. These data are presented in Table 2.

DISCUSSION

Acute administration of CyA resulted in marked decrease of

TABLE 1. EFFECTS OF CyA AND CyA+D ON GFR, SNGFR AND GPF.

	GFR (ml/min)	SNGFR (nl/min)	GPF (nl/min)
Group N	1.29±0.01	30.6±1.3	113.7±8.5
Group CyA	0.83±0.08*	18.7±1.8**	63.3±8.4**
Group CyA+D	1.46±0.25	31.5±2.8	106.2±9.7

* = $p < 0.05$ vs other groups; ** = $p < 0.01$ vs other groups.

565

TABLE 2. EFFECTS OF CyA AND CyA+D ON Ra, Re, P_G, P_T AND Kf.

	Ra	Re	P_G	P_T	Kf
	(dyne/sec/cm^{-5})		(mm Hg)		(nl/s/mm Hg)
Group N	2.39	1.59	46.8	13.7	0.029
	±0.22	±0.16	±0.7	±0.3	±0.001
Group CyA	3.83*	3.25**	49.5*	14.3	0.017**
	±0.50	±0.53	±1.5	±0.2	±0.002
Group CyA+D	2.31	1.46	45.3	16.6**	0.037
	±0.25	±0.22	±0.8	±0.6	±0.004

* = $p<0.05$ vs other groups; ** = $p<0.01$ vs other groups.

SNGFR, accounted for by a reduction of GPF and Kf. In this study we have tested whether D was effective in reversing the hemodynamic changes induced by CyA. Our results show that during D infusion, both GFR and SNGFR were completely normalized, as D was able to act on both pre- and post-glomerular resistances, restoring GPF. Moreover, SNGFR was normal despite a significant reduction in effective filtration pressure; such an effect is probably due to the striking increase of Kf which, in presence of filtration pressure disequilibrium (like in our rats), can influence SNGFR to a greater extent than in filtration pressure equilibrium (3). In conclusion, vasodilating doses of D are able to reverse the acute renal dysfunction induced by CyA.

REFERENCES

1. Sabbatini M, Esposito C, Uccello F, De Nicola L, Alba MM, Conte G, Dal Canton A, Andreucci VE. Transpl Proc, June 1988, in press.

2. Dal Canton A, Conte G, Esposito C, Fuiano G, Guasco R, Russo D, Sabbatini M, Uccello F, Andreucci VE. Kidney Int 22:608-612, 1982.

3. Tucker BJ, Blantz RC. Am J Physiol 232:F477-F483, 1977.

REVERSIBILITY OF ACUTE CYCLOSPORINE RENAL IMPAIRMENT BY DOPAMINE
IN HEALTHY SUBJECTS.

G. CONTE; M. SABBATINI, L. DE NICOLA, G. GIGLIOTTI, G. FUIANO,
A. TESTA, V. SEPE, P. IMPERATORE, A. DAL CANTON"and V.E. ANDREUCCI.
Departments of Nephrology, 2nd Faculty of Medicine of Naples and
Faculty of Medicine of Catanzaro; Italy.

INTRODUCTION

Up to now, no studies were designed to investigate the role of
renal hemodynamic abnormalities in relation to acute Cyclosporine A
(CsA) nephrotoxicity and to verify whether dopamine infusion could
cuonteract this acute renal disfunction in healthy subjects.

METHODS

Eight healthy male volunteers were studied by renal clearance
methods (with continous infusion of inulin and PAH) during maximal
water diuresis to evaluate the proximal tubular function (1). Two
different protocols were used: (A) After a steady urinary volume was
achieved, 4 basal clearance periods were performed before
administering per os CsA at the dosage of 12 mg/kg b.w., then three
clearances periods per hour were performed in the next four hours.
(B) On the basis of the data obtained by protocol A, a second study
was performed. Protocol B was identical to protocol A, with the only
addition of an i.v. infusion of dopamine(2 ug/kg b.w./min) which was
started at the beginning of the third hour after CsA administration
and continued for 60 min thereafter. After the end of D infusion, 3
further clearance periods were performed as in protocol A. In both
studies each clearance peiod lasted 20 min.

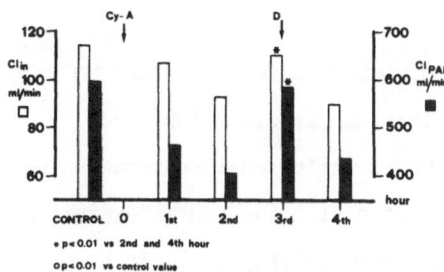

Fig. 1. Effects of a single dose of CsA without and with i.v. infusion of dopamine on C_{In} and C_{PAH}.

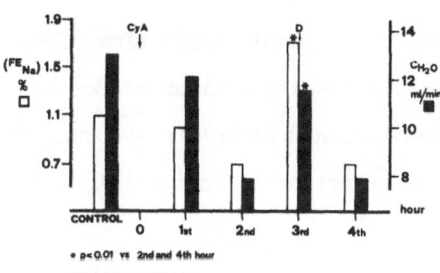

Fig. 2. Effects of a single dose of CsA without and with i.v. infusion of dopamine on fractional excretion of sodium and on free-water clearance.

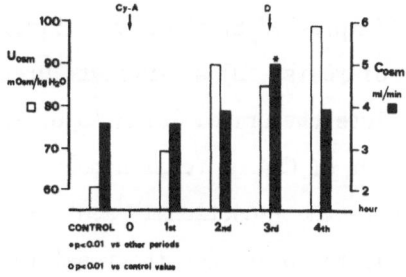

Fig. 3. Effects of a single dose of CsA without and with i.v. infusion of dopamine on urinary osmolality and osmolar clearance.

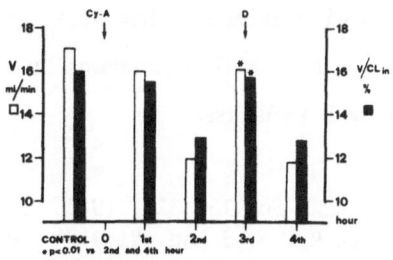

Fig. 4. Effects of a single dose of CsA without and with i.v. infusion of dopamine on urinary volume and fractional excretion of water.

RESULTS

In A, after CsA, inulin and PAH clearance fell, as maximum decrease, to 16% to 39%, so that filtration fraction increased (p<0.01). A slight hypertension occurred while renal resistances were markedly raised (p<0.001)(Fig.1). Fractional urine and Na excretion and CH_2O decreased and UOsm increased (p<0.01)(Fig.2,3). In B, D was infused from 120' to 180' after CsA, i.e. when the adverse effects of CsA on renal hemodynamics occurred. In B, D infusion was able to counteract completely the effects of CsA on renal plasma flow, GFR, fractional urine output and CH_2O (Fig.4) despite similar values of blood concentration of CsA; only UOsm remained higher than normal in conjunction with increased fractional excretion of sodium (p<0.01).

DISCUSSION

In this study, CsA administration determined a) a marked fall in renal plasma flow (RPF was expressed as CPAH), b) a moderate decrease of GFR, c) a fall in distal delivery (expressed by the lower urinary flow in a condition of maximal water diuresis), d) an antinatriuretic effect and e) a reduced ability to dilute the urine. Taken together, all these data indicate a primary effect of CsA on renal hemodynamics the renal hypoperfusion after CsA mimics the "functional" acute renal failure (2). Thus D appears a drug able to counteract the renal vaso-constriction caused by CsA. Our data indicate that D infusion at dopaminergic dosage restored RPF, GFR and urinary volume to normal basal values. In conclusion, our data give evidence that acute CsA nephrotoxicity in healthy humans is due to severe impairment in renal hemodynamics, which can be reversed by D infusion.

REFERENCES

1. Seldin DW, Eknoyan G, et al. Am NY Acad Sc. 139:328, 1966.
2. Palestine AG, Austin HA, Nussenblatt RB. Am J Med. 81:419, 1986.

RELATION BETWEEN GENGIVAL OVERGROWTH AND CYCLOSPORIN
(CyA) BLOOD LEVELS IN RENAL TRANSPLANTED PATIENTS

MATARASSO S, VAIA E, BOZZINI V,FEDERICO S°, PAPA A°,PACCHIANO G°,
FUIANO G°.
DEPT. OF ODONTOLOGY AND NEPHROLOGY°, II FACULTY OF MEDICINE, NAPLES,
ITALY.

Introduction. Gengival hypertrophy has been associated
with the use of several drugs (phenytoin, primidone, valproic acid,
nifedipine,nicardipine et al). Recently also CyA has been reported
to cause this side effect. The mechanisms by which CyA cause gengival
hypertrophy are little known: it has been hypothesized that, like
phenytoin, CyA may select a subpopulation of fibroblasts producing
highlevels of collagen, which accumulates causing gengival hyperplasia
Aim of this study is to see if the incidence and the severity of
gengival hyperplasia was related to the CyA blood levels.

Patients. The study was carried out on 24 patients. The patients
were grouped according the following criteria:A) Immunosuppressive
treatment. B) Blood CyA levels (mean of the last 2 months).
Control Group: Patients on immunosuppressive therapy other than CyA;
Group I: Patients with Cy blood levels (detected by polyclonal RIA)
steadily ≤ 300 ng/ml.
Group II: Patients with Cy blood levels steadily between 301 and 650
ng/ml.
The clinical and laboratory features of patients are summarized in
the following table.

CLINICAL FEATURES OF PATIENTS

	Pts n.	Age	Time after transplant (months)	C_{cr} (ml/min)	Blood CyA (ng/ml)	Dose of CyA (mg/kg/day)
Control	3	39.6	62 + 24	75 + 22		
Group I	10	34.0	19 + 11	65 + 18	290 + 21	4.1 + 1.4
Group II	11	37.7	16 ± 15	53 ± 19	481 ± 100	4.9 ± 2.4

METHODS.

Gengival overgrowth and bacterial plaque index were defined as follows: 1) Gengival overgrowth (hyperplasia): Essentially papillary process affecting labial, buccal, palatal and lingual tissues. It was scored (0-3) as indicated in the legends of figures 1,2,3,4.

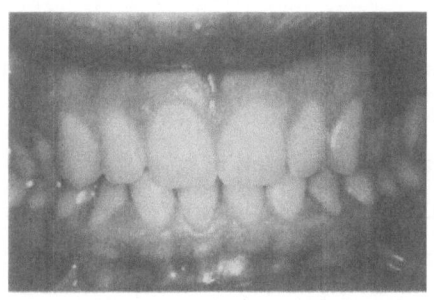

Fig.1)0: Normal

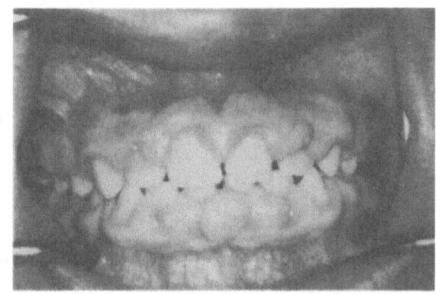

Fig.2) 1: Mild gengival overgrowhh

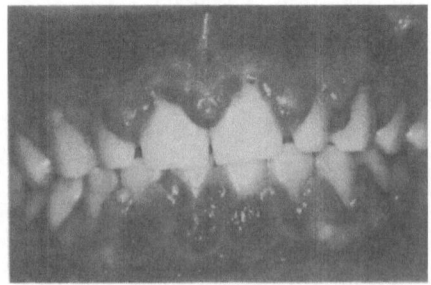

Fig.3) 2: Moderate gengival
overgrowth.

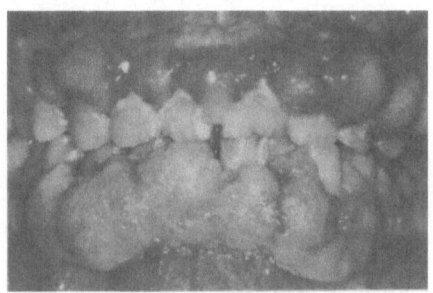

Fig.4) 3: Severe gengival
overgrowth.

2) Bacterial plaque index: According to Loe Silness, plaque bacterial index was scored, on the basis of local irritant factors, as follows: 0: Absence of dental plaque; 1: plaque evident only by dental instruments examination; 2: plaque evident by careful inspection; 3: obvious presence of large amount of plaque. All patients were carefully examined by one or more dentists ignoring their clinical and laboratory data and scored for dental overgrowth on the basis of the criteria above reported.

RESULTS.   The dosage of CyA was not different in Group I and Group II, averaging: 4.1 mg/kg:bw (SD 1.4) in Group I, 4.9 mg/kg/bw (SD 2.4) in Group II. In addition, 6 patients of Group II received calcium antagonists (3 diltiazem, 1 nicardipine, 2 nifedipine) to treat hypertension (3) or only to increase CyA bioavaibility.

In table 1 is reported the observed bacterial plaque scoring.

Table 1: Bacterial plaque index

	0	1	2	3
	% of patients			
Controls	0	33	33	23
Group I	0	30	60	10
Group II	0	37	50	13

In table 2 is reported the gengival overgrowth scoring.

Table 2: Gengival overgrowth

	0	1	2	3
	% of patients			
Controls	0	0	0	0
Group I	20	40	40	0
Group II	0	33	33	33

Incidence and severity of gengival overgrowth was significantly higher in Group II as compared with Group I (p 0.05). It is also of interest the observation that most patients presented higher localization of both bacterial plaque and gengival overgrowth on the dominant side: this is presumably in relation to a better oral hygiene obtained by brushing the handedness-contralateral teeth.

CONCLUSION.

Gengival overgrowth was absent in patients on immunosuppressive therapy other than CyA, whilst was present in both CyA Groups. In Group II it was more severe than in Group I; since oral hygiene, as assessed by plaque index, was similar in the two Groups, two factors (or probably the association of both) could account for this: a) Greater CyA blood levels in Group II; b) Ca++ antagonist (6 out of 8 patients of Group II were treated with these drugs). Recent studies show, in fact, reported that nifedipine could be associated with gengival hyperplasia. Our data confirm that CyA can cause moderate to severe gengival hyperplasia and suggest that the incidence is related with CyA Blood levels. To minimize the incidence of this side effect, the patients should be advised of brushing with great accuracy the teeth, particulary those on the dominant side.

REFERENCES

1. Rostock, Turnes. J. Periodontal 57:294, 1986.
2. Tyldesley, Rotter, British Dental J. November 10, 1984.

SUBJECT INDEX

AUTHOR INDEX